THE MANIC LINK

By Stuart William Marshall

'The Manic Link' explores the idea that Jesus was a manic depressive and that it is common for people with manic depression to hold the belief that they are Jesus, otherwise referred to as the messianic delusion. The book also explores how people with manic depression buy and sell things which relates to capitalism and advertising, how they tend to be grandiose, humorous, sometimes over sexual and believe in love. Unfortunately, people with manic depression can become paranoid and experience persecutory beliefs which can lead to them to become violent. The Manic Link concludes that the characteristics of manic depression/bipolar disorder are hardwired in religion, culture, advertising, capitalism, creativity, paranoia and chaos.

I sent a copy of *The Manic Link* to the following:

1.Professor Brendan Kelly - Professor of Psychiatry in Tallaght Hospital and Trinity College Dublin.

2. Eoghan Harris – Ex-Columnist Sunday Independent.

3. Dr Mark Dooley - Philosopher and writer. Ex-daily mail.

4. Pete Murphy - Writer and musician, columnist with The Irish Times.

5. John Waters - Ex-Irish Times Columnist.

And received back the following replies;

'The Manic Link' provides a unique insight into the experience of mania, the farther reaches of the human mind and the possibilities of the human condition. Few books have the courage to tackle these topics in the first place and fewer still do so with the passion, elegance and erudition of The Manic Link. This is an invaluable document, a timeless gift to students of the human mind.

Professor Brendan Kelly, Professor of Psychiatry, Trinity College Dublin. Books written by him include:

The Psychiatrist in the chair, official biography of Professor Anthony Clare, written with Muiriss Houston.

Hearing Voices: History of Psychiatry of Ireland.

Coping with Covid Virus.

The Doctor who sat for a year.

Dignity, mental health and human rights.

The science of happiness.

His latest book: Asylum, Inside Grangegorman

"What makes the mind of a mad tyrant tick? What subliminal psychic energies motivate religious revolutionaries, politicians and celebrities? And what happened when those traits go unrestrained? These are just some of the unsettling questions posed by Stuart Marshall in The Manic Link. Whether you love or loath it this challenging book will force you to think about contemporary society in novel ways. For that alone it is worth the risk"

Mark Dooley, Ex-columnist, The Irish Daily Mail, and author of 'Conversations with Roger Scruton', 2016

Roger Scruton: The philosopher of Dover beach, 2009

Conversations with Roger Scruton.

Why be a Catholic, 2011

The Roger Scruton reader: Questioning God.

The Philosopher (Derrida) 2006

The Politics of Exodus (Kierkegaard) 2001

The Sunday Independent December 1ˢᵗ 2002

The Reason Good Old Solomon Cursed Like a Sailor

To our detriment, we as a race have lost touch with the creative side of our brain, the side which abhors authority, writes Stuart William Marshall.

Men and women are indeed closest to animals physically. But what makes them special is the emotional differences between them, and how they express the emotions. Women like to touch a lot. The greatest mode of emotional expression is our skin. We have the same amount of hair as an ape but we only have 5% of its fur. Why we lost the fur is not clear, but in doing so, the greatest amounts of nerves were exposed to the environment.

Through skin we can sense light touch, deep touch, pleasure, pain, vibrations, two pint discrimination, hot and cold, and a sense of three dimensional space, which is technically called proprioception. It is through skin that we become intimate with each other.

UNTIL 5000 YEARS AGO ALMOST HALF THE POPULATION WAS LEFT HANDED SO THEY WERE IN TOUCH WITH THEIR CREATIVE SIDE – JOURNAL OF EVOULTION.

Lips and hands are the leaders in the touch field. In the brain we have two areas; one for touch (sensory use) and one for muscle (motor use). They lie side by side in the sense area. The lips and surrounding areas take up a quarter of the brain, the hands take up another quarter.

It is likely that touch led to language. The exposed skin presented the greatest organ to the environment and the complexities it revealed had to be expressed somehow. The expression is language.

Hand signing led to speech. That past lingers in the way the Italians and other Mediterranean people use their hands when they speak.

We lost some things too. We have become too right-handed, 85% of the population are right handed. Until 5000 years ago, almost half the population was left handed so they were in touch with their creative side. But of course, that side of the brain abhors authority. Cursing comes from the right musical brain, you can be sure Solomon cursed a lot.

An example of a chapter of 150 in the book that could be reviewed in a newspaper.

Bryan Appleyard review of *'A LIFE IN OUR PLANET MY WITNESS STATEMENT AND A VISION FROM THE FUTURE'* by David Attenborough with Johnnie Hughes.

There are three issues;

1. World population

2. Atmospheric carbon

3. Remaining wilderness.

In 1960 the population was 2.3 billion, atmospheric carbon was 280 parts per million and the remaining wilderness was 66%. In 2020 the population was 7.8 billion, atmospheric carbon 415 parts per million and remaining wilderness was 35%.

"96% of the mass of all mammals on earth is made up of our bodies and those of the animals we raise to eat". All wild mammals from whales and elephants to mice account for just 4%. We have to let more land to go wild and to become vegetarians. *28ᵗʰ of September 2020 Sunday Times Culture Section*

The levels of population, atmospheric carbon and remaining wilderness are unsustainable and are increasing/decreasing at exponential rates. This could be considered as sign of uncontrolled capitalism and mania.

A special thanks to my teacher Michael Carragher and to Eileen McElhinney and Leonora Doyle Hunt for typing.

PREFACE

At the donation by Warren Buffett of ($31bn) to the Bill Gates (Microsoft) Charity Mr Gates quoted from his personal copy of Adams Smiths "The Wealth of Nations" which he donated to Mr Buffett.

He recited the opening line *"However selfish so ever man may be supposed, there are evidently some principles in his nature which interest him in the fortunes of others and render their happiness necessary to him"* the world's wealthiest man told its second richest, 2006.

Samuel Beckett letters

"As for saying who I am, where I come from and what I'm doing, all this is quite beyond me"

"What makes the mind of a mad tyrant tick? What subliminal psychic energies motivate religious revolutionaries, politicians, and celebrities? And what happens when those traits go unrestrained? These are just some of the unsettling questions posed by Stuart Marshall in 'The Manic Link'. Whether you love or loathe it, this challenging book will force you to think about contemporary society in novel ways. For that alone, it is worth the risk."

Dr Mark Dooley (ex-*Irish Daily Mail* Columnist, Bibliographer of Robin Scruton)

Hypomania, some sociopathic personality disorder and obsessive compulsive disorder, supplies the most successful mixture in psychology.

Like a Gaia of the mind a system of evolutionary control of human thinking and emotion through a spectrum of mania, Schizophrenia, hypomania, schizoaffective Sociopathic, Obsessive Compulsive Disorder, Normality, Depression, Anxiety, Jealousy, Paranoia (Buying, selling, criminality, class) Religion (manic – Methodists Presbyterians) (Hypo manic - Protestant) (Depressive – Catholic). If two very intelligent people have children, they often have a manic child. I feel it is possible that the mix up of these conditions balance out into a Normal curve of origins.

Stuart Marshall

The Daily Telegraph, Friday 1ˢᵗ September 2023

Obituary of Richard Lynn

Richard Lynn was known as the "scientific racist." New Zealand political scientist James Flynn has thrown cold water on the "genetic deteriorations" theory of Richard Lynn by showing that notwithstanding welfare policies, in twenty-one countries, IQ had been rising by three points every decade since testing began.

Manic Depressive Illness

Mania is found in one in 100 people and is associated with overspending and selling and hence advertising and capitalism. People tend to become grandiose and spend more than they can afford. Their Ego is high and they have a lot of belief in themselves and this high confidence may be taken as a sign of the economy getting better. Things that make you manic and overspend are humour, sexuality, creativity, increased memory and possibly paranoia (hence the popularity of cleaning products). Mania is associated with increased emotion, intellect and physicality. Hypomania is found in 1 in 10-20 people and is a lower form of mania. It is my thesis that hypomania is increasing in modern society. Did Jesus have the messianic delusion? Was he a maniac depressive/Bipolar disorder? Did he think he was the son of god? Approximately one in twenty manic depressive patients have the messianic delusion.

I came first in my secondary school (high school) in the Leaving Certificate (A Levels) with A's in Biology and Chemistry and a B in Physics and a C in Honours Maths. I then studied medicine for seven years in Trinity and specialised in psychiatry. In my final year I wrote an essay for Professor McCormack. I had very little belief in myself but he said I was in the top three in the class; that put the spring back in my step. I spent two years in general psychiatry, six months in mental handicap care, six months in geriatric psychiatry, one year in child psychiatry, six months in community care, and a year working in a semi-secure psychiatric unit. I had passed the first part of two examinations for the Membership of the Royal College of Psychiatrists. My professional interest in schizophrenia and then manic-depressive illness, have given me an insight into the condition of hypomania that I developed after I had tried to stop a fight and was kicked unconscious outside a club.

In schizophrenia you have "positive symptoms", sensory phenomena such as seeing, hearing, smelling or tasting things that are not there, and also delusions, which can take many forms, e.g. telepathic, religious, sci-fi, grandiose, paranoid, persecutory or paranormal. In schizophrenia the disturbed perceptions are independent of the person's mood change, if any is present, and are not as understandable as those in manic depression.

Dr. Patrick McKeon divides "masked elation" into three types. The first is often referred to as dysphoric mania, meaning unpleasant high or "mixed mood". The second form of masked elation is where the patient is expressing paranoid ideas or other psychotic features and may be mistakenly diagnosed as having schizophrenia. Sometimes it can be difficult to distinguish between the paranoid delusions of mania and paranoid schizophrenia. It is only after a period of observation that a doctor is able to make a clearer diagnosis.

In the third masked elation type the hyperactive mental state of elation only becomes apparent when the person stops drinking or taking illicit drugs, or when sedative medication has been withdrawn.

In Manic-Depressive Illness (MDI) there are certain features of character, personality, and behaviour that are found by psychiatrists in the manic (high) phase of the illness. There are 40,000 MDI sufferers in Ireland, approximately one in every 100. Charles Dickens would certainly seem to be an M.D.I. sufferer: "He was vivacious and charming, charismatic and possessed superabundant energy. In 1838 he was writing *Oliver Twist* and *Nicholas Nickleby* simultaneously. His second American tour (1867) netted him profits of £20,000 (£1.5 million in modern day money). He also suffered from dysphoria (mania) being tormented, imperious, vindictive, and implacable once wronged"[1]

Mandela was charismatic, humorous, intelligent, and sexual and directed his paranoia in the search for truth.

A *manic high* means that the patient is physically, mentally, emotionally and intellectually overactive. For example a friend who was manic was overactive, funny, grandiose, charismatic, expressing love, inappropriately sexualised, thinking quickly, thought he had psychic abilities and could contact God and thought he was Jesus - all aspects of manic elation. Non linear thought, humour, emotion, intuition, faith in God come from the right brain (possibly characterised by being left-hand dominant). Charismatic emotion is getting people on your feel-good level and you inspire them. He was stabilised on Epilim, an antiepileptic and mood stabilizer, something that suggests his mania was related to electrical activity in the brain.

Some questions in this regard come to mind, and ought to be examined. Does "thinking love" come before "emotive loves"? In other words, do thoughts come before emotions? Is mania more left handed? Does thinking switch between left brain and right brain? Grandiose emotion makes you think high, depressive emotion makes you think low.

Emotion⇔Thinking

I believe that *manic archetypes* are hot-wired in the brain though not normally "turned on"; but when these manic archetypes are stimulated in people, both normal and manic, certain patterns of behaviour are expressed.

Manic Depressive Illness (MDI) is found in one percent of the populations of western developed countries in Socio-economic Class 1 and 2 where studies have been done. Of this one percent fifteen percent of close relatives (parents, brothers, sisters, and children) will also have MDI. MDI is higher in the natural parent than in the adoptive parent. In 100 identical twins with MDI, 70 of the other twin will have MDI. In a study of 100 non identical twins 15 will have MDI.[2]

But some traits of MDI are found in at least ten percent of people, maybe more in large cities, for example in New York where people talk and walk thirty percent more quickly than average. In cinema, the average length of a shot has declined from 10 seconds in the 30s and the 40s to less than 4 seconds. In pop music, not one act reached No1 with a debut single until 1994. (Saturday Night by Whigfield.) In 2014, 14 artists made the top slot in that one year. An increasing number of cities in the modern world have a population of 10 million or more; more slums and pollution also go with global urbanisation. This burgeoning has been relatively rapid - and is

---

1 William Boyd, *Charles Dickens: A Life*, by Clare Tomalin; reviewed in the *Irish Times* 8th Oct 2011.
[2] *Coping with Depression and Elation*, Dr. Patrick McKeon.

ongoing. Industrial cities are about 250 years old and developed quickly, but on a smaller scale than modern cities, where high birth rates are coupled to relatively low death rates.

Emotion and thinking are affected by the individual's position on a bipolar scale, people being more creative and productive toward the manic end. The same thing may occur on a societal level. Climate and 24-hour news dominate media.

In the First Industrial Revolution Britain supplied 60 percent of coal and 50 percent of iron in Europe, and the Revolution led to the development of canals and railways, with subtle but eventually powerful effects on society. Interestingly, the Duke of Wellington, as Prime Minister, was opposed to the railway industry because he felt that mobility of the masses would lead to people becoming dissatisfied - but it is such dissatisfaction that provokes and inspires change. Perhaps the duke could see the threat to his own class's position such change might effect.

In industrial Britain ideas and creativity were stimulated and there was very little censorship. In Bourbon France, by contrast, there was significant state control of ideas and perhaps in part because of this there was very little industrialisation – workshop - rather than factory-based. Furthermore, Great Britain had the biggest navy in the world up to the Second World War, the British Empire depending on sea power and on global trading in everything from tobacco, spices, tea and sugar to, in earlier times, slaves. This exposure to wider ideas may have helped foster hypomanic ideas as well as trade.

The Second Industrial Revolution was centred on Germany, and saw the industrial and technological advantage move away from Britain. New discoveries in technology, notably the Bessemer converter and the Open Hearth method - both invented by Englishmen, ironically - made cheap steel possible; in the old days of the crucible, it had always been expensive and seldom economic, but now it began to displace iron as the ubiquitous material of the age. The addition of limestone as a flux made commercial exploitation of the Lorraine iron fields possible; previously, a high level of phosphate had made Lorraine iron of little value, but now they were an enormous resource to the new Second Reich (something that made their loss felt all the more sharply by the French), a resource that was augmented by the value of the phosphate-and-lime slag as a chemical fertilizer.[3] Thanks not just to Lorraine's Iron ore, but to the huge war reparations - which provided for investment in infrastructure - the new Germany quickly became world leader in not just iron and steel production, but in chemical and electrical engineering, while her coal output also was prodigious.

As the First Industrial Revolution had energised English society and ideas, the same thing began to occur in Germany. Germany always had been a nation of artistic and scientific accomplishment, but now a new and sinister element began to emerge. Prussia always had been a powerful military power, disproportionate to its size, and the new Reich really was an extension of Prussian militaristic ideas across all of Germany. In addition to industrial development, the power of the Royal Navy had, arguably, boosted the energy levels of British society, and now something similar began to happen in Germany. As the Royal Navy was world leader by a wide margin, the Second Reich's military was by far and away the most powerful in the world.

Why did anti-Semitism get a grip on Germany more so than any other country? Is it because of Protestant mania associated with jealousy and paranoia?

Hypomania

Under certain circumstances a lower level of mania, hypomania, can be induced in almost the entire population; we saw this in Britain with the death of Princess Diana where people wept for their own death. (De Clerambault's Syndrome page 215) When people are made hypomanic they spend more money, because of a generally increased sense of well-being, confidence and self-love. People at auctions talk of the euphoria of buying and selling; EBay fans frequently spend more than they know to be prudent on things they don't even want. The most shocking examples may be found during tulip mania in Holland in the seventeenth century when one pound of bulbs allegedly sold for the price of a house.

---

[3] Alsace-Lorraine had been taken as part of the spoils after the Franco-Prussian War of 1870-71.

The spending of money is the basis of capitalism, and such neo- or hypomanic behaviour certainly stimulates the market and leads to the rapid turnover of a great deal of money. Furthermore, the more rapid the pace of activity the greater the urgency to pass the trade along: to buy *or* sell. And surely one of the most manic places is the stock exchange? The pace here is so intense that dealers allegedly get by on champagne and cocaine, and they are burned out by the age of thirty.

The market is further driven by advertising, which in turn seeks to stimulate emotional states in order to create a Pavlovian association between the commodity being advertised and the positive state that advertising seeks to create. Some advertisements set out to be funny (however predictable the punch line or tiresome the ad becomes after hearing it twice). Others shamelessly stoke our emotions - an excellent example, that works well year after year, is the ad for tea, which describes a father remembering his sense of childhood wonder as he shops for Santa's presents for his own children. Sexuality is all but ubiquitous in advertising, the subtle message being that the product or service advertised will enhance one's sexual desirability and make one more sexually desirable to others. Beautiful people and beautiful backdrops enhance the sexuality of the message, and so too does the suggestion of humour - everyone is smiling or laughing at the target buyer's implied wit or charm. Optimism and a certain grandiosity form a background mood.

Other advertising appeals not to the target buyer's subtle greed but to his fear, sometimes indeed stoking paranoia. Home protection products or services would be a typical example - but here, too, other emotions may be deployed. The burglars are amusingly stupid, something that highlights the target buyer's intelligence by contrast - but they still are a threat, so the service is needed, and, the target's intelligence having been subtly acknowledged, as an intelligent person he will feel subtly compelled to buy.

Appeal to paranoia rather than to fear per se may lie behind advertising for some products and services, notably hygiene goods and services, where one is led to believe that the threat from dirt and germs is everywhere.

It seems impossible to avoid concluding that advertising has driven the rampant consumerism of the present age. Given this consumerism and the casual way in which sex is presented in newspapers and on TV - despite the acknowledged dangers of promiscuous sex - it is worthwhile considering whether hypomania may be a semi-deliberately induced state across the Western world. Because of its association with consumption and "good times," hypomania could be described as the illness of success. The Prozac generation has possibly increased the numbers who "suffer" from this condition.

Manic Archetypes may be recognised - they are listed below. An archetype is, literally, an ancient pattern toward which subsequent manifestations tend. The pattern may be only dimly discernable in these manifestations yet it is the pattern, the archetype, which determines their form.

MANIC ARCHETYPES	GROUP PSYCHOLOGICAL CHARACTERISTICS	MYTHICAL CORRELATES
1. Love of self	Nationalism; Ego; Confidence; "Because you're worth it".[4]	Jesus
2. Love of others	Socialism; Super Ego; Parental support; "I'd like to teach the world to sing".[5]	God
3. Paranoia /Jealousy	National Socialism; Id; Killing without guilt.[6]	"Paranoid position" Kills ID Satan/ Antichrist
4. Energy	Work ethic; Persistence.	Workaholic
5. Charisma	Messianic delusion; "The best a man can get".	Ideas of grandeur
6. Creative	Seeks beauty	Narcissism; Apollo
7. Intellect	Seeks truth	Utopianism
8. Humour	Anarchy; Chaos; Sex	irresponsibility

---

[4] L'Oreal ad, and used in other words in many ads in a consumerist age.
[5] Lyrics that were adapted by Coca Cola to sell to consumerists.
[6] As in ads for products that "kill all germs".

9. Sexuality	Disinhibition; Sex addiction	Bi-sexuality
10. Spending	Capitalism; Advertising; Technology; Management.	Bankruptcy
11. Drugs (artificial mania)	Mass hysteria	Bacchus; *"in vino veritas"*
12.Competition	Aggression Sport; Fighting	Mars
13. Loquaciousness	Talking; rumour-mongering	Rapid speech
14. Emotional labiality	Happiness	Irritability

Archetypes are associated with Carl Gustav Jung's school of Analytical Psychology. Like those of all of the members of the "Vienna School" Jung's ideas cannot ever be proven or objectively analysed (for all the name he gave them). Nevertheless, many therapists have found the idea of the archetype a useful one in treatment, and the concept may be adapted to examination of hypomania.

Manic depressives are sometimes deluded that they are Jesus Christ i.e. the messianic delusion. I postulate that Jesus Christ was a deluded Manic Depressive and expressed a lot of its symptoms.

HYPOMANIA AND MANIC ARCHETYPES

Hypomania, between mania and normality, may be closer to the latter than its name would suggest. Sexuality, grandiosity, humour, intellect and creativity along with love and paranoia (which can include jealousy) are the main manic archetypes. In themselves these are harmless and indeed usually good and adaptive - even a degree of paranoia may be necessary in, say, a war situation, and grandiosity can impart adaptive self-confidence. However, they also may serve as strong indicators of mania.

The result of mania is often not positive. People spend money or set up grandiose schemes and go bankrupt. In the old days before there were drugs (tranquillisers) they could die of exhaustion. People with manic tendencies are often disinhibited and have a lot of casual relationships that can lead to marriage breakdown and the possibly fatal acquisition of STDs. They have amplified excitement and labile emotions. They also get paranoid and might think people are trying to kill or harm them. This paranoid position can lead to action that can result in them killing, being killed or being a danger to others or themselves.

With mania, too, there often is a cyclical mood swing toward depression; this can be very severe, bleak and lonely, sometimes resulting in suicide. In the depressive phase of MDI you get the following characteristics:

- Laziness; lethargy; lack of drive
- Poor motivation
- Spendthrift performance
- Low sex drive
- Lack of creativity
- Low self esteem
- Guilt/Shame
- Loathing self/others
- Suicidal impulses

When the brain is made hypomanic by stimulation of the manic archetypes we get expression of thoughts about law and order. The French Revolution's ideas of liberty, equality, fraternity, and American ideas about the pursuit of happiness would have grown out of hypomanic thoughts, the eye of illumination on the dollar bill with the triangle. Modern liberal democracy evolved from what then would have been regarded as delusions - of the manic mind - and one still lives more in the illusion of freedom than in a state of real freedom.

We may say that liberal democracy is an expression of manic-depressive delusions. Freedom is based on love - in theory at any rate - but often is controlled by paranoia: as Jack Nicholson said in *Easy Rider*, "everyone talks about individual freedom, but show them a free individual and they get scared" - then start killing and maiming to prove they aren't scared.

Aspects of hypomania may be adaptive, at the level of the individual, the community, and even the species – "super-normality" might be a better term? A capacity for hard work, resourcefulness and inventiveness may imply a certain manic application by the individual to his task or his perceived *raison d'être*. Thomas Edison, who spent only three years at school and started work selling newspapers, patented over 1,000 inventions, notably the phonograph and the electric light bulb. He slept, apparently, only as much as necessary, though when not under pressure typically slept eight hours a night; this suggests that he was "normal" - not hyperactive or compulsive. Edison's inventive mind expresses the creative hypomanic archetype.

A new study shows that highly creative artists have temperaments more akin to manic-depressives than the general public. A study by Stanford University suggests that healthy artists are more similar in personality to people with manic depression than they are to people in the general population. "My hunch is that emotional range, having an emotional broadband, is the bipolar patient's advantage," stated Dr. Strong, implying, at least, support for the thesis that hypomania is potentially adaptive. "It isn't the only thing going on, but something gives people with manic depression an edge, and I think it is emotional range."[7]

However, hypomania ultimately may be maladaptive. The degeneracy and collapse of the Greek and Roman empires may have been through hypomanic pursuit of greater and greater thrills such as alcohol, incest and voyeuristic excesses, and religious diversity, with an accompanying lack of moral restraint. Even in the field of religion a ruthless single-mindedness may overwhelm moral impulse, as with the Jim Jones cult. Jones was the American founder of the People's Temple that established Jonestown in Guyana. He led 914 of his followers to an act of mass suicide, the greatest mass suicide in modern times, in 1979. Dazzled by Jones's charisma, they fed cyanide in orangeade to 240 of their own children. He said, "If you want me to be your Jesus then I'll be your Jesus. If you want me to be your Lenin

---

[7] The *Irish Times*, 22 May 2002, p. 5.

I'll be your Lenin. If you want me to be your God, I'll be your God." Jones got very paranoid in the end in Guyana.

Another Messianic leader was David Corish who barricaded 119 of his followers, of whom 40 were children, into a farm house in Waco, Texas. They had 150 automatic guns and held out for 51 days. Corish was the only male allowed to sleep with the women in his cult and he had numerous children by them and by minors. The sect was a branch of the Seventh Day Adventists and they thought Corish was Jesus. Corish read Revelations to them all the time and said that the end of the world would be in their life time. Through the siege he released twenty hostages, mostly children, and nine escaped eventually. When the house was stormed by the police 74 died, killed it is thought by booby trap fires laid by Corish. Corish was found with a bullet hole to the head.

Another manic with the messianic delusion was Charles Manson. Less notorious is Wayne Bent, who was imprisoned in New Mexico for 18 years in 2009 for sleeping with minors; they thought he was Jesus. The F.B.I. estimate that there are 5,000 cults like this in America, all showing evidence of the manic archetype grandiosity. The National Security Agency U.S.A. spends 11 Billion dollars a year.

Some cult beliefs such as Khlysty are dystopic, where outlawed sects who believe that sin was a necessary step to redemption danced naked; self flagellated and had group sex. "Orlando Figes, Sunday Times 17 Feb. 14

At the Sun Moon University that he founded in Asan, South of Seoul, the Rev Sun Myung Moon blessed the biggest ever wedding on 14 Oct. 2009, when 40,000 people around the world were married, some doing it by satellite or the internet. The ceremony marked Moon's ninetieth birthday and his own fiftieth wedding anniversary. Many of the couples had only met two or three times, because of the church's controversial system of arranged marriages. It had been almost 50 years since the self-proclaimed messiah figure, who says he was called at 15 yrs to finish the work of Jesus Christ, had married his first 24 couples, picking the partners himself, in his Unification Church - the Moonies.

Though there is strong evidence that the pace of modern life fosters hypomania, the phenomenon is not new. The White Lotus Movement in

China resulted in the death of 15 million people. In 1836 Hong Su Twang had a nervous breakdown and a vision where it was revealed to him that he was Jesus' younger brother. He set out to rid China of Confucianism. His followers grew and grew and he marched on Northern China having taken control of Southern and Central China. In the Tipping Revolution, between 1850 and 1865, twenty million people died, twice as many as in the First World War. When Hong died they fired his ashes through a cannon.

Christianity was not widespread in late-nineteenth century China and in 1949 Mao expelled 10,000 missionaries. Mao killed 45 million of his own people. In earlier times China also had displayed hypomanic tendencies, and a parallel can be distinguished. In the third century BC Emperor Chin was autocratic and had a centrally controlled bureaucracy run under the philosophy of the long-dead Confucius, who advocated order, control and tradition. The good of the people, not the individual, came first, and Chin exerted tight control over academics and farmers - just as Mao did in the Cultural Revolution.

Fear of chaos persists as in the time of Confucius. Chinese leaders today have to control 1.3 billion people and stop the outbreak of war such as at the White Lotus Movement and Hong Su Twang disaster. Yet the Chinese have and since time immemorial have had a craze for gambling. The I Ching may be said to be a gambler's cryptic manual, and certainly this oracle is constantly consulted by businessmen. Mah Jong is another immemorial manifestation of gambling. One may speculate that this fixation on gambling is a substitute for religion, which the state outlaws.

The brain has I billion neurons,1 trillion synapses. Man is also optimistic.

Yet one does not need to venture as far as China to find manifestations of hypomania. Mabel Barlrop, aged 53, set up the Panacea Society in 1919 at her home in Bedford a market town in Southern England. The Panacea Society was seen as a New Jerusalem and a new Garden of Eden. Mabel preached that she was the daughter of God and was preparing for the Second Coming and that she could make up for Original Sin and achieve immortality on earth.

Mabel had 70 followers in the surrounding countryside, widows, spinsters and wives. Mabel recommended celibacy and claimed continuity with Joanna

Southcott, who had claimed 100 years previously that she was preparing for a Jesus that Mabel thought, was here. Using arcane reasoning and numerology Mabel claimed to be of the eighth generation since Joanna, and took the name Octavia. When she died they kept her body for three days and when it did not resurrect or be assumed to Heaven they buried her and broke up the commune.

Mabel spent two periods in mental hospitals, the second time for 18 months probably for mania and depression. Mania would explain the manic delusion of her being the daughter of God, but the manic archetype, grandiosity, may have manifested as hypomania before breakdown occurred.

Also, the Panacea Society needs to be seen in an historic context. During and after the Great War there was a pronounced rise in spiritualism, as bereaved parents and spouses sought meaning in their loved ones' deaths, and some sense of continuity and even purpose. The name itself may be significant in this light.

Stimulating the manic archetypes can induce hypomania. When people are hypomanic they express to some degree the manic archetypes - as, perhaps, Mabel expressed grandiosity - so that, for example, spending leads to more spending and sexual activity leads to sexual disinhibition or even hypersexuality and sex-addiction.

Expression of the manic archetypes reveals a person with good self-esteem, who likes other people, falls in love easily, spends money; one who is sexually disinhibited, funny, driven, creative, intellectual, ambitious, confident, decisive, charismatic and sometimes somewhat paranoid; one who shows perseverance and a strong work ethic, labile emotions, enthusiasm; one addicted to success, profit motive. A good memory is often a quality. The hypomanic may have ideas of grandeur but is not manic and often is successful in his undertakings.

The downside is that mania is associated with messianic belief, miracles and the dark sort of visions of the Book of Revelations. Out of such fixations can emerge paranoia? This is associated with schizophrenia but I think any presentation of schizophrenic or schizoid symptoms ought to be examined for evidence of mania. The Christian God is Manic paranoid.

This suggestion is indirectly supported by the psychiatric establishment. In some cases of paranoia and schizophrenia treatment may call for the sort of tranquillizing medication that depresses manic behaviour, e.g. Epilim, Tegertol (used in Epilepsy) and Lithium. This is hardly surprising as drugs that mimic mania and cause paranoia are amphetamines, ecstasy, cocaine, crystal meth and alcohol, most of these being stimulants. A new breed of drugs is the 2C1 family a psychedelic phenethylamine. Its side effects are paranoia and hallucinations. It is known as N bombs, Smiles and Solaris. In the case of alcohol, while this is a CNS depressant, the reaction in coming off can lead to a hypomanic "high" increased blood pressure - Joyce and Francis Bacon directed their hangovers toward creative endeavours.

We can see from this observation that, paradoxical as it may seem, antidepressants can cause mania. Medicalization of mania by the use of antidepressants has created an image of pharmacologically-happy, laid-back clients, but this may not always be the case. During a stay with a Mormon family in Utah, investigating how religion affects people's contentment, Whippman notes that the state is not only home to Provo, the poll-topping happiest town in America, but also the country's highest levels of antidepressant use. From "The Pursuit of Happiness" by Ruth Whippman. Review by Victoria Segal

Another aspect worthy of further investigation is that syphilis and multiple sclerosis can cause demyelisation of nerves, and this can lead to grandiosity, labile emotions and paranoia. Hypomania may therefore have physiological correlates.

Repetition helps memory and improves any skill, and hypomanics tend to be repetitious, repeating over and over, sometimes mantra-like, sometimes out of their sense of elation, whatever it is that exercises them. This repetitiousness may help account for their perceived greater intellectual powers.

But trying to find *the* cause for the condition is misguided, for likely there are many causes.

Manic Depressive Illness

Signs of Mania:

- Increased activity and gestures (pacing, foot-tapping)
- High self esteem
- Poor judgement
- Labile emotions
- Racing thoughts like a train speeding through the head
- Decreased need for sleep staying up without sleep. Research by the National Sleep Foundation shows that Americans have reduced their hours of sleep from eight in 1960 to just five or six today. Another sign of mania.
- Over work. Over a million Japanese employees regularly put in at least 100 hours monthly overtime. Under new legislation employers are supposed to monitor the 80-hour threshold, which is considered the point at which death from overwork- known as karoshi - becomes more likely. Japan's ministry of health released its first White Paper on karoshi prevention last month. In addition to revealing shockingly long working days the paper links over 2,000 suicides a year to exhaustion or other- related factors. David McNeill, Irish Times, 9th November 2016.
- In South Korea the main death rate among 10 to 30-year-olds is suicide. Study at school starts at 8am and goes for 7 hour classes to 4pm. Then home and a break for an hour then working to 11pm. TV and phones are often not allowed. Sian Griffiths Sunday Times Review 27 November 2016
- Poor temper control - from irritability to blazing anger
- Pressured speech - can't keep up with manic thoughts
- Increased activities with high risks of painful consequences - sexual affairs, gambling, risky investments, poor business decisions, buying and selling, humour, drugs.

Mania does not mean psychosis, but psychosis may include some of the symptoms of mania. Psychosis implies detachment from reality rather than the deluded perceptions of reality that the manic may have. Psychotic symptoms include delusions - notably grandiose delusions - and hallucinations, and these can induce paranoia (though this can also be a symptom of mania, as explained above).

Diagnostic and Statistical Manual of Mental Disorders (DSM) IV-TR

Bipolar Episode and Bipolar Disorder

Bipolar disorder is characterized by more than one bipolar episode. There are three types of bipolar disorder:

1. Bipolar 1 Disorder, in which the primary symptom presentation is manic, or rapid (daily) cycling episodes of mania and depression.

2. Bipolar 2 Disorder, in which the primary symptom presentation is recurrent depression accompanied by hypomanic episodes (a milder state of mania in which the symptoms are not severe enough to cause marked impairment in social or occupational functionally or need for hospitalization, but are sufficient to be observable by others.)

3. Cyclothymic Disorder, a chronic state of cycling between hypomanic and depressive episodes that do not reach the diagnostic standard for bipolar disorder.

Manic episodes are characterized by:

A. A distinct period of abnormally and persistently elevated, expansive, or irritable mood, lasting at least 1 week (or any duration if hospitalisation is necessary)

B. During the period of mood disturbance, three (or more) of the following symptoms have persisted (4 if the mood is only irritable) and have been present to a significant degree:

1. Increased self–esteem or **grandiosity**

I'm the best, I'm special, I'm the greatest, I'm superior, I'm brilliant. U2 song - Even better than the real thing.

U2 song - One Love; One left brain balanced by, Love right brain. Vowels signify emotions.

The best built cars in the world - Toyota

Carlsberg probably the best larger in the world.

Gillette-the best a man can get.

Chanel No 5- "I wear nothing else to bed" Marilyn Monroe

2. Decreased need for sleep (e.g., feels rested after only 3 hours of sleep)

3. More talkative than usual or pressure to keep talking (speech)

4. Flight of ideas or subjective experience that thoughts are racing (train in the head).

5. **Distractibility** (i.e., attention too easily drawn to unimportant or irrelevant external stimuli)

6. Increase in goal directed activity (either socially, at work or school, or sexually) or psychomotor agitation

7. **Disinhibition** - Excessive involvement in pleasurable activities that have a high potential for painful consequences (e.g., engaging in **unrestrained buying sprees,** sexual indiscretion, or foolish business investments)"

8. **Humour infectious mood Spike Milligan.**

9. **Paranoid Emotions, OCD** (Obsessive Compulsive Disorder) cleaning products. Killing wife or family member.

Substance-Induced Mood Disorder

The mood can manifest as manic (expansive, grandiose, irritable), depressed, or a mixture of mania and depression.ie. Cocaine, amphetamines, alcohol, antidepressants and ecstasy.

Ancient cultural correlates of hypomania may be discerned in both the Ten Commandments of the Old Testament, the fundamental two to which Christ reduced these, and the Seven Deadly Sins that have emerged from Christian-era Church scholarship.

Looking first at the Ten Commandments:

1. *"I am the Lord thy God! Thou shalt have no other Gods but me"*: this betrays grandiosity, paranoia and jealousy, hypomanic traits that have

marked the Abrahamic religions down the millennia. The wrath of the Old Testament God can be discerned in St Dominic's apocryphal remark at the massacre of the Albigensians: "Kill them all - God will know his own!" This in turn can be heard echoing in Colonel Chivington's admonition to his Colorado Volunteers at Sand Creek, when hundreds of peaceful Cheyenne were massacred: "Kill them all - nits make lice". The same fanatical intolerance is manifest in Islamists' butchery of "Kaffirs" and "Infidels", and in the automatic death penalty for apostasy in fundamentalist Moslem states. Excess and brutal intolerance are clearly manifest, and there is no perceived need to justify the hypomanic claims.

2. *"Thou shalt not take the name of the Lord thy God in vain"*: this follows from the first commandment, and adds control to the paranoia and jealousy. The spiritual delusions that may accompany hypomania - though more often mania or psychosis - is also apparent here.

3. *"Thou shalt keep the Sabbath day"*: routine is often a characteristic of the hypomanic (and of sufferers of associated afflictions). Church attendance is often associated with music and singing, the release of endorphins and bonding of community, and there may be much emotionality. This emotionality can manifest itself in many ways, from hymn singing and chanting of the Psalms to the hysteria of some fundamentalist Christian Churches in the Bible Belt, with "speaking in tongues", snake-handling in religious trance, "casting out of demons", when "sinners" are brought to such a point of excitement and sacred terror that they vomit "their demons" out.

4. *"Thou shalt honour thy father and thy mother"*: a good admonition in itself, but can lend itself to hypomanic fixation on tradition and setting an example, or preserving the blood line at all costs. This manifests hypomanically in Moslem honour killings.

5. *"Thou shalt not kill"*: murder is the most extreme crime a person can commit, a breaking of the ultimate taboo that holds societies together. But linguistic analysis of the original Commandment indicates that the verb is not *kill* but *murder* - i.e. thou shalt not murder one of your own tribe. When we examine some of the more appalling events of the Old Testament ("Break his teeth in his mouth Oh Lord. Let his children be

fatherless and his wife beg for her bread", for instance), we see how killing can be an actual divine-mandated virtue, one that the paranoid or grandiose hypomanic can all-too-easily invoke to justify his actions. We may also see this admonition in the holy wars of history and the *jihads* of today.

6. *"Thou shalt not commit adultery"*: again, this is good advice for individuals and society. Adultery undermines marriage and endangers the security of children. Sexual disinhibition is manic behaviour and when people sleep around paternity becomes dubious and the bond of the father with his (?) children is weakened. If men don't know who their children are the children are at greater risk of not being provided for and protected so the society which they help constitute is endangered. Another, darker sort of hypomanic interpretation of this commandment can be found in societies that can justify murder as punishment for adultery, from the "crime of passion" formerly in certain European legal systems to the Moslem honour killings of today.

7. *"Thou shalt not steal"*: again, a very commonsensical exhortation, but one that can accommodate the hypomanic love of money. Property rights can lead to a wide range of social ills, from rampant capitalism to the mutilation of offenders in many Moslem states, where Sharia law can see the "offending" hand cut off.

8. *"Thou shalt not bear false witness against thy neighbour"*: further good advice, and a warning against hypomanic indulgence in lying and injustice.

9. *"Do not let thyself lust after thy neighbour's wife"*: sexual disinhibition is a hypomanic trait, with the potential for community discord if indulged.

10. *"Thou shalt not covet thy neighbour's house, nor his farm, nor his cattle nor anything that is his"*: acquisitiveness and morbid jealousy are hypomanic traits, and this warning admonition about respect for property rights would have been particularly important in a farming community. In a herding or hunting community, which the Israelites still were, this admonition would have had even greater value, because the sense of honour, and the readiness to defend this, seems to be of a higher order in such communities where individual initiative and the readiness to defend

one's property are so much more important than in the more communal sedentary farming culture.

Jesus' two commandments can also be seen to have hypomanic elements in them:

"Love thy God with all thy strength and all thy might" can indicate grandiosity as Christ claimed to be the son of God.

"Love thy neighbour as thyself" could be interpreted, if one takes the exhortation literally, to be beyond the capacity of most people, and only possible for the manic or the hypomanic. The New Testament also contains the Pauline admonition that love is the "greatest" of the three virtues (faith, hope and charity, which emerges out of the sort of love for one's neighbour that Christ prescribed).

Seven Deadly Sins of Church teaching likewise have hypomanic elements in them.

Envy: elements of morbid jealousy and discontent at others' good fortune. Many murderers have preferred to see their partners dead than with someone else, even at the price to themselves of life-imprisonment or the death penalty. This is evident in "honour killings" but it is not at all unique to Islamic culture, and can be seen in "The Ballad of Frankie and Johnnie", where the woman kills the man "'cause he was doing her wrong".

Greed: excessive desire for money or possessions can create a manic boom in property, as we saw in the Noughties, one fuelled by advertising and all the risk-taking that capitalism thrives on.

Sloth: in many ways the opposite of hypomanic greed, it can also be a manifestation of the depression that goes with the bipolar form of mania.

Gluttony: the wish for excessive food or sensual indulgence can be a manic trait, and the problems modern society has with gluttony is further evidence that hypomania is becoming increasingly "the norm". Obesity and diabetes are on the increase across all age groups, and binge drinking is creating all sorts of social problems. The disinhibition that alcohol promotes can also foster other hypomanic behaviour, notably envy and wrath.

Wrath: intense anger can stem from paranoia or jealousy, and may lead to killing when in a drunk or jealous rage.

Pride: perhaps more accurately described as vanity - true pride tends to foster self-responsibility - this "deadly" form of pride is love of self, which fosters or stems from grandiosity. The feeling of pleasure and satisfaction when one has done well can be a good thing, but a too-high opinion of one's worth can lead to, say, making poor business decisions when over confident, discounting good advice and, in extreme cases, calamitously self-destructive behaviour.

Lust: any strong desire including (sexual) can lead to disinhibition and reckless behaviour. Extramarital affairs can result in STDs, children born out of wedlock, marriage break up and perhaps catastrophic loss of home, job, reputation and position.

In the **manic phase of MDI** you get the following characteristics;

MDI – Faster walking-talking-speaking

      Manic Depressive Illness. Biopolar Disorder – emotions: love-crying
      Intellect – intelligence – ideas quick
      Spiritual – God-Christ-Christianity – Oh Holy Brilliant God
      Forgiveness
      Heaven-high
      Humour-funny, witty – quick-laughing-infectious mood
      Sexual- physical/appetite
      Paranoia-evil/sickness/dirty-hell
      Charisma – spending – self love

Traits of manic drugs, i.e. cocaine and in a way LSD. Both can cause traits with paranoia.
Anti-epileptic drugs used in mania. Electrical suppression
Capitalism – buying and selling
Creativity - ideas art, beauty books painting
Culture – mainly expressed by mania
Advertising is based on culture and branding – music, humour, sexuality, beauty, intellect, Vowels – numbers, i.e. U2, intuition, transport, emotion, spatial awareness, dress sense, dance movements.
Christianity is a manic religion.

MDI – works through depression – such as Beckett's world

These manic traits are found in a lower level of hypomania which along with obsessive traits is the best way to be.

Jesus was a manic depressive who thought he was Jesus.

Grandiose, paranoid manic depressive hypo maniac, Hitler, Stalin, Mao & Putin.

The Celtic cross symbolises the sun and the cross the pagan Irish Christianity.

Socio-Economic Status

Observations on hypomania include:

> Those at high risk of bipolar disorder (MDI) were: single subjects, those in receipt of social assistance, pensioner sickness payments, unemployed, subjects with a shorter educational history, and subjects with lower income. Conversely, parental higher education and higher level of parental wealth were associated with increased risk. The associations of lower socio-economic indices of subjects may be explained as a consequence of the disease. The association of higher socio-economic indices of parents may be explained by socio-economic achievement in the family of origin.[8]

Bipolar patients slide down the social scale even though their parents are in the upper social strata. Examples of this are Van Gogh (painter) who was financially looked after by his brother Theo; he only sold one painting in his life time. Syd Barret (singer, lyricist) of Pink Floyd had a breakdown and James Joyce's daughter Lucia (dancer), whose letters Joyce is thought to have used to write *Finnegan's Wake*, also had a breakdown and ended up in a psychiatric hospital for years. Lucia had fancied Samuel Beckett. Tennessee Williams' sister Rose was diagnosed as a schizophrenic in 1937 and lobotomised in 1943; her brother was worried that he might go mad. Ray Davis of the band the Kinks was diagnosed as a MDI (bipolar disorder) in 1973 when he attempted suicide. Brian Wilson of the Beach Boys recorded

---

8 Tsuchiya KJ; Agerbo E; Byrne M; M Mortensen PB; *Psychological Medicine*, Jul 2004.

eleven albums between 1963-66 including *Pet Sounds* that is considered to be the best album ever. In 1978 he was diagnosed as a Bipolar Schizoaffective. He had abused cocaine, LSD and heroin. It is said that Dusty Springfield the singer was also a Manic Depressive. David Bowie was scared of mental illness as his stepbrother Terry was a psychiatric patient, he had three aunts with psychiatric illness and there was a history of family suicide.[9] Bowie admits to having been schizophrenic in the 1970s with a cocaine-induced drug psychosis resulting in his self-perception as a "rock messiah". Vince Taylor, who inspired Bowie's Ziggy Stardust, had taken LSD in the 1950s, resulting in a breakdown; he later claimed to have been reborn as one of the Apostles. Bowie met him in 1966 and Vince showed him a map showing were UFOs had landed in the U.K. Bruce Springsteen's father was diagnosed as a paranoid schizophrenic (autobiography- Born to Run) but was probably a dysphoric irritable manic depressive and Bruce suffered from creative depression, manic depression and attended psychotherapy and was treated with antidepressants that improved his creativity since 1982.

The University of Pittsburgh's UPMC says of bipolar disorder:

> While bipolar disorder is often romanticized since many highly creative people have suffered from highs and lows, this disease destroys many lives. The suicide rate among individuals with bipolar disorder is the highest of any psychiatric illness. Nearly half of all U.S. suicidal deaths each year are in patients with bipolar disorders. Their risk for suicide is more than 20 times that of the general population. Of particular concern is that attempts made by bipolar patients have about a one in five chance of being lethal, compared to a one in twenty chance within the general population. A variety of medication are used to treat bipolar disorder. Lithium has long been used as a first treatment. Treatment can be effective but unfortunately, many people do not comply with the prescribed treatment, particularly when they experience its manic phases.

This summary makes clear the "hazards of the high". Alcohol, coffee and nicotine make the user hypomanic by stimulating the Central Nervous

---

9 *Sunday Independent*, 10 March 2013.

System. Alcohol is seen as a depressive drug, but its suppression of negative inhibitory neurotransmitters can result in positive CNS stimulation on withdrawal when epileptic CNS fits, high pulse and high blood pressure can cause strokes, something that is also caused by cocaine and amphetamines.

Neurotransmitters are the chemicals in the brain that cause nervous stimulation; about 95 percent are negative (acetylcholine), five percent positive. Alcohol reduces inhibitions so people sing, dance, tell jokes, feel sexually attractive, but ultimately can get paranoid at perceived slights - all manic archetypes. The more people drink the less discriminatory they are in sexual and other ventures, such recklessness being part of a wider hypomanic behaviour syndrome.

The role played by alcohol, however, can be difficult to define. Some alcoholics report an apparently contradictory sense of high Ego coupled to low self esteem. This may be accounted for by the disinhibitory effect of the depressant, the disinhibition leading to Egoism, the depressant itself, coupled to the alcoholic's semi-subconscious awareness of the negative consequences of alcoholic indulgence, together lowering the sufferer's esteem.

Hypomania stimulates ambitious thought about what might once have been considered off-limits ideas: law and order and equality. The American belief in life liberty and the pursuit of happiness, as penned by Thomas Jefferson, in the 1776 Declaration of American Independence, expresses the thinking that today runs the world, but these and the concept of liberal democracy itself may be, ultimately, products of the manic mind.

"We hold these truths to be self-evident, that all men are created equal, that they are endowed by their Creator with certain unalienable Rights that among these are Life, Liberty and the pursuit of Happiness ...."

Serfs of the Middle Ages, even slum-dwellers of the early nineteenth century, could hardly imagine the conditions their descendants live in - and could anyone deny the possibility at least that people like Jim Larkin, Padraig Pearse and maybe Charles Dickens (with his bewildering output and his passion for social reform) were hypomanic?

It is interesting to speculate on the extent to which the French Revolutionary belief in Liberty, Fraternity and Equality was influenced by those drugs (alcohol, coffee and nicotine), that were part and parcel of the revolutionaries' lifestyle in coffee shops and bars. For the first time tea, coffee and nicotine were available to the masses; in the seventeenth century a caddy of tea would have cost a labourer's month's wages. *"The first coffee shop in Europe opened up in Oxford in 1650 and 50 yrs later there were hundreds in London alone. Fredrick the Great banned them in 1769 because he felt they were corrupting. Coffee is more popular the furtherer you go north in Europe. In 1913 the world's keenest coffee drinkers were the Dutch the Danes and the Swedes who drank at least eight times as much as the Italians. Even today nobody drinks more coffee than the Finns".* 7 February 2016 Empire of Things: How We Became a World of Consumers, from the Fifteenth Century to the Twenty-First by Frank Trentmann reviewed by Dominic Sandbrook.

The influences of Enlightenment ideas, and the economic constraints imposed by war and taxation, are of course acknowledged as major factors, but it took human agency, perhaps hypomanic activity, to bring them to Revolution. It would seem that the difference between the American Independence and the French Revolution was the paranoia and anger in France and the pursuit of fairness and independence (positive mania) in America. In the French Reign of Terror perhaps 16,594 were guillotined.

In 1996, professors David Lykken and Auke Tellegen from the University of Minnesota analysed long-term satisfaction rates of identical and non-identical twins, some of whom had been raised together and some who had not, and concluded happiness was almost 100 percent genetic. "Trying to be happier is like trying to be taller" they reported.[10]

Many sufferers of MDI have the messianic delusion, thinking they're Jesus or God. Approximately half of those found Guilty but Insane have killed, often parents, children or family members, sometimes under messianic delusion. Jesus might have been a manic-depressive, many of whom believe they are the messiah. In the "Jerusalem Syndrome" one psychiatrist in Jerusalem had 50 cases of messianic delusions in a year.[11] Jerusalem from "Yeru" meaning "foundation of" and the name of the ancient god of the evening star ;Shalem.

---

[10] David T Lykken and Auke Tellegen, "Happiness is a Stochastic Phenomenon" in *Psychological Science*, Vol 7, No 3, May 1996.

In 1840 in the psychiatric hospital Bicetre in Paris one in four diagnoses were delusions of grandeur who thought they were Napoleon. Women thought they were Joan of Arc. London review of Books 21 May 15 Laura Murat; "The man who thought he was Napoleon" review Mick Jay

The messianic delusion incorporates the various claims made by Jesus Christ, who thought he was the son of God; believed in the rising of his body to heaven; believed in love and an all-powerful God who forgives sins and with whom all who subscribe to the belief-system will live happily ever after. He also preached miracles and invoked the dead. All this could be interpreted as a very saleable religious manic commodity that is the Christian brand, which spreads across the MD spectrum of archetypes, from the more restrained Roman and Anglican Catholicism to the more normal Protestantism who have Bishops and no Popes and manic forms of Protestantism: The following sects have no Popes or no Bishops/ Presbyterianism (chosen people), Baptism (singing and preaching), Quakerism (talking aloud), Methodism (charity), / Lutherans (work ethic). Born-again Christians tend to get more and more manic as we go along.

To judge from his own trial under Judaic law, it seems that around the time of Jesus other people may have been executed for making the blasphemous claim that they were the messiah. For anyone to make such a dangerous claim would seem to suggest mania, or at least hypomania. Significantly, perhaps, Jesus reduced the Ten Commandments of Moses to two: "Thou shalt love the Lord thy God with all thy heart and with all thy soul and with thy entire mind. This is the first and greatest Commandment. And the second is like unto it. Thou shalt love thy neighbour as thyself. On these two Commandments hang all the law and the prophets" (Matt. 22.37- 40).

Love is a manic archetype that is embedded mainly in the right brain, and Jesus used aphorisms and parables rich in metaphor that also is embedded in the right brain. It may be significant that Jesus did not say to love everybody but to love "thy neighbour". This suggests the same sort of tribalism that that underlies Mosaic Law and that Jesus was as paranoid and suspicious of outsiders as most of his contemporaries. The parable of the Good Samaritan

---

[11] *Found in the Pilgrimage*, BBC 2, 17 December 2013.

does undercut this interpretation but the warning, "I bring not peace but the sword", may offer support.

This exploration of Jesus-as-hypomanic, though speculative, illustrates accurately enough the confidence to take on apparently superhuman tasks that the hypomanic often has - making the ultimate sacrifice, in Jesus' case. Also, some of what Jesus had to say about love fits the hypomanic pattern. On the one hand he offers the unconditional love of the child; on the other he threatens the direst consequences for those who do not love him (or at least his divine father). When we are in love there is, at some level, a fear - paranoia when it reaches unhealthy levels - of losing the love of our partner.

Fear and love are different sides of the same coin. We fear what we find dangerous and threatening, and the loss of love is very high on this totem. When we are paranoid in a relationship we check up where our partner has been and maybe check underwear for signs of sexual activity. This level of paranoia is dangerous, and some of Jesus' actions suggest that he was capable of unreasonable violence (apart from the eternal violence threatened against those who did not love him): his whipping the moneychangers off the temple steps is hard to understand, given that these men performed an essential and even sacred service, the graven images on Roman coins being forbidden in the temple itself, yet money being necessary to purchase sacrificial animals. **It is not the money that is the problem but the love of money that leads to jealousy of wealth.**

Would Jesus have been jealous of the Apostles liking Mary Magdalene? Though two geniuses of the twentieth century, Sigmund Freud and James Joyce, suffered from morbid jealousy, showing that it is not strictly a clinical condition, the mindset of morbid jealousy more typically is found in the paranoid manic. John Keats (born 1795) was jealous of Fanny Brawne his fiancée: "I am sickened at the brute world which you are smiling with". Jealousy is found in man and, in manifest actions at least, in animals. A husband has to know whether his wife's children are his, and sometimes male animals such as silverback gorillas and lions kill the earlier male's infants when they themselves take over nursing females.

Morbid jealousy is dangerous and in mankind can lead to murder. Recently I met a man who killed his wife because she had started to socialise after years of being kept at home by him. A successful businessman, he expressed no regret or remorse: "I prefer her to be dead than going out." They had moved from house to house maybe to stop her going out. He also murdered his two children as they pleaded, "Why are you killing us daddy?" With paranoia you tend to have polarised vision - the perfect wife and the whore - and this man was not about to allow his perfect wife to make a whore of herself.

Daphne du Maurier said about the 1938 cinematic hit, *Rebecca*, that it was all about jealousy not a romantic novel. Producer Dino de Laurentiis pulled out of Fellini's 1959 film *La Dolce Vita* because as a father he couldn't stomach the murder scene of two children by their father.

But as jealousy is so universal a trait, it must be an adaptive, not maladaptive, trait. Does jealousy serve a constructive purpose? Presumably so, if it evolved in apparently every species - the more jealous males ensured propagation of their own genes, to the point of murdering young they could not be sure of. Does jealousy keep partners together? Does jealousy suit monogamy? Possibly yes - but at what point does an adaptive trait become destructive?

Apparently the wife of the morbidly jealous man referred to above was a pretty woman, and across years and cultures proverbs warn against marrying a beautiful woman. But legal codes, in patriarchal societies anyway, go some way to providing safeguards: *"Thou shalt not covet thy neighbour's wife."*

Machiavelli said there are two ways of controlling people, love and fear, and he said that fear of punishment was the more successful control. If there is an element of fear in the conventionally jealous man that makes him prefer to live in the bliss of ignorance as to the exact parentage of his child, might it be folly of society to make itself wise in the ways of DNA testing? Or does this technology merely extend the possibilities for adaptive - in the long-term - jealousy?

The hypomanic perhaps has more reason than most for doubting the fatherhood of his children, as he himself is more disinhibited sexually and this leads to promiscuousness. Especially if paranoia develops, he is likely to project similar behaviour onto others, making his suspicion seems good sense if not proven fact. Their persistence in sexual promiscuity, even though hypomanics are as aware of AIDS as any other, is another manifestation of the reckless confidence that is a feature of the condition.

The Pony Express, trains, boats, cars, Morse code wireless messages telephone, coal, oil planes steel stronger ships computers, face book and the internet. The Paranoid Position may be seen increasingly as a social phenomenon as society itself moves at a faster pace, stimulates itself with everything from factual matters to trivia to perversion, thanks to the Internet and ubiquitous, twenty-four-hour television saturation, and works itself up to reckless levels of impatience and bravado with drink and drugs and frantic schedules of consumption. Every week we see on our streets a frenzy and savagery that seem psychotic and hear of people being murdered, often such people are killed for little or no reason.

Such manifestation of the Paranoid Position is far from new. The faster pace of life dates from the middle of the First Industrial Revolution with the steam-train, which increased both the speed and range of travel. Up until then the fastest speed available was that of a galloping horse, and such a speed could be sustained only for a short, exhilarating while. There was dark speculation at the time that any speed greater than 25 miles an hour would cause death, as God had not created the human body to withstand such speeds. Interestingly, the Duke of Wellington, then Prime Minister, was opposed to the idea of travel for the "lower orders", probably aware of how travel would broaden their minds, put them in contact with new and "dangerous" ideas, and subvert the existing social order.

Until then the only manifestation of hypomania discernable from today's vantage was in the upper class, which had the wealth to afford horses and to travel widely, and to indulge in horseracing and in such drugs as laudanum. The "lower orders" walked everywhere, which alone constrained their exposure to the world, slowed their pace of living, and left them too tired to indulge in hypomanic pursuits - even if they could have afforded to.

After the Second Transport Revolution - the spread of railways - the pace of life picked up, and what we can call hypomania becomes more discernable. The church bell was the closest most people got; instead they went more by the seasons, birdsong, blossom, harvest time, sunset and moonrise. To uniform day-month-year format that our computers command from us today across different time zones. Perhaps the Iron Duke was onto something: the "lower orders" did indeed become more dissatisfied as the nineteenth century progressed, with the emergence of trade unionism and a widespread rise in nationalism across Europe. From this dissatisfaction, one could argue, came a great range of social reforms, from extension of the franchise through factory legislation to implementation of state-socialism.

It would be wrong to impute a definite chain of causation here, yet it is interesting that the Reform Bill of 1832 came barely a decade after George Stephenson inaugurated the Railway Age with the Stockton and Darlington Railway, and Bismarck introduced state socialism a couple of years into what's now regarded as the Second Industrial Revolution, whose most important effects, in Europe at any rate, were in Germany.

Furthermore, the "lower orders" came to be manifestly affected by hypomania as the century wore on, especially toward its end in the years of "High Imperialism" and the "yellow press", which emerged from developments of the Second Industrial Revolution - cheap paper and printing - coupled to the more widespread literacy brought about by the various Education Acts. "Jingoism," an aggressive nationalism expressed in music hall songs, and the yellow press, were driven by the working class and to a very great extent underpinned British Imperial thinking and perhaps the very Empire, for all that it was the working class that suffered in sustaining the Empire through the soldiers it supplied to colonial wars and through the monetary sacrifices the metropolitan made to sustain its foreign presence. In one form and another hypomania can be discerned through the New Imperial age, and it helped to unleash the First World War and all the manic destructiveness of that.

A new transatlantic fibre optic cable with High Frequency Trading is 6 thousands of 59.5 thousands of a second quicker than normal fibre optic cables trading. The fastest service could cost up to $20 million for 5 years of access or $333.333 a month. A slower option which takes 62ms to complete the trip costs about $35.000 a month. HFT makes up 50 percent of USA trading and 40 percent of Euperone trading and makes millions of dollars in a market of multi trillion equity markets of automated stock-market trading. The miniscule time saved will bring in millions of dollars; Microwave is faster but cannot be used at sea.

Rory Mulholland Irish Times 3th October 2015.

In a computer world you have more people, you see increased speed, more frequency, decreased cost. Two billion people have e mail addresses, one billion are on Facebook and there are a billion credit cards in circulation in the USA.

Today, however, paranoia seems to be occurring more on a personal than on a cultural level, perhaps because now hypomania's public endorsement is more that of universal love in the PC agenda than the publicly endorsed xenophobia it was associated with in the Imperial age. But there are many other reasons for this personal expression of the Paranoid Position.

An important part of modern Western culture is advertising, which tries to make people buy more - i.e. it makes them more hypomanic, more ready to accept, with zest or with less critical questioning, what otherwise they might question or reject. Adverts sell things that clean because we are programmed to be paranoid of germs and dirt. In fact, evidence suggests that lack of exposure to dirt may result in asthma, which in Ireland affects twenty percent of children (25 percent in the UK).

But while it has become part of our culture, advertising conversely can be used to dictate, or at least influence, how our culture develops. Advertisers want people to buy their products; many of them (advertisers) use cannabis, cocaine, amphetamines, L.S.D. and Ecstasy to make themselves more creative. Coca-Cola, the most successful drink in the world, used to have cocaine in it and this made people manic. Coke kept the idea of manic, happy, smiling people and put it in their advertisements. In today's more nuanced times brand names such as Levis, Pepsi, Nike and Coca-Cola can be sold in advertising that is "culturally sensitive" and promises to lead to social and individual fulfilment. Pepsi used "the Pepsi Generation" for years before Coca Cola caught up with "It's the real thing".

Psychiatry recognises two types of people who spend without control: those in the manic phase of manic-depressive illness, and those suffering from compulsive buying disorder.

Kellet, S., and Bolton J. V. (2009) Compulsive buying disorder. Clinical Psychology and Psychotherapy 16,83-99 say that compulsive buying disorder "is experienced as an a irresistible - uncontrollable urge in excessive and time consuming retail activity that is typically prompted by negative affectivity" and results in "gross social, personal and/or financial difficulties" CBD is found in 5.8 percent of the United States population. Male similar to female. CBD is characterized by an obsession with shopping and buying behaviour that causes adverse consequences. People spend more and get into trouble with the banks. Materialist values, consumer culture, capitalism and advertising drives their spending. It is similar to, but distinguished from, OCD hoarding and mania.

People drink and spend more money when they are manic, and spending money is the root of capitalism and advertising. The things that make people manic and spend are self-love, love of other,[12] humour, sexuality, paranoia, intellect, creativity, and over activity - the various manic archetypes. Ogilvy, the advertising guru, said sex and humour don't sell. He was obviously wrong, in the light of subsequent discoveries.[13] The manic archetype theory can go a long way to account for advertising and its success in selling sex, cars, chocolate, coffee, drink, pole dancing, phone porn, cigarettes etc.

Multinational conglomerates that see profit and consumerism as the only parameter of cultural success form the driving force in modern capitalist society and surpass the force of democracy. Their aim is control of the market through advertising in order to maximise their profits. "In the 15th century rich people were splashing out on spoons, forks, eggcups and drinking glasses. By the 1700 a typical Dutch farm house was stuffed with a "clock, carpets and curtains, paintings, books and some porcelain dishes" Today an average German owns 10,000 different things. Consumerism has actually been one of the great liberating forces of the modern age. The characteristic consumer durable of the 1950's and the 1960's was the washing machine".

Maybe society can be manipulated so that it controls the id and expresses it in an acceptable way. If advertising can influence our outlook and our culture, perhaps it could be made to do this toward the benefit of the world if advertisers could be made socially responsible; the Benetton ads have made

---

[12] Love-of-other was well expressed in the old Coca Cola jingle by the New Seekers: "I'd like to teach the world to sing / In perfect harmony / ... / I'd like to buy the world a Coke..."

[13] "Sex Sells" by the Tulips expresses the actuality in song.

some headway in portraying a peaceful, inclusive world in recent years. However, given that their raison d'être is to encourage spending, a hypomanic activity, it seems difficult to imagine advertisers developing a vested interest in social responsibility. Benetton may only be taking advantage of the current popularity of political correctness.

Humanity tends toward chaos unless restrained by rules and regulations, and hypomania tends to reject all regulation, subjugating everything to gratification of the id. Hypomania eventually leads to cultural and social chaos. Control of sexuality, morality, thinking and creativity is lost; people get more and more manic with a loss of focus; e.g. with hypomanic pursuit of ambition, the extended family gives way to the so-called nuclear family, and this, after easier access to divorce and lowered social censure of personal morals, to the single-parent family. The satisfaction of the id is one of the means by which we measure success in modern cultures; hence, ironically, society tends toward a primitive state under hypomania, where murder becomes more prevalent. Basic instincts are satisfied and the domestication of man is reversed.

Simultaneously, because of its predilection for unconditional love of fellow-man, hypomania has been in part responsible for a far less punitive judicial system and penal regime. This may be all to the good - provided that the changes lead to improvement in the well-being of society and enhance the good of the majority. But it is at very best debatable that this has been the result. Anyone of middle age or older can recall a time when a murder made for shocking news in Ireland; today there may be several in a single week. Up to a third such murders may be carried out by people on bail for violent crime; many are committed by men sentenced to "life in prison" for previous murders but released on licence, on average after fourteen years and often less.

Thus greater social tolerance is exacerbated by greater reluctance to punish violent deviancy from the social norm, accelerating the trend toward primitiveness. As good-living people see their safety imperilled with all-but impunity they are forced toward greater self-reliance. In recent weeks, in response to a spate of brutal burglaries, vigilante groups have been set up in rural Donegal. Some years ago an isolated farmer, Padraig Nally, shot and killed his tormentor, a violent career criminal for whose arrest five bench warrants had been issued while he carried out a spate of burglaries across the West of Ireland.

But, if hypomanic rejection of regulation leads toward chaos in which ultimately nothing can thrive, reaction must come - the Donegal vigilante patrols may be an early manifestation of this. Even the multinational companies may come to agree that, if there is no more to life on this planet than profit, a market is necessary for profit to be extracted, and markets cannot thrive in anarchy; thus they will subscribe to rules and regulations that will protect man from himself. Thomas Mann claimed that "to maintain in masses respect for reason and truth and in so doing honour their longing for justice is far better than implanting mass myths and turning loose upon mankind hordes dominated by powerful illusions" - whether these be that social reform can be effected by removal of the punitive element from the penal system, that things go better with Coke, or that Guinness is good for you.

How we advertise ourselves is how, on a species-level, we sell our genes: through buying and selling in the market place, where we live, what job we have, our type of car, class, accent, cultural values, school, religion and clothes. People are attracted to the glamour of films, modelling, money, music and gossip, but such jobs and positions may not actually pay, may be "powerful illusions." For example, a friend's father was very successful with two pubs in working class areas but, wanting a more glamorous location, with a richer clientele, he bought a pub in a middle class area and lost thousands.

Advertising is the most modern form of art we have. It might shape our lives more than common culture, or old culture derived from parables, stories and myth. Today advertising has taken over myth and reshaped it. Films now have product placement. Culture is changing all the time especially over the last hundred years. But mankind could not have changed over a few thousands of years compared to the millions of years of evolution. The hardwiring of hundreds of thousands of years cannot be easily changed or manipulated. Nurture cannot be more important than nature outside of individual cases. Essentially we have changed very little in wants and needs emotionally, physically, and intellectually over the last ten thousand years; but in recent decades, a hundred years or so at most, we have changed our society to a degree and at a pace that is utterly unprecedented, such a pace, indeed, that is figuratively just one step ahead of overwhelming us. AI (Artificial Intelligence) is the next problem on the list. (2015)

We are social animals, and, almost by definition, chaos in society must lead to that society's breakdown. Darwinism claims that random mutation may lead to either adaptive or maladaptive developments, and natural selection then remorselessly and disinterestedly destroys the maladaptive ones. Though selection is always of the individual organism, and Social Darwinism has been discredited, change nevertheless occurs in society as well as in individual organisms; the difference is that such change is not completely random but consequent to earlier developments. But if change is not random, can selection dispense with maladaptive change?

Such selection cannot be natural, in the Darwinian way, for each change has its advocates and detractors and the interplay between these determines the fate of the change. But whether the change is adaptive or otherwise will affect the amount of support that it garners, and the relative number of its advocates and detractors. Ultimately the longer-term result is that all social change is dispensed with, but some can last a very long time indeed: events have proved that Communism clearly does not work, yet Marxism thrives. Fads quickly burn out in the same flame that forged them. Those that endure have been given the name memes by the eminent Darwinian, Richard Dawkins.

Memes are dealt with later; for the moment we may say that change ultimately may affect society no less than the individuals who make up that society.

It is possible that hypomania, per se, is neutral. In Edison's case it led to success for the individual and great advancements for the society of which that individual was a component; in Jim Jones's case it led to self-destruction of both the individual and the society, as the hypomanic belief in Manifest Destiny led to genocide of whole native tribes in the New World. But in all cases, whether of individual, species, or society, the niche that is left by extinction will be filled by others better adapted to fill it.

Hypomania may even lead to both extinction and the emergence of new "forms": if hypomanic excess was what eventually led to the fall of the

Roman empire, it was equally hypomanic cultures that filled the niche left; firstly the manic hordes of Ostrogoths, Visigoths and Huns, later a repressive, obsessive Christianity.

In our own society we see some signs of the hypomanic degeneracy that afflicted the empires of the ancient world. In addition to alcohol we have many other drugs. In place of chariot races and gladiatorial slaughter we have the Super Bowl, Grandstand, personality prize-fighters like Muhammad Ali, and war on CNN. We have cars easily capable of doing twice the speed limit and the children of small farmers and factory workers broken by the purchase of holiday homes in exotic locations. We have frantic spending, keeping up with the Joneses, capital as a measure of overall worth and, at national level, the pursuit of economic growth for its own sake.

Much of this demand and expenditure is fuelled by advertising, which creates and fosters a need that is more artificial than real. This is at both individual and cultural level: the USSR was brought down by spending on a Star Wars programme that was sold to them as a "need" they had to meet or perish - a Darwinian model of survival of the fittest.

As in the fifth century, might our own Western society, already speeded up to manic levels by technology, as well as by degeneracy, implode, or be brought down by manic hordes of Muslim and Third World "barbarians," its empty niche filled by repressive, obsessive fundamentalist Islam?

Again here we may see hypomanic love for our fellow man, which insists that all refugees, genuine or spurious, be welcomed into Western society, even though such people openly proclaim their hatred for Western values. The accompanying hypomanic sense of grandiosity creates a sense of invulnerability to "primitive" values and beliefs, which our hubris convinces us we can overcome. The two hypomanic beliefs create a positive feedback loop that may prove perilous for our society.

If hypomania can be maladaptive, society must devise mechanisms of selection that root out such maladaptive changes. But how can such selection be agreed in any society that is put in a state of flux by the very changes it seeks to regulate?

Totalitarian societies could impose such selection without society's agreement - and it is worth considering whether the growth of democracy is the fundamental force behind such rapid and dramatic change as we have witnessed in the past 200 years or so. If this is true, is there any way that democracy can control maladaptive change in the way authoritarian societies could?

The short answer would seem to be No - for two reasons: first, democratic consensus is difficult to obtain, as proved by the ongoing debate over climate change and the necessary responses to it; and second, we can only know if change has been adaptive or otherwise with hindsight. Even if climate change is taking place, how much is man-made?

It is sometimes remarked that recent years has seen the West enter a post-democratic phase. Evidence for this purportedly ranges from secret surveillance of its citizens by the USA to the gradual erosion of national autonomy in the EU - for instance, the Irish being "asked" to re-run referenda until the "right" result is obtained. Such anti-democratic measures are excused on the grounds that world events and resources are now controlled by large blocs rather than countries, and that national independence needs to be subsumed into one of these blocs.

Such blocs, controlled by a relatively small number of individuals, would be better able to come to consensus on what they judged to be maladaptive, hypomanic behaviour. We see this already in the countless EU directives issued over the years, controlling and regulating ordinary people. One can understand building regulations and safety standards, but to make use of imperial measures illegal in trade seems disquieting.

Nevertheless, imposing certain checks and balances could dampen down hypomanic activity to the benefit of all. A good example would be drug tests on stockbrokers and dealers, who could bring about, in an extreme situation, collapse of the world economy in an afternoon.

However, one could argue that national democracies being subsumed into international blocs is itself evidence of hypomanic activity, and it would seem to take hypomania for the small cabals in power to sustain control of these blocs, so it becomes hard to place faith in these same cabals dampening down hypomania in society at large.

Hypomania has to be controlled in some way or else society collapses into chaos. One could argue that such collapse already is well advanced. There were five murders in Ireland in 1960; today there are over 100 per year and often several a week. Not infrequently, such murders are committed by murderers who had been sentenced to "life" for previous murders. Between a quarter and a third of violent crime is committed by people on probation, leniency by the courts allowing such offenders to continue to bring society deeper into chaos. In 2013 one such offender was sentenced to three years for assaulting two gardaí with a golf-club, when they apprehended him housebreaking - but 34 months of the three years were suspended.

The pitfalls of such a hypomanic society are evident. How did other societies deal with them? The lawlessness of the nineteenth-century American West is legendary. It was dealt with by rough justice. However, was lynching, and the severity of "Hanging Judge" Parker, not perhaps other evidence of hypomania?

North of the border Her Majesty's government in Canada took a different approach: law, in the form of the Royal Canadian Mounted Police, preceded settlement beyond the frontier. Thus the hypomanic violence of the American West was not allowed to emerge.

Going back further, the Roman Catholic Church was well aware of the pitfalls of a manic society and developed ways of dampening manic traits. After the Reformation "Improvement" the Protestant Churches continued such dampening in their flocks. It can be argued that Catholicism was more constricting of hypomania than any of the Protestant Churches, but in the matter of sexual repression Protestant Victorian England was the exemplar.

Such repression was, in fact, adaptive and benevolent in the round. Before social security was available promiscuous sex would have been disastrous for society. Children needed two parents to have any chance of thriving, or even surviving, and an unmarried mother would have to both look after her child and work to support it and her, all but impossible when long hours' toil was the working day. "Baby farms", which cared for the children of such women, at a high cost to the mothers, survived into the twentieth century. Harsh societal penalties were imposed to deter premarital sex, and while these seem to have been much harder on women than on men, this in part was because an abandoned pregnant woman stood to suffer a hard fate when the man could easily evade his duties and lose himself in industrial cities, or the army or the navy.

With the social changes that followed the two world wars, and especially after the development of the contraceptive pill, women were freed, to a great extent, of the dangers of single motherhood; and with further changes in societal attitudes, and better social welfare support, the stigma of illegitimacy was gradually removed. The "permissive society", very hypomanic, was a consequence.

But the loss of the previously rigidly-enforced sense of duty was seen immediately in breakdown of the traditional family, as the emphasis changed from responsibility to rights, the latter quickly coming to be seen as divorced from the former and being sacrosanct and unconditional. Family breakdown, with children reared without a male role model, fosters juvenile delinquency, which exacerbates hypomania, and the courts' reluctance to interfere with the "rights" of offenders accelerates social breakdown.

Trying to control contraception and abortion is clearly futile if not ill advised in an overpopulated world, yet one can see the social advantages in supporting marriage and monogamy. 8,500 abortions in the Republic of Ireland in 2022.

Yet how effective might any attempt to reinstate earlier attitudes be, in a zeitgeist that increasingly divorces rights from responsibilities? Indeed, there is all but a disavowal of responsibilities in faux-liberals' fight to have prisoners given conjugal visits, the responsible members of society being left to rear more children that result.

Can we, indeed, ever legislate effectively for moral behaviour? The idea that the Ten Commandments indicates that we can so legislate may be misleading. Originally the Commandments were more a civil than a moral code, adapted to a tribal society: textual analysis suggests that the Fifth/Sixth Commandment originally meant "Thou shalt not murder" - i.e. not kill a member of the tribe. The Commandments gained wider acceptance as Judaism gave rise to Christianity and this became a world religion rather than a tribal one; but now increasingly once-universal precepts are being questioned in a society that rejects, if not the very existence of God, any divine right to "Command" anyone in the laws of a secular land where everyone has the right not to be commanded or coerced by anyone else (and little concomitant responsibility to command or control oneself).

The permissive society made extramarital relationships almost respectable, and certainly no longer the scandalous thing they would have been.

What happens in those societies that reject modern values is almost worse. The recent kidnapping of little girls by Boko Harum in Nigeria is typical of what happens when rights are made subservient to perceived divine command. Islamists' attempts to bring about a modern caliphate are truly terrifying in their capacity for rolling back the Enlightenment and destroying the rights of almost everyone, certainly those of women. Wahabbism endorses barbaric practises from slavery to infibulation and the charismatic and/or frenzied proclamations of its adherents are clearly hypomanical if not totally maniacal.

Boko Haram and Wahabbism in general seek to "legislate for morality" as the Victorians did, but in a far more extreme and brutal way, controlling women by physical enslavement and in a more intimately physical way by excision of part of their genitals in order to make sexual intercourse not merely bereft of pleasure but positively painful for them. This all but ensures, in a virulently patriarchal society, that the man's line will be unquestionably legitimate, more unambiguously than any social disapproval could.

Female promiscuity is seen in many species and can be accounted for by better ensuring genetic continuance, by "spreading the risk" so to speak, in conjunction with the genes of several partners. In some species, domestic cats, for instance, multiple matings and super-fecundity sees kittens of the same litter with obviously different parental characteristics. Other species, man for instance, manages the "risk" of ensuring genetic continuance by partnership in a monogamous relationship. Monogamy assures the father that it's for his own children he's working and providing, and he best ensures their well-being by securing that of their mother.

But the two systems of gene-propagation are not mutually exclusive - or at any rate nominally-monogamous arrangements are frequently departed from. Men were, traditionally, more inclined to "stray", but today women are as free to do so, after being liberated from their fertility by modern contraception.

But even in the past it was cynically remarked, "It's a wise child knows its father". Women have always gone outside the confines of monogamy and often brought the consequences back with them to the monogamous relationship, thereby ensuring that their genetic heritage was strengthened by maximum immersion in the gene pool, combined with the protection of a husband. In many and maybe most cases, the husband may have suspected or known the truth but gone along, out of pragmatism (a child was less a mouth to feed than a potential asset, and indeed a real asset from a quite young age), love, or societal pressure stemming from the fear of public humiliation and the scandal of marriage breakdown.

Today DNA testing can determine paternity, but with what consequences for relationships and social organisations? Will it pander to greater hypomania? What we know about human nature, coupled to the prevailing zeitgeist that elevates rights almost to fetishism, and discounts responsibilities, suggests that greater societal instability will be the consequence of greater knowledge in this matter.

Both promiscuity and monogamy offer advantages in propagating the genes, and the genetic legacy may have consequences for subsequent behaviour. The choosing of our partner on sexual, physical, emotional and intellectual grounds must be one of the most important characteristics that we express seeing as it leads to our genetic heritage that is left behind when we leave. What are the characteristics of man that make him succeed physically, mentally and emotionally? If hypomania results in promiscuity, which results in more offspring, is hypomania therefore a species-adaptive trait? Alternatively, if hypomania results in carelessness and irresponsibility then will fewer of the hypomanic's offspring survive to sexual maturity and the trait prove maladaptive?

This thesis, that hypomania may be adaptive, at the level of the individual, the community, and even the species, must be regarded as tentative. The collapse of the USSR may have been due to ideological blinding rather than cultural hypomania, a delusional belief that no other system could be better, which resulted in Soviet agriculture, to take one example, suffering from ideological constraints from the 1930s to the very end - food shortages were a regular feature of Soviet life, ranging from the terrible famines of the 1920s and 30s to well-founded jokes. ("What's two miles long and eats cabbage?

A Moscow meat queue.") The Victorians had a similar belief in the British Empire, the Americas in Manifest Destiny; ideological blinding must have been a factor when the scions of Empire worried about the decline in the physical strength and moral fibre of the Empire's defenders - the working class, which provided the rank and file of the British Army - when the cost of maintaining the very Empire impoverished the lower classes of the cosmopolitan. When the economist JA Hobson pointed this out in 1902 he was ignored.

The nineteenth century saw, in addition to New Imperialism and the Gilded Age, the invention of modern advertising attempts to make products more available to the consumer and to dictate consumer spending. Do we buy things we do not want or need? Does advertising control us and change our behaviour? Does it change what we think and feel is it such a pervasive effect on us as consumers? Mothers testify to "pester power": problems at the checkout where sweets are displayed and the children become demanding.

The law of elasticity says that you can only sell a certain amount of product, after which there is substitution; the money spent is the same but the products bought change. Advertising complicates this by trying to change the brands bought. People buy a BMW or Armani clothes or Chanel No.5 in order to reflect, in some way and to some extent, the way they see themselves and the image they wish to present to the world. People laugh and say the car is a penis extension but they are not very wrong. A salesman claims that the BMW car is only a badge; that we believe in the badge that is advertised. We look at each other in the traffic. The Volvo is safe; the Saab is for the driver who does not want to stand out; the Merc is for posers.

The old saying has it that only fifty percent of advertising works but unfortunately no one knows which fifty. By stimulating the manic archetypes you stimulate spending and due to advertising you get greater capitalism. It was in the latter part of the twentieth century that advertising took over the front page of magazines and journals, and advertising supplements appeared; proto-environmentalists were complaining about hoardings and billboards in nineteenth-century England.

It seems safe to say that while the Victorians had advertising they were not hypomanic. Yet is this true? The Victorians en masse were deeply concerned with social problems and in a relatively short period changed the workplace in many sweeping ways. They saw not just Britain but most of the world covered by railways, speeding up beyond previous imagination the speed and extent of travel (an aspect of hypomania) and they brought British Christian rule to a fifth of the world and a quarter of its people, including more than 100 million Moslems and even more Hindus. Individuals like Dickens and Brunel were incredibly driven people, creative and hard-working and socially engaged. In the USA the personal and business wealth of JP Morgan has been calculated as equal to all the real estate between the Mississippi and the West Coast. Philanthropy, in its modern form, emerged in the Victorian age.

One might say that their use of drugs was another hypomanic trait of the Victorians, who had virtually unrestricted access to any drug then known (opium and absinthe being particularly popular, though the fictive Sherlock Holmes used cocaine). Again, however, there may be a difference in the type of drugs used that makes direct comparison hazardous: cocaine, hash, E, speed and LSD all have paranoia-inducing qualities. Also, while individual Victorians had drug problems, Victorian society had no sort of "drug problem" such as our society has.

"Problem" may be an inadequate word; perhaps even misleading. Not alone is recreational drug use widespread today, drug use may be intrinsic to modern economies. Stockbrokers testify to use of cocaine on the stock exchange floor, stimulating frenetic trading, as well as a "champagne and cocaine" lifestyle after work. Such is the pace that many stockbrokers are burned out inside ten years, but in those few manic years they may make enough to keep them for the rest of their lives.

Similarly, drug usage is said to be widespread in the advertising industry. There's a certain logic here in that advertising induces mania in society, and this mania may be reflected in the use of drugs, especially cocaine, that mimics the mania found in the advertising industry.

Hypomanic traits seem to reveal what is potentially successful in at least some people's lives. Whether such traits will be beneficial in the case of any one person we cannot know in advance, but intuitively hypomania does seem to offer some positive effect on human life, culture and creativity both individually and collectively.

MANIA, PARANOIA, HYPOMANIA

In manic depression certain characteristics are found that I call the manic archetypes. These archetypes are found in the manic phase of manic-depressive illness. Lower levels of the manic archetypes are found in people who do not have manic-depressive illness. These archetypes can be stimulated to make the person hypomanic.

A manic high means that the patient is physically, mentally, emotionally and intellectually overactive. This over activity is objectively and clinically definable, and readily apparent to the layperson, even if only by comparison to "normal" behaviour.

However, below the manic threshold is a state called hypomania, where the patient's energy, physical, mental, emotional and intellectual, is between normal and manic Bipolar Disorder 2 in DSM5 (*Diagnostic and Statistical Manual 5*). Throughout this paper the term *hypomania* is used in a somewhat looser sense than its current strict clinical definition, which is usually over-activity of physical, mental, emotional and intellectual faculties, high pressure of speech and thought, grandiose delusions, labile emotions, loosening of association and consequent increased creativity, extending over a period of two weeks or longer. But this looser definition need not negate the value of the paper, for the lines that are drawn between "normal" and "hypomanic" behaviour are not lines cut in scientific stone. "Tending toward hypomania" is a cumbersome phrase, and it is this tendency, latent or manifest to different degrees, that this paper seeks to explore and examine.

Also, this paper associates paranoia with mania, where paranoia is normally associated with schizophrenia, especially if there are religious delusions especially concerning Jesus (messianic delusions). Freud felt that schizophrenia should be treated as separate from either mania or paranoia; this paper rather sees the condition (paranoia) as interpenetrative of both the others. The more one goes forward, exploring new worlds - in mania - the more one looks behind - with paranoia - to ensure security in the new territory.

Paranoia is related to jealousy. The jealous nature does not trust and this may lead to paranoia, fear that something will be taken away. Paranoia lends itself to capitalism through the advertising of products such as cleaning agents and insurance policies: don't leave the family penniless; the germs are out to get you and your house should be clean or the neighbours will sneer and you need a house alarm. Consequently, many housewives spend a good part of the day cleaning the house and their husbands clean the car at weekends.

The drive to clean has an Obsessive Compulsive Disorder quality and it may have negative effects. Excessive cleaning may lead to more asthma in children due to less exposure to dirt, and it may impose an unnecessary burden of labour. It is calculated that despite the conveniences of mechanisation and piped water, housewives still spend as much time doing the laundry as their grandmothers and great-grandmothers did. The range of products to deal with the toilet, the laundry, the windows, the sink, the dishes, the clothes are myriad: bleach, soap, shampoo, perfume, deodorant; Persil, Ariel, Daz, Cif, VO5, OMO Brasso, Silvo, Fairy Liquid, Cosmetics, Shake and Vac, Flash, Ajax, Harpic, Domestos ("Big Dom"). Everything must be shiny and clean. Quentin Crisp once said that you did not notice the dust after four years, and while he was joking the point is made that one does not need to be obsessive-compulsively clean to succeed.

On 19 July 2014 BBC2 broadcast *The Men who Made us Spend*, by Jacque Peretti. Fear/Paranoia makes us spend. People buy SUVs because their size makes their drivers feel safer even though they turn over more easily. People are scared of cholesterol and use statins more and more. Antibacterial soaps and hand-cleaners are more common and Dettol is now used in clothes cleaning. There is frequent germ panic prompted by such things as Asian flu. We are bombarded with new drinks including "vitiman water". Fear of aging affects a lot of people and they exercise more and get face lifts. Fear of death is a big business. Health insurance capitalises on this and on the fear of sickness. One of the first products with built-in obsolescence was the light bulb: after the Second World War bulbs with a ten-year life span were shelved in order to ensure rapid turnover. Buying is getting easier with credit cards causing less pain. Internet buying is done by Pay Pal. Games sell more than music and video put together.

Paranoia is a manic archetype. The paranoid fear of being killed by an animal or another human being is a basic fear in man. Early man lived in continual fear of being killed or having offspring, relatives, friends, peers and tribe killed - a paranoid state. As he set out to hunt, or to defend his territory, he travelled forward carefully (mania) but was sure to look over his shoulder (paranoia). Perhaps because of this original association between hunting and defending with paranoia there evolved the ability to kill without guilt. Unfortunately psychiatrists usually lump paranoia under schizophrenia or schizoaffective disorder. This is not necessarily the appropriate classification for it.

Mania and paranoia go hand in hand and to an extent, in some cases at least, are indistinguishable: mania comprises anxiety, fear and paranoia. During the Cold War the USA and USSR were paranoid about each other; today's paranoia is of drugs, terrorists or an endangered natural ecosystem.

From a cultural perspective, however, paranoia may be adaptive in the long term. The most enormous and impressive advances have been made during wartime, and between the two world wars the rate of advance in, certainly, aero technology slowed greatly. The Spitfire, the Messerschmit Bf109 and even the fabric-fuselage Hurricane were enormous advances on the aeroplanes of the Great War, but it was Fairey Swordfishes, open-cockpit biplanes, that took out the *Bismarck* in 1941. Of course, this is true only to a point, as the potential for nuclear war proves. Six out of 10 people in the U.K. in the sixties believed that nuclear war was a possibility.

When people have manic-depressive illness they can be in different emotional states. Hypomania is a similar affective condition that can be stimulated in most "ordinary" people, sometimes toward a particular end. Typically patients show a stylised mood swing pattern, from mania through "normality" to depression and back up again; but really there may be no regularity or cyclicity to mood changes. Some people will be hypomanic virtually all the time, and it is these people that this paper is mostly concerned with.

DIAGNOSTIC CRITERIA FOR MANIC EPISODES

Before diagnosis of mania, at least three of the following must be present to a significant degree for at least one week:

Grandiosity
Decreased need for sleep
Pressured speech
Flight of ideas
Distractibility
Psychomotor agitation
Excessive involvement in pleasurable activities without regard for negative consequences e.g. sexual relations.

Characteristics (the manic archetypes themselves) that advertising may use to promote hypomania - and thereby advance the advertiser's product/service - are:

GRANDIOSE DELUSIONS - God, Jesus, Space Traveller, Most people think their O.K/special but not brilliant.

HUMOUR – anarchy, infectious mood

SEXUALITY - disinhibition

SELF LOVE - ego, nationalism, "the best a man can get"

LOVE OF OTHERS - super ego, Socialism

PARANOIA - id, Paranoid position, National Socialism

CHARISMA - enthralling

SPENDING - capitalism

COMPETITION - sport

ENERGY - work ethic

INTELLECT - seeks truth and finds beauty

CREATIVITY - seeks beauty and finds truth

EGO - shame/laws of the self.

SUPER EGO - guilt/ parents/laws/church/morality

ID - instinct

SLEEP - some people thrive on less sleep. They tend to be more ambitious, outgoing, optimistic and even more energetic. Famous workaholics are Leonardo da Vinci, Thomas Jefferson, Margaret Thatcher and Benjamin Franklin. (Jamie McGinnes, *Sunday Times* 10 April 2011). All of these were manic in their own different ways, but perhaps of special note in the part played by Franklin and Jefferson in the Declaration of Independence, a very manic document that proclaims "Life Liberty and the pursuit of Happiness".

Other signs of mania are;

High activity, high esteem, poor judgement, poor anger control, irritability, gambling, poor business decisions, grandiose delusions and hallucinations (notably of Jesus and/or the Devil) and racing thoughts.

Humour: absurdity and anarchy campaigns against self-control and critical evaluation, and stimulates acceptance of the advertised product/service/belief-system.

Sex: disinhibition stimulates demand. The increasing prevalence, or at least social acceptability, especially on T.V of heterosexuality may reflect a more hypomanic society. Freud tried to make the connection between sex and humour but he never had a psychotic manic patient and therefore never saw the connection even though he developed cocaine as a local anaesthetic and took cocaine socially as a euphoric stimulant that was legal at the time. Freuds early conviction that cocaine was a universal panacea for mental and physical distress. He became addicted himself explaining hallucinations he endured and he caused addiction in others by blithely dispensing the drug. We are never so defenceless against suffering as when we love. That work, love and taking responsibility are the most important things in life. FREUD. The Making of an Illusion by Frederick Crews Sunday times 27 August 2017 review by Bryan Appleyard.

Self love: self esteem: narcissism obviously leads to greater purchasing readiness, but may also be used to promote nationalistic causes; a function of the Freudian ego.

Self-love is the basis of humanity. Drugs such as cocaine increase self-love and they also make you like other people; they also sexualise people and make them paranoid. Hash and other drugs are used in advertising brainstorming. A friend of mine was doped with a cocaine sandwich by a guy who then raped her. Fortunately she went to a doctor and he did blood tests on her. A solution was found and the people involved were satisfied with the outcome.

Self-help books try to stimulate self-love; they use mantras such as "I'm the best" that reinforce self-love. Tina Turner sings about "Simply the Best." Other commodities, like Oil of Olay say, "Because you're worth it". Forgiving yourself is important in self-love. Catholics have confession in a way that Protestants do not. Does this increase the control of the RC Church?

Love of others (a function of the Freudian super-ego), in a hypomanic state may be used to promote socialism: love of family, friends, society, country and world. Jesus said love your neighbour as you love yourself; he did not say love everybody. Can you love yourself as well as other people without bringing on paranoia? Is self-love a prerequisite for the love of others?

Jung believed in a world consciousness and this arguably is now emerging in such global organisations as Greenpeace and Amnesty International. Perhaps world consciousness was also shown by the grieving for Princess Diana - though this also was a function of the power of TV, something that was also shown by 9/11. People live their lives through TV-prompted emotion - "Telemotion."

Catholicism seems to control by fostering poor self-esteem, fear, guilt, loving a fearsome God, and deferring wishes for happiness until we get to heaven. Having asexual priests and nuns in the church leads to a manic depressive mood environment around the church and a lack of hypomania but not as manic as non-Catholic churches such as Presbyterian, Baptist, Pentecostal, Protestant, Born Again and Methodist.

Intelligent Catholic manic people may be attracted to the church as priests or nuns because of its manic qualities, and over time their genes are lost to the gene pool, as they do not have children. The absolute infallibility of the Pope during "ex cathedra" expression of church doctrine is hard to believe in, in the modern world, as is the belief in transubstantiation. In this regard hypomania may be a way of social control that has developed in the Church. Priests are attracted to God and this may be a sign of hypomania as is the delusion that you're Jesus or God, and they would have been watched and controlled by the Vatican.

Even though there might be manic priests there are fewer manic bishops and fewer manic archbishops, the manic tendency being progressively weeded out so that we do not get a manic pope. The fact that the Borgias were supremely hypomanic doesn't belie this claim: Alexander VI bribed his way into the papacy, in a very different, non-democratic age. All popes in recent centuries have been conservative if not reactionary, with the exceptions of John XXIII and possibly John-Paul I.

Paranoia, fear, anxiety are all manifestations of the Freudian id state. In the "paranoid position", when paranoia is induced, a hypomanic may be able to kill without guilt.

Yet the id has to be expressed if an individual and even a society is to function; all these primitive actions and atavistic emotions have to be experienced. People's basic fantasies like the Oedipus complex, murder, and patricide are expressed under certain understood environments whether this is real or fiction. Underlying the facade of middle class beliefs in the civilised West is a cauldron of opposite emotions. In extreme societies like the Islamic State such expression may be not merely easier, but positively socially laudable.

Paranoia requires an object of hate, which may be traced to human survival instinct but manifests in such rivalry as Coke -v- Pepsi; Celtic -v- Rangers. Studies indicate that xenophobia is individually and culturally adaptive: driving strangers away, or having as little as possible to do with them, reduces the risk of attack by enemies. In a modern global world, with various legal and security safeguards that were absent in tribal societies, the danger is far less, and the gains to be made from trade or cross-cultural interchange may even make xenophobia an individual and cultural liability. But this change is in most cases mere centuries old, in many places it may be only decades old, and in some places it may never have taken place at all. Even in the civilised West, as HG Wells put it, scratch the most urbane of us and the hot red eyes of the caveman will soon begin to glare.

Our predilection for xenophobia may be used by governments (or terrorist organisations) to promote war or such causes as National Socialism. In Ireland we traditionally hated the British whereas the German National Socialists hated the Jews. The Jews, a stateless, transnational community for centuries, survived many years of xenophobic persecution as a wandering tribe. An obstacle that tested their perseverance and their religion was the nationalism that they themselves now nurture in their homeland, Israel. But their own newfound nationalism may lead to a different sort of xenophobia and confrontation - indeed it already has - and perhaps, eventually, annihilation by the surrounding Moslem lands.

Charisma: promoting hypomania within a personality culture may be used to advance the cause of the leader of a country, cause, etc. This may be for good – Churchill - or ill - Hitler (though obviously good and ill are subjective terms). There is a connection here with sex: when people are manic their sex drive increases; they become more charming, have great self-esteem and are sexually attractive.

Spending: people may enjoy spending, and if this trait can be encouraged by stimulating hypomania through advertising, capitalism benefits. In part to appeal to the hypomania of the marketplace, many products are advertised as "new and improved", thereby stimulating demand in people for what they haven't got and are encouraged to believe they're entitled to.

Energy: hypomania may promote the work ethic. When people are manic or in the grip of an idea they can be workaholics and never even notice time passing. In times of war or national emergency, such as in New York in 2001 - indeed, across the USA then - we see it at a macro-level. In the film, *Sink the Bismarck*, the protagonist and his staff work so wholeheartedly at their task that they lose track of time and at the end go for dinner at breakfast time.

Intellect: The left-brain tends to promote intellectual, rational, linguistic, analytical, reason, science and linear strengths. These are deployed to discover objective facts, or "truth", with alternating right-brain checking and synthesising of discoveries or imagined discoveries of emotion and sentiment.

This approach may be constructive, but the intuitive impulses of the right-brain may be misleading and in the final analysis "truth" also may be spurious. Eugenics was a respected science, widespread in American universities up into the 1940s, and no one doubted its validity or "truth".

It must be admitted, however, that the ideas of eugenics are as valid as they ever were - or as invalid. Richard Dawkins recently caused outrage when he claimed that there is a moral obligation to abort a foetus with Downs Syndrome. What has changed is less the facts of the matter than the "truth", which is not a purely intellectual matter.

Creativity: manic-depressive people tend to be more creative than the average; hypomania, perhaps artificially stimulated, may help "ordinary" people to better appreciate and create beauty (drama, writing, singing). Wittgenstein was analytical, left-brained, and language-based in his early years, and right-brained, synthetic, intuitive, imaging, musical, aesthetic, mystical and religious in his latter days. At the end he said that language had multiple meanings, suggestive that he may have integrated left- and right-brain functioning. Wittgenstein came from a dysfunctional family. Three of his brothers committed suicide. He was probably hypomanic. His family owned half a percent of all the gold in Austria and had to pay off the Nazi's with it to get their freedom.

Competitiveness: this, a natural and species-adaptive trait, may be used hypomanically to simulate war, say in sports - which seem to be getting more aggressive and dangerous, reflected in the need for, say, helmets in American Football and more recently hurling. But competitiveness may be used more destructively to promote violent behaviour, deliberately or otherwise: most fatal fights occur after drinking hours, when alcohol-induced hypomania and paranoia/jealousy affects a greater number of people. One punch and bang head off the ground and die.

Grandiose delusions: hypomanic people think they are the very best; they might imagine themselves God, Jesus, Napoleon, or better writers, businessmen or inventors than they are. Nero, clearly hypomanic if not fully manic, is supposed to have imagined himself a great artist, though if he had been it is likely that at least some of his works would have survived.

MEMES

Such emphasis on advertising as has been made here suggests that humanity is affected exclusively by outside circumstances, and threatens to discount inner urges; and clearly this is too sweeping a claim. The argument between nature and nurture is impossible to conclusively resolve. People's emotional make-up is determined in part by their genetic inheritance, but it also bears a close relationship with the nurturing environment in which a child develops. Richard Dawkins speaks of "memes," values and attitudes that are recognisably the same within a culture, and which are "inherited" - just as genes are, though in a different way. Thus the child may genetically inherit a large or small build, and a calm or nervous disposition from one or both parents, but she will also "inherit" religion, social and racial attitudes, political beliefs, etc. Obviously, in an adoption scenario, the memes a child "inherits" may be very different from those of her genetic siblings.

Memes may lead to a predisposition toward or away from hypomania: a child reared in New York City, say, may become hypomanic whereas a sibling reared on a farm in Connemara may not.

Natural selection works for memes because what is important in the emotional, intellectual and physical states in human evolution is selected. People support and patronise those inventors, composers and playwrights whose ideas they like, and these artists, etc, thrive while others, and those others' ideas, fail, like natural selection. Consumerism dictates culture.

Sometimes the balance found in evolution over a long time is disrupted by the rapid appearance and adoption of memes that result in huge changes in social expression. This occurred in the decades of and following the Enlightenment, and in our own time by the rise of feminism and the cult of the individual.

Scott Fitzgerald said of his wife Zelda. "I wouldn't care if she died, but I couldn't stand to have anyone else marry her". They had rows fuelled by alcohol and sexual jealousy. He died a "failure" at 44 and only 30 people attended his funeral even though he had been very famous. Pollock the artist also died an alcoholic at a young age.

Fitzgerald's paranoid sexual jealousy is captured in the lyrics of Sting's song about a paranoid stalker, a favourite at weddings: "Every step you take, every move you make, I'll be watching you". The idea of stalking and control of the spouse or girlfriend is more common than people think and is dangerous.

Changes in culture may find expression in manic traits such as marriage in decline, divorce on the rise, contraception, foetal termination, the demise of the nuclear family and parenting by the state controlled by social workers.[14] These are arguably manic traits and they also express the increasing power of feminism in society. The rise of feminism has been accompanied by increase in breakdown of traditional structures, and while there is much that is good in feminism, breakdown of traditional structures has also had negative consequences.

Germaine Greer said in 1970 "Once that [the family] withers away Marx will have come true willy-nilly, so let's get on with it." With greater maturity she seems to have realised how wrong she was. Children from broken marriages and broken homes have an increased rate of admission to prisons and mental institutions.

In addition, parenting by the state might be better than by seriously dysfunctional parents, but the increased power of the state to intervene in family matters is fraught with danger and the potential to made problems, on a societal level, far worse. At the height of the "Satanic Panic" in the 1990s, children were forcibly removed from their parents in the Orkneys and in Yorkshire on what turned out to be entirely imaginary grounds. The trauma suffered by parents and children alike must have been dreadful.

This handing over of greater authority to social workers is itself perhaps a manifestation of increasing hypomania in society; certainly it can increase the power of some who have hypomanic traits. While social workers may be well-intentioned, at least some of them have grandiose notions of their own beliefs, and may be dogmatic and intolerant, and convinced that they know better than anyone else.

The rise in adultery, divorce and family breakdown has been followed in more recent years by a rise in hyper-sexuality and sex addictions. According to the European Federation of Married Catholic Priests more than 100,000 men have left the priesthood to get married.

---

[14] See *The Metamorphoses of Kinship*, by Maurice Godelier.

Fifty Shades of Grey by El James is a soft porn novel that has sold 30 million copies. Like all such novels it stimulates the sexual archetype of mania. The difference wrought in society in only a couple of generations is illustrated by the scandal caused by D.H. Lawrence's novel *Lady Chatterley's Lover*. In the early 1960s, more than 30 years after its author's death, it was tested in court as obscene, and - in another instance of societal change - the prosecuting barrister asked the jury, "Is it a novel you would even wish your wife or servant to read?"

Deleterious effects of hypomania can also be discerned in the money market, with all the changes that can bring to society and even culture. John Coates describes how making profits in a rising market brings on powerful feelings of euphoria and omnipotence in successful stockbrokers.[15] These also may experience racing thoughts, need less sleep and seem to be more sexually confident. With higher levels of testosterone (the success hormone), their confidence and readiness to take risks morph into overconfidence and reckless behaviour. This is driven by drugs, cocaine, crystal meth and speed as well as alcohol - classically after a successful deal, champagne. Male dealers in technology stocks had huge gains in the late 1990's leading to "displayed manic behaviour and a sense of infallibility" it was equally telling that women "appeared relatively unaffected". Men in the west are much more likely than women to get caught up in deranged market bubbles such as the bitcoin a testosterone fuelled bubble.

On the other hand, Steve Jobs was described as being charismatic, funny and highly intelligent, all signs of hypomania, and he had the manic energy to found Apple, worth two trillion dollars.

The 1916 Irish rebel James Connolly was described as having energy, enthusiasm and high intelligence, all features of mania /hypomania.

Bob Geldof described the Band Aid 30 yr 2014 single sales and down loading as going manic, "That's the digital age."

Taken in toto, these changes all express how social and cultural changes may be driven by mania / hypomania. As the culture is made more manic it buys

---

[15] "The Hour Between Dog and Wolf", in *The Sunday Times*, 6 May 2012.

and sells more, gets more grandiose (variations on the "you deserve the best" advertising line is widespread), high Ego, hyper sexuality, humour, paranoia all building to chaos and loss of control.

RED, BLACK and WHITE

We see these "primary" colours in the red of the lips and blood; the apparent black of the nipple, the pupil and the mouth; the white of the teeth and the eyes. These are the colours of childhood. Ancient Egyptians had kohl and rouge lips and cheeks, emerald–green eyelids and liquorice-black kohl-rimmed eyes and nail colour. In ancient Egypt and Rome when women were treated well they made red lipstick from blending fat with red ochre and Romans made rouge to colour their cheeks Elizabeth 1 used rouge on the face with lead white cosmetics and in mid 18th century in France painting your face was part of life in court especially in the upper classes. Queen Victoria declaration that make-up was vulgar meant that a pale, virtuous look was now preferred. Gabrielle Chanel maintained that lip stick was a women's prime weapon of seduction. From Face Paint: The Story of Makeup by Lisa Eldridge.11 October 2015 Sunday Times Style magazine

Red, Black and White are the main colours. They sell Coca Cola (biggest selling soft drink), the manic car has to be the Rosso red Ferrari, Marlboro (biggest selling cigarette - itself arguably a psychological substitute for the displaced nipple), and Heinz (biggest selling ketchup). Santa wears a red suit and black belt and has a white beard, and in this guise the Coca-Cola Company created him. Manchester United F.C. wears a strip of red, black and white. They are the most popular team in football and the best and young footballers want to play for them. Over the last twenty years teams in the ascendancy have been red i.e. Liverpool, Arsenal, Man United, Nottingham Forest and Cork City. The colour scheme is a main element of their popularity. Chicago Bulls, Air Jordan Trainers.

Some other products that use Red, Black and White are from CULT, Masterpieces. Icons of our generation (Tecium Publishers) 2008. Coca Cola, Stop Sign, Texaco, McDonalds, Nutella, Kit Kat, Tabasco, Wrigley's Spearmint, Mickey Mouse, Kinder, Nintendo Game Boy, Chanel Rouge nail varnish, Levi's, Ray Bans, American Flag, Lacoste, VW Camper Van, UK

Bus, UK Post Box, Mont Blanc, Swiss Army Knife, Bic Lighter, Pritt Stick, Haagen Dazs, Heinz Tomato Ketchup, Toblerone and Mars.

More sinisterly, red, black and white is the colour-combination of the Nazi party, the colours having been adapted from the flag of the Second Reich and, before that, of Prussia, said by Napoleon to have been "hatched from a cannonball".

RIGHT BRAIN, LEFT BRAIN

Roger W. Sperry, an American psycho biologist discovered in the late1960's that the human brain had a right brain – left brain way of thinking. Sperry got the Noble prize in 1981.

While the left brain (right hand) is analytical and linear, the right brain (left hand) is intuitive and may skip in a non-sequential activity. Hence it is believed that creativity comes from the right brain, which tends toward synthesis, parallel thinking putting different ideas beside each other in a way that encourages cross-fertilisation. Intuition comes from the right brain and allows people to follow thoughts that are different from left-brain logical thoughts. However, if the intellectual, in seeking truth, overloads the left brain she may flip into right brain activity and experience beauty.

At the risk of over-simplification, the left brain seeks truth whereas the right brain seeks beauty, the beauty of harmonic synthesis that accommodates all factors.

During the First World War some soldiers did not know their left from their right leg. They put a band of hay on the left leg and a band of straw on the right leg so the commander could shout out hay straw, left right.

People are more creative when they are high/manic and when a creative person gets depressed he may talk of writing block. One of the ways out of this is to drink heavily. Alcohol can break writer's block in more than one way. For many artists the disinhibition caused by intoxication makes it easier to write through the block - in much the same way as it may enable a normally shy person to socialise.

For the manic-depressive there may be another mechanism: alcohol suppresses brain activity but the next day it speeds up as a reaction to having been temporarily tranquillised, thus when in a hangover you are more sensitive to noise and ideas. Francis Bacon (painter): "I often like working with a hangover because my mind is crackling with energy and I can think very clearly. I love living in chaos." and James Joyce (writer) and Brendan Kennelly (poet) used to create on hangovers. Musicians and artists who get rich may stop working on hangovers because they can afford to stay in bed with some Solpadine. Muslims do not drink alcohol and do not get hangovers. Neither do they take heroin, cocaine or speeds which are associated with creativity. These factors help account for the fact that Moslems tend to be less creative and more rigid.

Effective integration of both hemispheres is the ideal.

Yves Carcelle, former controller of fashion group LVMH, was said by Antoine Arnault, the son of the owner of LVMH and CEO of the Berluti brand, to have had the perfect mix of the left brain/ right brain that is what top managers need.[16] U2 is a good name double vowel emotion,U Right brain Left hand,2 Left brain right hand

Angela Ahrendts, CEO of Apple, was said by one of **her early employers**, Donna Karan, that she merges the left brain of a number cruncher with the right brain of an artist. "She knows how to balance a collection, taking into account the business needs while always protecting the integrity of the designer".[17]Professor John Hunt of London Business School "The belief was that managers could produce a rational, bureaucratic scientific system, whereas in fact we all know it is about emotion, irrationality and the creative side, about love and hate." Obituary Sunday Independent 8th Nov 2015. Gucci CEO, Marco Bizzarri said "Fashion is about creating emotion - it's not necessarily rational" Style Magazine Sunday Times 8th Nov 2015.

They dream because they have models Bill Gates, Larry Page and Mark Zuckerberg.

---

[16] Obituary, *Irish Times*, 6 September 2014.

[17] Profile, Sunday Times, 7 September 2014.

The association between the brain hemisphere and the opposite side of the body is long known, and it is possible to thus identify which hemisphere is dominant in any individual. Left-handed people are often credited with being more intuitive, creative and musical, the reason being that normally dominance switches from the brain hemispheres to the sides of the body, so a left-handed person would usually be "right-brain dominant." Clinical tests reveal that this rule does not always hold; that some people may have these capacities located in the left hemisphere. Nevertheless in general it seems fair to say that with the right hemisphere are associated powers of synthesis, spatial awareness (cubism) and appreciation, dress sense, dance movements, and what are generally held to be "creative abilities" such as art and music.

When old skulls are examined from thousands of years ago (Mesolithic) it can be shown by the way the teeth have been ground down what percentage of the people were right-handed (50%) or left-handed (50%) - *Journal of Evolution.*

The rock at the entrance to Newgrange has two carved left-handed circles on one side and three right-handed circles on the other side. This may reflect nothing more than mirror-image symmetry but it also may reflect that there was an approximately equal number of right-and left-handed people at the time. It has been shown elsewhere that people of celtic origin 5,000 BC were 40 percent left handed as opposed to today where 10-15 percent are left-handed. Interestingly, however, the proportion is much higher in the case of twins, one third of who are left handed.[18] Like a disproportionate number of recent US presidents, Obama is left-handed.

Approximate rate of left-handedness in selected countries:

China – 3%   India – 4%   Japan – 5%   USA & Europe – 10-15%

Aboriginals - 50% left-handed & 50% right-handed. Aboriginals are considered more creative, musical and spiritual.

---

[18] *Journal of Evolution.*

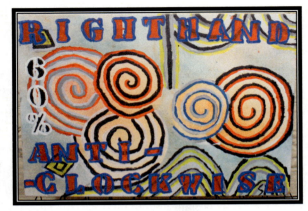

*60% - Right handed
(Anticlockwise)*

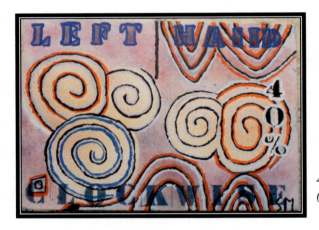

*40% - left-handed
(Clockwise)*

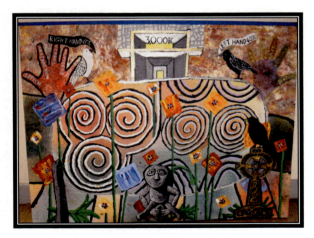

Newgrange by S. W. Marshall

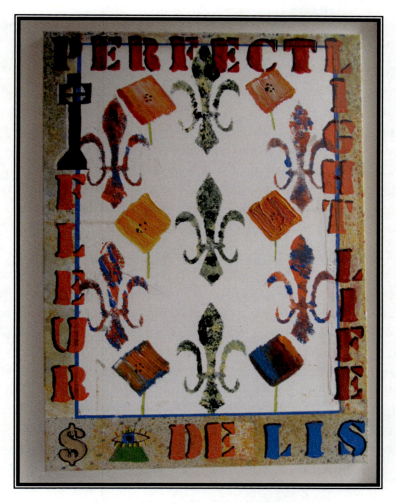

Fleur de Lis by S.W. Marshall

Such a difference in ancient peoples would have resulted in a different society. Australian Aborigines are 50% right-handed and 50% left-handed and have a different culture that does not fit into western culture. Partially trying to survive the dominant culture they find themselves in Aborigines drink alcohol to excess but spend a lot of time being creative.

If left-handed Aboriginal society is more manic, musical, intuitive and creative, the society that existed thousands of years ago would be different to the right-handed society of today. There would have been a different value system. People would have done different jobs, being more creative even in "non-creative" work.

The division of the brain is reflected in the division of work in society. The division between Arts and Science is artificial, and relatively easily bridged, but it is real enough for society as a whole. A famous left-handed musician was Jimi Hendrix, considered to have been the best guitarist of his generation. John Lydon (Johnny Rotten singer with the Sex Pistols) was beaten at school for writing with his left hand. Fay Weldon the writer finds morning work to stem from the creative, woolly, right hand side of the brain, often just an effusive ramble. She edits in the afternoon what she writes in the morning, after she lets the left side of the brain, the one that wields the red editorial pen, take over.

But with their intuition and creativity, it is possible that left-handers may be more likely to undermine society - or at any rate this is the perception, if for more cloudy reasons. In former times children were beaten at school and at home for using their left hand, *left* coming from the Latin for *sinister*, which acquired connotations of evil. Protestants are called "left footers," allegedly because their turf-cutting spade had a left-sided foot-brace on the blade; Catholics used a right-sided brace. Arabs are insulted if you shake them with the left hand as the left hand is used for dirty jobs such as going to the toilet. Jesus Christ is said to sit on the right hand of his father, God. This may be a mere aberration, or it may be the remnant of a more widespread appreciation of left-handedness.

Karen Pine, a psychologist at Hertfordshire University who specialises in shopping behaviour, believes that problem-spending - "I want it now" - can be tackled in more straightforward ways. "When we go shopping we tend to take the emotional impulsive sides of our brains with us," she says. "What we ought to take is the logical, sensible side."

The Pope on his visit to the UK talked about Science and Faith coming together i.e. left and right hand being more equal. Even the modern pop culture is not immune with the Script calling their album *Science and Faith*. The golfer Rory McIlroy talks about being in "the zone" when he plays well. Dan Brown says, "The deeper I've got into science, the more I've come to understand that science and religion are two different languages trying to tell the same story."[19]

I believe that the dialectic of touch between the left and right hand led to development of language where touch was expressed by vocalisation when stroked nicely (*ah*) and pinched/ hurt (*ouch*). The difference between a hairy ape and man with a 5-percent remnant of its fur is language. Through skin we can sense light touch, deep touch, pleasure, pain, vibration, two point discrimination, hot-cold and a sense of three-dimensional spaces which is called proprioception and spatial awareness. It is through touch that we become intimate.

Iggy Pop the singer says that people need to be touched and held, and admired, and those three things are really, really hard to get unless you've got some sort of partisan to fake it for you. Like if you're a little kid, your parents fawn over you, until that takes so much energy that they get divorced or something, it ruins their relationship. Sunday Independent 9 November 2014 interviewed by Emily Hourican

Non-linear and Synthetic language such as what Brian Eno uses with Coldplay the band are "Cook like an Italian" i.e. be simple " Don't use every colour in every painting"; "You must be fishers of men, not too proud to use simple hooks".[20]

---

[19] Dan Brown in interview with Matt Rudd, *The Sunday Times*, 12 May 2013.

[20] Matt Munday, *The Sunday Times Magazine*, 18 September 2011.

Left Brain/Right Hand	Right Brain/Left Hand
Linear	Non linear
Analysis	Synthesis
Doing	Being
Speech	Music appreciation
Abstraction	Spatial
Numbers	Emotion (integrates feelings)
	Humour
	Aesthetic appreciation
	Face recognition
	Intuition
Verbal	Non verbal, Inflection,
	Spontaneity,
	Slip of the tongue
	Images
	Body stance
	Language of cries, Gestures,
	Cuddling
	Suckling, Touching,
	Faith in God
	Patriotic fever
	Driving, skiing, dancing

CREATIVITY

In any event, emotion (right brain) needs a creative environment to blossom and bloom. The emotional level of expression would seem to be more developed in humans than is rational linear thinking: About two thirds of communication is non-verbal, and much of the remainder depends on paralinguistic factors (tone, pitch, loudness) rather than words themselves. It's what is felt and expressed at an emotional level that is important, more than what is said. When people communicate it is primarily the emotional intuitive right hemisphere of the brain that understands. People remember the emotional expression and this defines man. Intuition is the seeking for beauty and synthesis.

Creative people find more ideas to work with, and often have a lot of energy to bring to these ideas (though we tend to associate the work ethic with the dour Protestant mindset that seems more concerned with conformity than innovation). They can work longer, harder hours and they succeed where others fail. Thus Churchill was able, at over sixty, to marshal the energies and enthusiasms of Britain, and later the free world, against Nazism, despite the apparently overwhelming odds. His creativity extended from painting to writing multi-volume histories of the Great War and of the English-speaking peoples, to seeing the psychological and emotive potential of a big cigar and his famous V-for-victory sign. "Churchill and Ireland" by Paul Bew said that Michael Collins and Churchill shared a similar manic depressive temperament

But the creative person is often emotionally labile, going from ups to downs, as did Churchill, haunted by his "black dog" of depression that was driven away by alcohol. Creativity is sometimes associated with bipolar illness - well-known examples of such maniacally creative people include Spike Milligan, Steven Fry, Paul Merton, David Williams, Dolores O'Riordan, John Cleese, Peter Seller's wife Brit Ekland thought he was bipolar, Marie Carey, Charles Dickens, Dylan Thomas, Ernest Hemmingway, Brendan Behan, Virginia Wolfe, Theodore Roosevelt and Van Gogh. King George 3 was bipolar / hypomanic kept in a straight jacket, over talkative, restless, irritable and grandiose. When well he was a prodigious writer and studied many topics. (BBC2-30 January 17. The Genius of the Mad King) Others who might have had MDI are Robin Williams, Lenny Bruce and Richie Pryor. Manic Depressives have over-inclusive thinking that leads to new associations and creativity.

Ezra Pound was charged with treason but incarcerated for being insane and mentally unfit for trial. He was incarcerated in St. Elizabeth asylum Washington for the criminally insane for 12 years from 1946-1958. He had praised the Axis powers and condemned the allies' forces and damned the "kikes" on 200 radio shows from Rome from Jan 1941 to July 1943. He was released on April 18; 1958. When asked what it was like to be released from a mental hospital. He replied "All America is an insane asylum." THE BUGHOUSE, The Poetry, Politics and Madness of Ezra Pound by Daniel Swift reviewed by John Walsh. Culture Magazine Sunday Times, 5

March 2017. In 1954 Hemmingway won the Nobel prize for literature and with other artists called for Pound's release such as Jean Cocteau and Igor Stravinsky.

Robert Lowell had a diagnosis of mania, manic depression and then bipolar depression. Robert Lowell; Setting the River on Fire by Kay Redfield Jamison. A Study of Genius, Mania and Character. As Reviewed by John Banville (Irish Times) and Helen Vendler. (The New York Review) 20 April 2017.

Jamison a professor of psychiatry at the John Hopkins School of Medicine, an honorary professor of English at the University of St. Andrews in Scotland and a memoir An Unquiet Mind (1995) on her own experience of manic depression is the best person to write Lowell's life story. His illness caused him to behave with violent unpredictability; he would go without sleep or rest for many nights and days, drinking and smoking incessantly, and indulging in the wildest fantasies and the most outrageous behaviour, haranguing everyone he met with outlandish accounts of his own divinity-he often saw himself as Christ (messianic delusion) -or issuing Napoleon or Papal commands, and talking, talking, talking , a tempestuous "conversion" to an exaggerated Roman Catholicism soon abandoned; the imprisonment for several months as a conscientious objector in World War 2, classic examples of bipolar disorder symptoms. Psychiatric treatment beginning at fifteen and continuing intermitting through adulthood. Education at Harvard and then teaching there, the cascade of prize winning volumes of verse from 1944 to 1977; the many enterprises in drama and travels abroad.

It is about the poetic imagination and how mania and imagination come together to create great art. The manic strain was on the maternal side-Robert's great-great-grandmother died insane in the mid-19th century. Norman Mailer said "All flaws considered, Lowell was still a fine, good, and honourable man." He was also, we might add, a great poet, as Kay Jamison's book resoundingly affirms.

Jamison has long argued for a strong relation between manic depressive illness and creativity. Although the extent of the connection is still under debate, the stimulus given by mania to certain writers, painters, and composers has been observed historically since classical times. Jamison cites two recent studies that examine large populations and attest to a link between bipolar disorder and creativity in artists. Lowell "The two horses, one is lying down immobile the other is galloping." He was born in 1917 and his mother died in 1954 following which he underwent nearly twenty electric shocks in Cincinnati.

Selfie: by Will Storr: How we Became So Self-Obsessed and What It's doing to Us: reviewed by Richard Godwin Sunday Times Culture section; 4 June 2017

The neuroscientist Robert Sapolsky notes: If you devote your time to thinking about what the brain, hormones, genes, evolution, childhood, foetal environment and so on have to do with behaviour as I do, it seems impossible to think there is free will. Storr owes much to Adam Curtis, whose BBC documentary (2002) The Century of the Self has something approaching genius for marshalling his material.

As distinct from MDI sufferers, consider the people with hypomania who lived in the (Chelsea Hotel:[21] The owner from 1964 to 2007 Stanley Bard who died in February 2017 at 82 years liked artists to stay there. Leonard Cohen, Brendan Behan, and Johnny Thunders of the New York Dolls, Arthur Miller, Sid Vicious. In one room, William Burroughs(wrote The Naked Lunch), Mark Twain, Jackson Pollock, Janis Joplin, Bob Dylan, Gore Vidal, Dylan Thomas(worked on the final version of Under Milk Wood there drinking 18 glasses of whiskey in a row a record, in his room before falling into a coma and dying in a nearby hospital),Sunday Independent 19 February 2017 Stanley Bard @ Telegraph, Patti Smith, Dee Dee Ramone, and in other rooms Thomas Wolfe (wrote You Can't Go Home Again), Arthur C Clarke (wrote 2001:A Space Odyssey) and Jack Kerouac (wrote On The Road). Numerous songs were written in and about the hotel. Andy Warhol filmed Chelsea Girls there.

Ernest Hemmingway, another hypomanic, died in1961 at his own hand shortly after having ECT. His father and brother also killed themselves. Gregory, Ernest's youngest son, didn't like himself and required 98 ECTs for what must have been drug resistant depression or intractable mania. Gregory was an addict and divorcee, all factors pointing to manic delusions.

Jonah Lehrer the author of "Proust was a Neuroscientist" talks about Virginia Wolfe getting high and being creative after a depressive episode. He did not realise the importance of M.D.I. in her life and many other creative people's lives. I was at a meal with Patrick Guinness of brewing fame who said his grandmother was a paranoid schizophrenic and this seemed to worry him and I said she was probably a manic paranoid and tried to relieve him.

A particular form of mania is dysphoric elation, when the sufferer does not enjoy his high but becomes irritable, aggressive and unhappy - Nirvana's singer Kurt Cobain suffered from such dysphoria, and may have given a certain cachet to such a disorder among teenagers since his death by suicide. The creative person also may suffer from grandiose delusions, which may be, in part at least, what drives his creative engine, but which clearly constitutes a hypomanic trait.

Creative people are more likely to hear voices and see visions than the normal population. They often have first degree relatives that have a psychotic illness. For example, David Bowie - manic-depressive brother; James Joyce - schizophrenic daughter; Tennessee Williams - manic depressive sister. Mott the Hoople's singer Hunter had a physical and nervous breakdown in 1974. Creative people are often the children of religious people - e.g. Van Gogh was bipolar also a priest as was his father, Nina Simone's father was a travelling preacher and she had a diagnosis of bipolar disorder, Divine Comedy singer Neil Hannon's father is a bishop, Lemmy's of Motor Head, Brandon Flower's of the Killers, Tori Amos's, Katy Perry's, John Hurt and Alice Cooper's fathers were pastors. Tom Cruise and Brian Friel spent two years in seminaries as Gabriel Byrne spent four years. Creative people tend to be over sexed: Picasso, Sartre, Rodin and Mozart, Liszt as well as lesser-known people like James Dickey. Politicians such as Theresa May, Angel Merkel, Gordon Brown and David Steel had fathers who were priests.

Creative hypomanics are often sensitive and spiritual and can see the world in a different perspective. They have the emotional talent that allows them to express their feelings, and sharing emotion can be very good for the psyche. The shared experience at a play binds the actor and the audience so that they can experience emotions such as love and hate.

[21] Suzanne Harrington, *Irish Independent*, 1 March 2014.

Sharing of manic emotions helps us to deal with people and an increasingly hypomanic society; sharing access to problems helps us further - however artificial, even spurious the problems an actor's portrays may be.

The minds of creative people are racing; they have more energy, are more highly sexualised. Rodin used to make love to his female model during the sitting. He did a statue of Balzac with a large coat that allegedly hides an erection, a joke between two creative, highly-sexualised men. Ernest Hemmingway was as famous in earlier life for his libido as he was toward the end for depression, due in part to his sexual impotence, and in part too to his creative impotence, the latter perhaps following from the former though both may be traced to alcoholism where you have a large ego and a low self-esteem. This combination sounds strange but when you add the "Higher Power" to the mix it can work out. Edna St Vincent Millay was one of the most successful poets of the early twentieth century, and notoriously promiscuous - when her sexual libido began to flag the quality of her poetry took a nosedive, as Hemmingway's did.

While generalisations are always risky, it appears that mathematicians are perceived as remote, almost lifeless people, and if their logical faculties are indeed more highly developed than those of the average it is feasible that this development may have been at the cost of their emotional (right brain) faculties.

Analysing analysis itself is seeking "fact", which one might define as truth without emotion, and such "facts" can too easily lead to lies - as in lies, damn lies, and statistics. Thus the crisis in the Irish government (in 2008) saw ministers arguing semantically to "prove" that a secret document advocating economic "cuts" really was only concerned with projected "extra expenditure." Analysis then synthesis is the basis for empirical scientific study.

The predominance of nurture and nature may depend on the relative focus in the right and left brain. However, their perceived remoteness does not imply that mathematicians are any less exempt from meme influence than anyone else, or from the influence of emotion: the most rampantly nationalistic Irish leader of the twentieth century, Eamon de Valera, was a mathematics teacher and, according to anecdote, credited by Einstein as being one of the few people in the world who actually understood the theory of relativity.

You can be creative without being intellectual. Socrates felt that artists he encountered did not know much about the meaning of their art. People with Manic Depressive Illness and to a lesser extent hypomania are in a unique position as they experience highs (mania) and lows (depression) and tend to create culture that reflects the mental set of the hypomanic person. People tend to be more creative when they are high.

Evidence suggests that up to half the people in creative spheres may have what we may group as "mental difficulties" - anything on the spectrum from schizophrenia to bouts of moodiness. Though poets comprise the largest group here, followed by musicians, creative scientists also suffer from "mental difficulties." Newton may have been borderline schizophrenic, and Einstein also suffered. Isaac Newton said "If I have seen further it is by standing on the shoulders of giants".

Recent scholarship by Dr Ruth Richards of Harvard has taken an unusual approach to exploring the adaptive aspects of this apparent connection between "madness" and "genius," by studying patients in psychiatric hospitals and looking for family patterns. She found that patients were, as a group, more creative than the normal population; but she also found a consistent pattern of "mental difficulties," albeit less severe, in families of those patients. This suggests, if not all but proves, that there is a genetic component to madness, and some authorities tentatively conclude that there is a spectrum of behaviour that ranges from maladaptive madness to selectively adaptive creativity that enables those who inherit aspects of the condition to see more effective ways of dealing with life's challenges. The inheritance seems to be a group of genes, rather than a single one, and because of the overall adaptively endowed by this group of genes a predisposition toward madness tends to be inherited along with, on a group scale, adaptive endowments. Those who inherit the full spectrum tend to go mad; those who inherit only components of it are more creatively adaptive than the average.

Mania may exist, therefore, because it works for the benefit of the species; however we do not know exactly how. The gene, or rather part or the entire genetic package is passed on from the sufferers, but more likely from the sufferer's siblings (who are more likely to be successful). Culture may even be driven by mania: a Book of the Month Club survey suggested that 70 percent of its authors suffered from manic-depression.

THE MANIC ARCHETYPES

These may be the products of nature, nurture or both. Drugs can change your attitude to adverts and even your beliefs. The French Revolution might not have happened if coffee, nicotine and alcohol had not been available: coffee shops and bars were meeting place for revolutionaries, and coffee, nicotine and alcohol may have made them intellectually hypomanic (Liberty, Fraternity and Equality) or even manic. Drink leads to manic archetypes being expressed, for example in jokes, conversation, sexual disinhibition, dancing, comradeship, self-confidence and spending. Happiness can be a manic trait - a disease, if it is part of the manic high, or merely debilitating, if we look on the past with rose tinted glasses.

Our memories tend to be optimistic, but the "good old days" may not have been, objectively, so good at all, and insisting on looking on them as such may rob us of our ability to live in the present and make the best of life. Socialism, of which such behaviour as that described is the pre-political expression, is a political manic archetype. Cocaine and speed will make a normal person go manic; Sartre is said to have written on speed and had two girlfriends on the go at the same time, and Hitler used it as part of his daily medication.

Self-belief and nationalism can make a country go a bit mad, Nazi Germany being perhaps the most infamous example; but this hypomanic cultural state was found in Ireland during successive soccer world cup competitions, when people took out loans and painted houses and cars and vans in the national colours, and followed the team all over the world at great expense. Nationalism is thus a manic archetype that may be expressed politically or personally, or in both modes.

People who are manic often feel that they are very important; some may think they are Jesus (messianic delusion-Jesus thought he was the Son of God) or some other figure of history. At the time of Jesus other people had claimed to be messiahs, and like him were put to death as blasphemers. Jesus may have been manic-depressive. His long sojourn in the desert, ending with a deranged account of being tempted by the devil, and his assault on the moneychangers on the temple steps, men who performed an essential service in keeping graven images (on coins) out of the temple itself, might indicate such a condition.

Christianity could be seen as a hypomanic religion. You have the ideal to live up to and the paranoia of the devil to overcome. Roman Catholicism (and certain other denominations) is depressive in that it is steeped in guilt. Presbyterianism is hypomanic because its adherents feel they are chosen by God from among all others and they attract those who are manic (high) and who think they are special to their manic preaching.

For some people, perhaps even most, religion may be adaptive and a positive force. The freedom championed by the American Constitution, whose fifteen authors included eleven Scots-Ulster Presbyterians, illustrates the potential benefits of a hypomanic culture: the American constitution is the basis of all liberal democracies and the pursuit of happiness.

The archetypes are reflected in the gods that people pray to. Gods are reflections of our intellectual, emotional and physical self, and sufferers from manic delusion often project themselves onto God - as deluded Christians may think they are Christ, Muslims may think they are Mohammed. Apollo, Zeus, Bacchus, Mars, Venus, like Christian saints, have their place as projected power figures in society.

The idea of one God and a saviour goes back to pre-Christian times. A lot of Christian belief and ritual such as communion and a saviour are based on pagan belief. The Eucharist originally was a pagan feast in which the king, willingly sacrificed for his people and their land, was eaten in a cannibalistic ritual. The preserved bodies found in bogs in Ireland with cracks in their skulls. The idea of a saviour is very manic: the idea that God himself personally died for me.

Is the very idea of one God a manic belief? Increasingly, as science explains what once was regarded as supernatural, gods come to be seen as projections of the mind and especially of the manic mind.

In *The Decline and Fall of the Roman Empire*, Gibbons speaks about the proliferation of religious sects that occur at the end of a civilisation. Manic cultures have many belief systems; thus we see the Islamic Taliban, and in Christianity the Branch Davidians and the James Jones cult, all committed to a messianic figure. Less extreme but still fundamentalist systems of belief may deny science and common sense in the name of a particular "received truth"; thus Pentecostalists, as well as most Baptists and Church of Christ adherents in the USA, deny evolution.

As civilisation is seen by many to be in its last days quasi-religious sects have emerged; these include Amnesty, Greenpeace, NATO, Vegans, the United Nations, and the Olympic Foundation. By contrast, the nineteenth century, which saw western civilisation as the "Manifest Destiny" of the world, was characterised by missionary zeal in the cause of mainstream Christianity, and great intolerance for minority sects such as Mormonism and, in the Islamic world, Ba'ahi.

MANIC SOCIETY

Football and golf for example are intuitive: you need an empty head and a feel for the ball, the spacio-visual intelligence. Soccer started as a street game between working-class men in the Industrial Revolution, when arguably the world began to become hypomanic - certainly life was being lived at a faster pace than it had been for centuries before.

Like soccer, over the years things with a manic nature have been accepted by society and some have come to dictate society's norms. Hitler's quasi-scientific notions of racial superiority quickly came to dominate German culture and determine the standards acceptable and applicable even to those who did not subscribe to the ideas.

Manic ideas may come to be accepted as the norm because they stimulate the mind in a way that is agreeable: it's agreeable to think that because I'm an Aryan I'm a member of a super-race; it's agreeable to think that because I'm a woman or Hispanic or African-American or Native American – I deserve special consideration by the establishment; it's even more agreeable to think that this special consideration is nothing more than what is owed to me as a woman or whatever, because of the way my antecedents or ancestors were discriminated against by WASP male-dominated culture.

For all that culture is a co-operative, shared, social construct, it is created by individual manic minds, by those who have the ideas and the creativity, and the drive and perseverance to express these new ideas. A society, therefore, can and indeed must be able to accommodate hypomania at the individual level; but as a society as an entity gets more manic it loses control of itself and chaos takes over from surrealism. Francis Bacon said he lived and created in chaos. The social controls and dampers become weakened and are overcome as more and more individuals assert their independence, withdraw their voluntary submission to consensus, the super-ego of society. The confidence of the self is increased and the interest of individuals is considered greater than the common good.

Furthermore, as society becomes less traditional, as the "extended family" is replaced by the supposedly natural entity of the nuclear family (probably, in anthropological terms, a "restricted family"), the checks and balances imposed by older, wiser grandparents, and the greater free time these have to discreetly police society, become lost. Normal morals are thrown out and everybody is fighting for the self.

With the moral glue left out society becomes a free-for-all. There is an increase in anarchy, humour of the wilder variety, and disinhibitionism in sexuality. "I'm the best"; "No one can stop me"; "I'm above the law." At best, there emerges the notion that anyone is entitled to "express himself" in whatever way seems right. Along with this goes justification in other attendant forms: paedophiles are notorious for justifying their behaviour by claiming that their victims really wanted and invited sexual attention.

Ayn Rand wrote in *The Fountainhead*, "I will not die; it is the world that will end". The basis of her philosophy was "Self-esteem and your own happiness, totally free society, and you are the world". Altruism was wrong. Rand's became the philosophy of Silicon Valley. Paul Ryan, Romney's running mate was an early follower of Rand; he stopped following her because she was an atheist.

In such a frantic, self-centred anything-goes world, we become obsessed with speed. We want the fastest car, plane, boat, coffee, religion, and food. We demand convenience food like McDonalds, where the food is waiting and ready in seconds. We have less patience. Whether by letters, phone or computer (Google, Face book, E mail, Internet browser, Amazon and EBay) communication has to be fast. What hypomanics communicate is speeded up even more, as their neural impulses are, with iPhones and other technology, which evolves at a faster and faster pace - technology itself has become hypomanic.

As a response to such individualism and narcissism, paranoia increases and eventually becomes rampant. It manifests, as always, more in social groups One and Two, but people lower down the ladder, with less power in society, tend to suffer disproportionately from the damage inflicted by such paranoiacs. In parallel with this, and reinforced by the inflictions on those down the social ladder, bourgeois fear of the proletariat feeds more paranoia into the social loop. Taken to its logical conclusion, such a process ultimately isolates the individual from society, rather than accommodating him and dampening his hypomanic urges, far less channel these into advancing the common social weal.

In recent years the Internet has opened opportunities to the most deviant. Even cannibals can now find, not merely kindred souls, but others who actually may want to be killed and eaten, as the recent case in Germany illustrates.

MANIC CULTURE

Manic culture is a culture of extremes - love, hate; old, young; black, white; sex; sin. As the world gets more manic things speed up: thoughts race and conversation hurries to catch them; music, ads, drama, drugs, cars etc, all follow. We are surrounded by advertising in papers, magazines, TV, radio and billboards, as well as on product-labels in the shops. Music sells emotion and is all-pervasive in the background. People spend more, drink more, and have more sex. Fast cars cost more and are much sought after, as is the comfort of the Rolls Royce - both speed and luxury reflections of mania. Basic features of the id are expressed in soap operas i.e. killing and drugs. Many stock market dealers are fuelled by cocaine and alcohol (often, tellingly, champagne); these dealers make decisions about billions every day.

Productivity will increase but as the market sways from one side to the other it runs the risk of crashing.

People who work for 48 weeks a year may understandably on their holidays go a little wild: they drink more, talk more, have more sex and do creative things. They may, alternatively, have drinking competitions and go to late bars and discos. There is no Super Ego (parent) to tell them to behave. Holidays promise to fulfil our wishes. People put up with mundane jobs by looking forward to their manic break. People tend to make friends easily on holidays, when other people are more open and friendly. On holidays, people are often in a different culture, and assimilate local idiosyncrasies. The downside of this manic activity is violence, accidents, unwanted pregnancies and venereal infections.

As well as holidaying abroad, people go and work abroad where, perhaps for the first time, they have to think for themselves and not have to worry about what family and friends think. Also, with the success of the Celtic Tiger (2005) more and more foreigners are coming here and the emigrants who left in the depressed Eighties are returning. Now (2009 foreigners are going home and unemployment is going up and we have to borrow €400 million a week to pay our bills. The people who left in the 80's typically went to large cities like London and New York, where the pace and pressures of life are much higher than elsewhere and this is where they are going again. They are also going to Australia and Canada. Dublin is turning into a cosmopolitan European capital city. Irish people are being affected by other, traditionally more manic, cultures. De Valera was worried that emigrants would return in the 1950's and 60's mainly from the U.K. with ideas that were more liberal and didn't suit his idea of Ireland dancing at the crossroads.

CIVILISATION

The Greek and Roman cultures became very manic before they broke down. Be thyself; know thyself. When the Roman Empire was working it had 59 million people with 10,000 civil servants compared to the modern day U.K. with a population of 65 million and 500,000 civil servants. Life was cheap and citizens, especially the wealthy ones, had slaves to do the work, leaving them time for art, drama, singing, dancing and poetry. But people became soft from society's emphasis on culture, rather than, as in the case of Sparta, warfare. They became more manic as the culture speeded up; they drank more and were more pornographic as they sought new forms of stimulation.

In Classic Grecian times it was quite normal for a man to have a young male lover, often the relationship being that of teacher and pupil. Both this and Ancient Roman society were markedly misogynistic, women being regarded by many as for breeding purposes, the finest sort of love that of homosexuality. The most feared regiment in the Greek army was comprised of lovers, who, it was reckoned correctly, would fight ferociously for each other. A hint of this relationship may be seen in the love between Achilles and Patroclus in *The Iliad*.

The "plebs" had to be satisfied by the leaders with games and chariot races and ritualised murders in the Coliseum, stimulating their jaded senses and filling their empty lives. "Bread and circuses" was the slogan in the decadent days of the Roman empire, and in one celebrated incident, when the economy and administration were so far gone that a choice had to be made between importing grain from north Africa for bread, or fine sand for the Coliseum, Nero's tribune immediately opted for the sand. They would have had a frenzied market place with people increasingly buying on credit as the empires essentially lived on credit past their time.

To their gods of drink and madness, Bacchus and Dionysus, they had bars and brothels and many of them decorated their homes with nude pictures (Picasso was influenced by the cubist nude pictures in Pompeii, not just African art). Dionysus was also the God of fertility and sex (mania) celebrated on St Bridgets day on the first of February the beginning of Spring. Emperors were believed to be gods, killing people in the Coliseum with a turned-down thumb. Caligula not only made a god of himself but a senator of his horse. In a similar vein we see Hitler and other dictators of the modern day; the parallels with classic times, as we struggle to stimulate our increasingly jaded senses, to fill our increasing leisure time, to spend our increasing disposable income, seem significant.

As part of the planning for D Day the Allies met in Bretton Woods in 1944 to draw up a plan, "Snakebite", which would create the lasting economic settlement that, had eluded them after the Great War. John Maynard Keynes, one of the most vociferous critics of the Versailles settlement, was one of the main movers. UNIVERSAL MAN The Seven Lives of John Maynard Keynes by Richard Davenport-Hines He believed in capitalism, he hated socialism and he effectively sacrificed himself to win a life and death loan from the Americans, after the war without which Britain would have plunged into an economic disaster. His libido drove his intellect, progressive Liberal democratic, rooted in a rationalistic, tolerant and optimistic view of the world. Snakebite eventually resulted hypomanicly in the International Monetary Fund and the World Bank; the World Trade Organisation; The Marshall Plan; the Organisation for European Economic Co-Operation; the General Agreement of Traffic and Trade and the European Coal and Steal Community, whose six members in 1951 became the 28-nation EU today.

These organisations were driven by manic co-operation where economics were shared and stimulated and people were given a positive outlook. Around this time the UN (the successor to the League of Nations) was established with peace (mania) as its aim. Mania was evident in the various friendly agreements as in the fear of war (paranoia) as the Cold War hardened and NATO was set up. The manic rivalry of the various organisations resulted in the fall of the USSR in 1989, after the Soviet economy was bankrupted by having to spend 45 percent of GDP on defence in fear of Star Wars. The USA had funded 8 percent of NATO.[22]

GOD

The Christian God shares facets with other gods, such as the Egyptian Sun God Ra; also, Christ is similar to Horus in his resurrection from the dead, assuring us of our resurrection from the dead when we will be together one day with those who have died before us, a manic belief. Akhenaton the pharaoh made a monotheistic state subsuming 2,000 gods into one God, the Sun God, (but with him and his wife Nefertate made living Gods, a manic notion). Like other megalomaniacs he built great palaces and tombs that would make him live forever.

---

[22] The *Financial Times*, the *Irish Times*, Martin Wolf 11.6.14.

The oldest Egyptian love poem from 1,500 B.C tells of a brother and sister who sleep together, a usual event in Pharaohonic dynasties but which upset the puritanical translator in the 1950s.[23] This poem is held in the Chester Beatty Library which also holds one of the world's oldest printed documents, a Japanese Buddhist charm or prayer printed on paper in AD 764 long before Gutenberg developed the printing press in the 1400s. It holds some of the earliest-known copies of the Gospels and the Acts of the Apostles, including Letters of St. Paul to the Corinthians, written in Greek. While Europe was in the dark middle ages, the Middle East was going through a learning burst especially in mathematics, astronomy and medicine. Beatty collected 30,000 items from 2,700BC up to when he died in 1968 when he got a state funeral the only citizen non politician to get one. Beatty made a lot of money and only collected the best items and this was manic in its own way.

Under the first Christian Emperor, Constantine, the Christian Church in 325 A.D at Nicea proclaimed "We believe in one God the maker of Heaven and Earth etc" - a monotheistic belief. Belief in living for ever and belief in the resurrection of Jesus are the ultimate manic delusions. What was the messianic delusion before Jesus Christ?

The Egyptian Empire (4,500BC-500BC) lasted 100 generations; the last phase of the Christian British Empire lasted merely five generations. But is there a connection? Is there a difference between early Egyptian thought Old Testament and Greek, Roman and modern day psychology?

In general people do not believe in death. Sin develops into guilt which develops into the manic belief of forgiveness which is mainly found in Roman Catholics in a regimented way in confessions. Even the suicide bombers do not believe in death; they believe in 75 virgins in heaven. No matter what you do you are free.

The suggestion from this may be that there are common psychological urges toward deism, or simply that local beliefs travel and are accommodated to other beliefs: the biblical flood features also in the earlier Epic of Gilgamesh. Atheist writers like Richard Dawkins would support the contention that we all share an urge toward what might be defined as morality, but which

[23] Dick Ahlstrom, The *Irish Times*, 6 March 2014.

Dawkins himself would analyse as a system that ensures the best chance of transmission of "the selfish gene" to the next generation.

If a hundred Moseses were sent up a mountain they probably would all produce the same Ten Commandments - a moral code that was urgently needed now in a community no longer under the legal aegis of Egypt. But perhaps such a code is actually hotwired in our brains, needing formal framing more to create a social contract than to impose anything new on any individual. Dawkins might say that, insofar as we have invented a God to ensure that we will be rewarded for keeping the tribal moral code and punished for breaking it, we have created God essentially in our image and likeness.

The Christian God is the God of creativity: he creates the earth, gives it light. He creates man in his image and then he creates woman from man's rib. God creates music, poetry, love etc. However, Egyptian gods are supposed to have been made from blood, sweat, tears and semen - made in man's image, rather than vice versa - so perhaps the creativity ascribed to God is misplaced. Mortals have remarked that they are closest to God when being creative. Michelangelo came close to God on a scaffolding in the Sistine Chapel painting God arcing life into Adam; John McGahern remarks that if art is to survive or even matter, the artist must leave something of his blood, sweat, tears or semen in his work - which makes the artist rather like an Egyptian god in this regard?

In another sense, we make gods of those who create: rock stars, film stars, Celebes, writers and painters. We make gods of people at the extreme: the rich, the fast (athletes), models and exponents of haute couture. We make gods of people in the media: journalists, TV personalities and radio presenters. The medium is the God (the message; Marshall McLuhan).

Many dictators made gods of themselves. The images of Hitler, Stalin, Mao, Franco, Ataturk, the Shah' and Saddam Hussein images were all over their states; they ruled and they controlled the media's image of themselves on radio, T.V, statues, big pictures and grandiose palaces. The more exposure and brain washing, the greater their following. They were not immune from paranoia: Saddam killed two of his sons-in-law and Stalin thought everybody was against him. He was the typical hypomanic with paranoia.

The manic archetype God is that of creativity and love which is found in the manic phase of MDI. God created love, the love drug, the ultimate manic trip (archetype) that is mimicked by ecstasy when it is taken for the first time and you get the love hit, the best feeling you ever have when you want to dance and hug each other. To believe this is, to an extent, evidence of mania - faith itself is manic.

Optimism and happiness are manic traits - they can exist without high self-esteem. In an intriguing study, the psychologist and neuroscientist Tali Sharot explains that we are all hotwired with the "optimism bias", and examines the evolutionary reasons why the human brain, contrary to rational experience, repeatedly demonstrates the capacity to expect positive outcomes. She sees optimism as "one of the greatest deceptions of which the human mind is capable".[24] Monty Python's crucified Brian, in the song written by Graham Chapman, famously exhorted us to "always look on the bright side of life". This was the late Jonathan Philbin Bowman's favourite song, played at a lot of people's funerals including his own.

Psychology Professor Seligman from the University of Pennsylvania has carried out a study of the speeches of American presidents. His theory was that voters would not feel attracted to pessimists but would welcome the sense of hope imparted by an optimist. Seligman found that in nineteen out of twenty-four presidential elections between 1900 and 1984 the more optimistic candidates won regardless of whether they were Republican or Democrat. The link between optimism and success was strongest in underdogs who came from behind to win: Truman in 1948, Kennedy in 1960, and Regan in 1980.[25] The phenomenon was repeated in 2016, when Donald Trump's aggressive cheerfulness defeated Hilary Clinton's glum earnestness.

We remain optimistic even when not aware of it and perhaps even when we suspect we're deceiving ourselves, because the alternative might be that we would never do anything at all, but our very optimism may bring us to strange places. When an economy is doing well there are less checks and balances. People who are good salesmen i.e., charismatic, intelligent and

---

[24] See *The Optimism Bias* by Tali Sharot.
[25] *Sunday Times*, Review Section, 30 June 2002.

funny do well. But they can front companies that are just a front, and serve no good or even real purpose.

Jesus died for us, the manic idea of sacrifice by a father (God) of his son. The promise of everlasting life and reincarnation are optimistic thoughts that help us through life.

People may seem depressed but feel high - dysphoria, an "irritable high" where the sufferer's mood does not correspond to the symptoms. Religious fervour may in many instances manifest as dysphoric, when fear of God's wrath, the end of the world, the "rapture," may conceal the secret belief that the religious person may be among the elect who will gain heaven at such an awful time.

Reviewer Tony Allen of American Apocalypse; A History of Modern Evangelicalism by Matthew Avery Sutton.

Only after the world is in flames can the faithful be rewarded with the second coming of Jesus going up to heaven whether by angels, spaceships or passing clouds "The Rapture". Past polls in the U.S.A. say 79 percent of U.S. Christians still believe in the second coming and 41 percent of all Americans think Jesus will get here by 2050.

Dysphoria may become delusion. A man set fire to a church causing 3 million Euros damage, because he was, he said, God Almighty and called himself Jesus Christ. "I burnt the church down." After a few months he was normal.

A depressed husband who had stopped taking his antidepressant medication for two months was discharged from court having hit his wife a manic depressive on the head with a hammer because she would not stop talking (a sign of mania). She was paranoid and was having hallucinations (hearing voices) and could not sleep because she thought there were people outside the house who wanted to get her. The defendant got a five-year suspended sentence and was ordered to take his medication and follow his treatment plan.[26]

---

[26] The *Sun*, 31 July 2010.

David Ikea is a rather high-profile example of Messianic Delusion. He was a football goalie turned sports-newscaster who wanted to save the world. He was ridiculed on TV but he was only a manic-depressive who would not take his lithium. Case histories of Messianic Delusion known to me personally include one man who became ill on visiting London. On returning to Ireland he was put into a psychiatric hospital. He felt that the nurses were waiting to present him to the world. Clearly manic, he was hard to stabilize and after a while he was discharged.

Another man who thought he was Jesus. He drove around waving to the people who he thought were waving at him. He grew a beard and long hair and wore long flowing white clothes, blessing people. He became very paranoid and killed a relative.

Another used to carry a bible and go up the local hill and pretend that he was preaching to the people. He also thought that he was Jesus, and he killed a relative.

One patient who killed a relative had thought he was Jesus for a year and wore hippy clothes with beads. He killed his relative because he thought the relative was the devil.

Another case illustrates both Messianic and commercial delusion. While attending bible classes and thinking he was Jesus, he was blessing people. Diagnosed as manic-depressive, he was settled on tranquillisers and Lithium mood stabilisers.

Another patient had slept with his girlfriend, her sister and her mother. One night his girlfriend and he got a bottle of vodka. The next day she accused him of rape. He was a pushover. He spent eight years in a secure unit and later he overdosed a few months after his release.

Another friend lay down on railway tracks to test God. He lost one of his legs but felt closer to God. Peter Sutcliffe, the Yorkshire Ripper who killed 13 women and attacked others, is locked up in Broadmoor Forensic hospital. He had tested God by driving off cliffs twice thinking delusionally that if he survived he would be 'doing God's will' by killing the women, Psychiatric lecture by a Garda in St. Patrick's Hospital.

Part of the reason religion features in psychotic episodes is that Christianity does not have enough to appease the spiritual needs of many who number themselves Christian. It does not satisfy the psyche of all people at all times of stress and the shortfall may focus the sufferer's attention on the core elements of the belief system. Forgiveness, reincarnation, the Eucharist and Jesus (the son of "God the Sun") are hot wired in the brain.

Though religion consoles and strengthens some people, the human spirit may demand more than a formal belief system it offers. The Gods in the mind are not satisfied; they need a more complex, imaginative, intriguing hypothesis that integrates human higher aspirations with more basic needs; something that will reconcile the superego and the id, in Freudian terms. Though Marx despised religion as "the opium of the people," he believed in higher states of mind and was not against spirituality. Patrick Kavanagh captures the need for such integration in "The Great Hunger".

As Kavanagh's great poem illustrates, sexuality is an essential human quality and one that needs healthy expression for fulfilled living. The great tragedy in Kavanagh's Ireland was that sexuality is demonised by Christianity, and Ireland at the time was truly priest-ridden.

Furthermore - and of equal danger - sex was denied to a priest or nun. If these people, especially those inside a closed order, become sexualised, the order may become in danger of imploding in chaos. The Murphy Report has opened a can of worms in the Roman Catholic Church exposing horrific abuse among its priests and cover-ups by the bishops.

Why there was so much abuse is hard to know but frustrated sexuality, in more than one sense, is a critical component. Recent testimony suggests that a significant number of priests were closet homosexuals and in a time that saw homosexuality criminalised and derided these men could have been understandably attracted to a spiritual job that is also powerful. The "vocation" they probably embraced with sincerity offered them the opportunity to make some sort of atonement for what they would have seen as their loathsomely sinful makeup; but the power that went with this job also compensated for any sense of inadequacy engendered by their "perverted" sexuality.

But that very power was terrifying, and corrupted some priests. They were well-served by the almost-superstitious awe in which simple, largely-uneducated Irish people saw priests, men of God whose holy hands touched the very body and blood of Christ. How could such holy hands possibly fondle little boy's genitalia? What priests - indeed, what man - could be attracted to young boys?

Priests were untouchables who thought they would never be found out. The first public sign that they were mortal emerged with the heterosexual Bishop Casey who had a lover and a son whom he tried to cover up and to whom he gave €70,000 from the diocesan funds.

The Irish people' faith was rocked to the national foundations. After the Casey affair evidence of far more odious affairs began to surface. Fathers Brendan Smith and Sean Fortune were revealed to be monstrous, violent pederasts who had abused and raped scores of children each, and there were many, many more offenders of lesser magnitude.

Manic people can be very dangerous. John D, a patient of mine, was a very large, intimidating man who would force girls to go out with him. He would stop cars and get people out and drive off, and often went into hotels and ate without paying. A doctor in his local psychiatric hospital felt so endangered that he carried a shotgun in the boot of his car. John was on Largactil 400 mg, four times a day, an elephantine dose. He broke up an office in his local psychiatric hospital and set fire to a room in another. His former teacher who was 100 years old said that he was uncontrollable at a young age. He hung himself after being released from the CMH.

Another patient who had been a jazz singer in London was seduced by an English gangster and they married even though she was warned about him - he used to beat her up. He had a canary that he could get to jump from bar to bar in the cage. He used to bet on this with people. One day the bird flew out the window. She was terrified. She got another canary from the pet shop but the bird did not jump and he lost his bets with his friends. He did not notice the new canary. She was thrilled to have tricked him: "It made the beatings worthwhile".

ECT (Electro-Convulsive Therapy) is one response to mental illness. It was formerly used quite widely; then, in the 1970s, following its disturbing portrayal in the film version of Ken Kesey's anti-establishment novel, *One Flew Over the Cuckoo's Nest*, it came to be seen as barbaric, even though some sufferers claimed that they had benefited from it. (In the film it is portrayed as violent and agonising; in fact muscle-relaxants prevent violent seizures.) In recent years the method seems to have become warily rehabilitated (though while it can lift depression it may also cause memory loss and mania it is seen as the preferred treatment for puerperal psychosis.).

In her book *Shockaholic*, Carrie Fisher (Princess Leia in *Star Wars*) talks of having ECT every few months, antidepressants didn't work, psychotherapy didn't work, "a tune-up whenever I notice the onset of depression"; her problems may have been caused by drug abuse that might also have affected her short-term memory. "Your whole life you hear about this terrifying treatment that turns you into a vegetable, only to finally find out that it had all the charming qualities of no big deal. Sort of like getting your nails done".

Lou Reed also had ECT, though in his case at the behest of his parents when he was 17 yrs in 1959. Because his parents thought he was a deviant (a homosexual) and in those days ECT was seen as a cure. He did a very manic album called *Transformer* in 1972 with the help of David Bowie and his guitarist Mick Ronson. Lou died in October 2013.

Vivien Leigh was bipolar and allegedly a nymphomaniac. Steve McQueen's biographer Marc Eliot claims that in the late 60's McQueen was abusing pot, LSD, cocaine, peyote and amyl nitrate. All this drug abuse made him paranoid and manic and he beat his wife Neile up, claiming she had been unfaithful, a classic manic paranoid presentation. As in mania he was sexually indiscreet and slept around.[27] (There is evidence that a history of psychological control is worse than one of violence when it comes to killing of a spouse or partner).

Sporting events have been seen as a means of social control. In the days of bread and circuses the Romans might see sand for the arenas as a more important means of keeping the people content than feeding them. In Ireland Gaelic games are robust affairs and in the past they were even more so - hurling may have developed from weapons practise, the ball being the lime-hardened brain of a defeated enemy, which was made into a projectile

---

[27] BBC, *Panorama*, 8 December 2014; Marc Elliott, *Steve McQueen: A Biography.*

designed to kill someone else. Sports "were passed down from an elite" and to this day the successful GAA player becomes one of a semi-exclusive elite, with career paths open that might be closed to others.

After the foundation of the Gaelic Athletic Association in 1884 "There was vast coverage of sporting activity available in a print media that was servicing a largely literate population." With literacy and exposure to wider cultural influences, "After a while blood sports were deemed to be undesirable."[28]

However, blood sports, while illegal now, are still played. Dog-fighting has a huge following and in some states like Louisiana cock-fighting is still legal. Sports are arguably getting more dangerous as even amateur sports like Gaelic football and hurling go for intensive training regimes and as performance-enhancing drug abuse is found in virtually every sport. In previous years American football players might be sent out onto the field after novocaine injections to their shoulders; today they and hurlers wear helmets to prevent concussion that players may sue for. Now there's cage fighting with mixed martial arts where everything goes from more violent boxing, wrestling and kick boxing.

CHOSEN PEOPLE

The search for a homeland, a Promised Land, brings with it nationalism, mania and paranoia. If one can see oneself as the person who will make this ideal a reality, one may fall prey to messianic delusions, in which "the other" is seen as the irreconcilable enemy, diabolic, to be overcome at whatever cost and without conscience's restraint. Examples of such messianic delusion may be discerned in Padraig Pearse, who unambiguously saw himself as a Christ-like figure and welcomed his execution as martyrdom, and perhaps Ian Paisley, who saw any concession to the enemy, Irish nationalism, as unacceptable and to be resisted by force of arms or any other means.

Paisley often likened the Ulster Protestants to the Lost Tribe of Israel, Ulster itself as their sacred homeland to be defended to the death. He frankly

---

[28] Michael Cronin in a review of James Kelly's *Sport in Ireland 1600-1840*, the *Irish Times*, 9 August 2014.

claimed that the pope is a demonic agent, if not the devil incarnate. Unusually Paisley made peace with Sinn Fein and was seen as a pal of Martin McGuinness in the end, but many of his followers would wish to have nothing whatsoever to do with Catholics or Irish nationalists of any hue, seeing them as they do from a paranoid perspective.

Similar attitudes can be seen in the various militia movements of the United States. Like the Paisleyites, these groups tend to have a fundamentalist Protestant ethos and see themselves as the keepers of the sacred flame, the real true believers of a promise allegedly made thousands of years ago by a tribal god to a warrior-shepherd surrounded by tribal enemies. Like Ulster, America has also been described as a Promised Land by such paranoid delusionals as lead the various movements. As always, anyone who does not share their views becomes "the enemy," and fair game - George Bush Jr claimed that "anyone not with us is against us," when he launched his "crusade" against terrorism. To use the word crusader upsets the Muslims as it reminds them of the slaughter in the medieval crusades, another manifestation of hypomania. Such people may shoot up synagogues, murder people at abortion clinics, and blow up federal buildings without a doubt that they are doing right and will find divine reward for their acts. The late Osama Bin Laden did the same in the name of an Islamic fundamentalist god, and his followers literally go to death to fulfil their messiah's wishes, drawn by the promise of heavenly bliss after a martyr's death. Bin Laden communicated with his followers through poetry.

THE AMERICAN DREAM

The American Dream is the dream of the Promised Land, the land of plenty. You can do anything. Work hard enough and you'll get it. Dreams are meant to be lived. Fame and fortune can be had. Anyone can build a business, write a best seller, and make a million. Ego grows, leading to belief in the self, the manic energy exploding into love and conflict. We want to be stars and if we can't do that we can look up to the stars and listen to gossip about them.

Of course the dream has a price. People divorce because they don't feel fulfilled - you're holding me back. Hollywood is manic, with enormous amounts of drinking, sex and drug abuse. Like New York it attracts people who are manic and are willing to travel there to pursue their dream. It would seem that half the waiters and waitresses in LA and New York say that their real profession is acting, playing in a band or some sort of artistic endeavour.

The American dream makes people believe that they can achieve their goals, acting in this case, by working hard and being serious and focused. But hard work and a sense of focus are not the only price. A New York friend of mine broke up a five-year otherwise happy marriage because she wanted to achieve her goal to become an actress. Divorce is rampant in the USA as people seek their "real" love.

The victims of these break ups are the children, who need both parents so that they can learn to express emotions, the expression of which is a core component of artistry. A mother gives expression (language, art) to the child and the father gives a father-archetype of strength and rationality. Ironically the artistic ideal, as propounded by Hollywood, compromises the most important art of all, creating a real human being.

America has made gods out of not just famous actors, but writers, sportsmen, singers - anyone with a public profile, however fleeting their career. "Ordinary" people read about these "super" "successful" people in magazines and look at them on TV. They are totally immersed in the dream and are hypnotised by the screen. People live the dream of a Superman as a part of their education.

AMERICA AND MDI

Manic depression works; otherwise it would have been bred out of the gene pool. The same holds true for schizophrenia. What in them is positive? The spectrum of emotional and intellectual energy from the fast positive to the slow negative drives MDI and the thinking is over-inclusive making it more creative.

Hollywood has become the pervasive hypomanic modern day frontier in the Wild West culture of creativity in music, painting, film and money. American cultural icons such as clothes (Levi's), soft drinks (Coke), cigarettes (Marlboro), restaurants (McDonalds), cars (Ford) and planes (Boeing) for example are found all over the world.

The air that liberal democracy lives on is controlled by lawyers and powered by the hypomanic nature of its leaders in the western world. J.F.K, Reagan, Clinton, Blair and Bush did not have a great quota of paranoia as did Stalin and Hitler who were in a full blown delusional psychotic paranoid position that resulted in them killing millions. In 1932-33 Stalin deliberately caused mass famine in Russia and the Ukraine when he enforced collectivisation by doing away with the *kulak* class of prosperous peasant. The best estimate of the number starved is about 5 million families; as kulaks tended to have large families anything between 15 and 40 million people died. Cannibalism was widespread.

Famine and cannibalism has been a feature of Communist rule. There had been the same mass-starvation, though on a smaller scale, ten years earlier during Lenin's "War Communism" phase, and the same was to occur on a far greater scale in Maoist China during the Great Leap Forward - from 1958 to 1961 - and from the Cultural Revolution - from 1966 to Mao's death in 1976. Frank Dikotter got unprecedented access to the Chinese archives and discovered that Mao starved 45 million peasants in a push for industrialisation. Jung Chang estimates that the figure may be as high as 100 million, making Mao the greatest mass-murderer in history.

Dikotter claims that between 1 million and 2 million Chinese committed suicide and as many as 2.5 million were beaten to death by party comrades "because they didn't work hard enough … because they spoke out, because they were accused of dragging their feet, because they didn't turn up in the morning, because in some cases they were considered too old or too sick and what are you going to do, continue to feed this person?"

Dikotter describes how "Some sold their children for a bowl of rice or ate grass, bark, mud and corpses in their desperation to stay alive." Responsibility for it, insists Dikotter, lies almost wholly with one man, Chairman Mao, who said "religion is poison". It was almost entirely a man made catastrophe, which happened after the Communist party herded the country's hundreds of millions of villagers into communes to boost agriculture and industry and compete with the world's super powers, and is something of a reprise of Stalin's mass-murder of the kulaks. As in the USSR in the 1930s, "This radical collectivisation simply destroyed any incentive to work". Agriculture output collapsed, hence the famine.

To exacerbate the problems, at this time cheap pork was sold to East Germany to help the fantasy of the Chinese's Marxist fellow travellers. What gets to Dikotter in particular is the silence surrounding the tragedy: "That to me is the real emotional point, that kind of silence, that way of tiptoeing around those massive black holes in twentieth-century history."[29] Such tiptoeing characterises the faux-liberals who do so much to set Western standards of acceptability. Modern day socialists feel that these deaths were necessary to build a socialist ideal and despite the fact that anything up to 100 million people were murdered through the Cultural Revolution, they revere Mao as a champion in the fight against capitalism.

People were thought to be happy in China but gangs, rape, looting and anarchy were rampant. With MAO's gleeful approval the country turned into civil war. The countries intellectuals were made slaves. "Bombard the headquarters!" was MAO's own edict to millions of ardent and bored young people-school children who played truant, students who beat up their lectures and workers who went on strike. CHAOS(mania) was glorious playing with and enjoying subordinates fear and seldom can one man have toyed with the psyches of so many. MAO left a legacy in China of paranoia (mania) that still grips its modern dictatorship under the latest autocrat, Xi Jinping. Dikotter. (A Peoples History). Waving their "Little Red Book" of MAO's thoughts. Red Guards, leftist students and school children were told to destroy the "Four Olds" old customs, old culture, old habits and old ideas. MAO's face on every bank note.

There is some evidence that Ronald Reagan was hypomanic - though this does not mean he was psychotically paranoid. He came very close to death when he was shot in an attempted assassination; as a consequence of his survival he may have felt a sense of being preserved by God, a sense of destiny, and this sense may have enabled him to make the big decision that brought down the USSR. He was the only Western leader since the Second World War who felt it was possible to actually beat the USSR, not merely co-exist alongside in a state of Mutually Assured Destruction (MAD). This supreme confidence suggests hypomania and the Star Wars strategy, which toppled the USSR, was certainly grandiose enough to suggest hypomania.

---

[29] Andrew Holgate interview, the *Sunday Times*, 10 July 2011.

In recently released tapes covering the Cuban crisis it is shown that J.F. Kennedy was confused, inarticulate and surprisingly ill informed, maybe due to the side effects of the amphetamines he was rumoured to have injected. Kennedy got bad advice over the Bay of Pigs; Castro had found out about the planned invasion and the counter-revolutionaries landed under a full moon, easy fodder for the Cubans.

Like JFK, Clinton was known to be sexually indiscreet. Obama's father died in a car crash after drinking and was a serial womaniser, something his son has to watch as he is also charismatic and this would point to hypomania.

Through the 1990s America was going through a boom and people were spending huge amounts of money. Despite the good times, though, the savings base was lower than it had been for decades and sub-prime mortgages were like confetti. This boom was driven by mania in the U.S.A. and Europe, particularly in Ireland. This is suggestive of manic irresponsibility, and is, of course, fuelled by extensive advertising.

That the American culture is getting more manic is suggested by the sexual and moral disinhibition we see on such popular shows as Jerry Springer, and even less trashy ones like Judge Judy. Pornography makes up 30 percent of internet use. Further evidence of American hypomania may be seen in the fact that people are having more hyper-sexual experiences and boasting about these - on Springer and other such shows - and in an expanding drug culture. According to some estimates, marijuana is now the second cash crop in the USA (after corn). Drug intoxication may lead to more killing without guilt, as many killings derive from both the drug wars and the paranoia of drug-fuelled city gangs. Rap musicians often encourage lawlessness and violence in their lyrics and in fashion they don't wear belts or laces like prisoners, encouraging identification by their fans and followers with criminals. After leaving Robben Island, Mandela had forgotten how to tie his shoelaces or his tie.

Another cause of violence is the widespread use of computer games that simulate death from afar. According to David Grossman, this was the most effective technique used by the US armed forces to improve their "kill score" in the years after the Korean War, when it was noted that through all the wars fought (insofar as it could be established) only one soldier in four actually aimed his gun at his foe, so deep-seated is the taboo against killing our fellow-men. By means of a variety of methods, video games being the most effective, the armed forces were able to get this proportion up to over 90 percent in the Vietnam War. Nowadays children are being brought up with such games almost as the "default drive" of many of them; Grossman has no doubt that such game-playing leads directly to violence in society.[30]

The more manic the USA gets the more paranoid will be the culture. This increases the risk of more McCarthyism, with Islam, not Communism, as the target of the next pogrom.

THE ORIGINAL PROMISED LAND

Israel is seen as the Jewish homeland, and is the focus of Zionism's most paranoid posturing. In the distant past, the Jews fought for this land that was allegedly promised them by God, repeatedly lost and regained it, and were eventually scattered across the ancient world after the Roman sacking of Jerusalem in AD 70. Has the existence of the modern Jewish state of Israel been detrimental to the Jewish religion? Did Jewish nationalism exist when Jews had no homeland, and did Zionism undermine "real" Judaism, for all that Judaism was founded on the promise of a Jewish homeland? Nationalism, after all, as a modern phenomenon dates only from the decades after the French Revolution. Were Jews more Jewish without a homeland?

The Kibbutz is a socialist ideal compounded with nationalism, a potentially paranoid mindset in which many Jews spend considerable time, and that may lead to killing without guilt. We see a capacity for genocide in the Zionist reaction to the Palestinian "problem," and a non-egalitarian approach to sharing land and power with the "other," the enemy. The inability to empathise with that enemy from their own experience under the Nazi regime suggests something almost psychopathic, brought about by the notion of themselves as a Chosen People, and therefore exempt from divine censure - mortal censure would hardly count against such an attitude.

That said, a full picture needs to include the fact that the Jews are the focus of persecution still. The Khartoum Declaration, signed by most Arab and

---

[30] David Grossman, *On Killing*, passim.

some non-Arab Moslem nations, commits its signatories to destroy Israel and "drive the Jews into the sea". Anti-Semitic attacks are increasing across Europe and the USA for many years now. As the old saying has it, you're not really paranoid if "they" really are out to get you, and the idea of a Jewish Homeland, where the Jews can protect themselves, needs to be seen in this light.

EMIGRATION

For almost two thousand years the Jews were an example of people who travel to other countries. It was during their Diaspora that they acquired the cultural characteristics the world tends to associate with them, clichéd though these characteristics may be. But as so often in ancient days, they were looking for a Promised Land, and perhaps it was this search that was their cultural definition. Moses was an itinerant; he travelled with his people into the desert and died before his people found their Promised Land.

But the Jews are not the only ones with a Diaspora. An urge to travel may reflect economic pressure, as it did in Ireland for 150 years after the Famine, but it also may suggest mania. People head into the unknown, assured of the hand of God on their endeavours (though whether people get high and travel, or travel and get high, is a moot point). Immigrants to USA brought out twice as many patents as American-born people.

All cultures have their mythical beliefs; e.g. the English have King Arthur and the Holy Grail and magic and love. The chosen ones go to the Promised Land, a belief than many had when they landed in America, the Puritans to build their biblical City on a Hill. But having got there, their descendants often look back wistfully toward their ancestral homelands. Irish Americans are, to use a cliché, more Irish than the Irish themselves. St. Patrick's Day is a major day in the USA, even more so than in Ireland. The Americans look to the Irish and the Irish look to the Celts. We have our own rose-tinted view of the past. Why do people need a mythical vision?

When people are manic (high) they tend to travel, sometimes flying on impulse, on their credit cards, to obscure or outlandish destinations. There is plausible circumstantial evidence that perhaps the majority of people who emigrated of their own choice were more manic than the average; it stands to reason that they were more adventurous and courageous. Australia is quite unusual in that a lot of criminals were sent there, people who, almost by definition, were manic. During the First World War, the ANZAC troops gained an enduring reputation for courage to the point of recklessness - they also were the most insubordinate and law-breaking of all the Imperial forces. Modern Australians' language is cruder, sexist and disinhibited than that of, say Britain - quite manic.

The Pilgrims who went to Western America in the 1700s and 1800s were probably more manic than the general population and believed in both the Kingdom of God and freedom of the individual on earth; they had been in the forefront of the Parliamentary forces in the English Civil War and had ideals of a Promised Land. Some had been displaced by the Civil War and after the Restoration they were victimised again by the Test Act and other penal laws. They fled religious persecution, first to the Netherlands, then quickly to the New World. Here they found not an earthy paradise but a hard land where they were surrounded by enemies, actual and potential, native tribes they regarded, very literally, as being slaves of Satan. A huge number of these Pilgrims had been traumatised and brutalised by their experiences and were manic by any standards, the place they fled to one of hard work and boredom punctuated by periods of intense danger. Genocidal pograms against the Indians were matched by manic intolerance of dissent in their own communities, something that reached its nadir with the Salem Witch Trials.

The moot consideration in the context of Diasporas, and belief in being a chosen people is whether hypomania - of which such beliefs, and such searching for a promised land, are symptoms - is an ancient affliction, rather than something that is of relatively recent emergence.

Though being chosen by God is often thought to be a Judeo-Christian-Muslim belief, the name many if not most so-called primitive people have for themselves translates roughly as The People. The Japanese, though of Buddhist and animist Shinto belief, also bought into the Chosen People mythology, and not just in the Imperial period of the first half of the twentieth century. Might this suggest that we all tend to see ourselves as divinely chosen, and set apart from all of those others?

Another consideration: might the idea of being divinely chosen be a species-adaptive one, reassuring each member of all tribes of the success of the tribal endeavour, until such time as the conflicting and mutually exclusive belief systems come up against each other (perhaps most ironically, as well as tragically, when the Nazi Super-race came up against the Chosen People)? At this point either one side defeats and displaces the other, which then must move to a more inhospitable environment and re-establish itself there, ensuring both expansion of the species into new niches and weeding out of weakness, or the entire and mutually supportive belief system collapses in anarchy and hypomania, such as we saw in New York and Afghanistan in 2001.

Xenophobia is actually a "good thing" in that it's species-adaptive - to a point at any rate. Suspicion of strangers means that one is less likely to be surprised by a sudden or treacherous attack by those who may be enemies. On the other hand, excessive xenophobia leads to insularity, which in turn leads to everything from ignorance to a depleted gene pool.

Hypomania may manifest as either xenophobia, as in Nazi Germany, or anti-xenophobia, as in the currently popular faux-liberal Marxist support for a borderless world, in which unfettered passage of people takes place. This multicultural opposite of the Chosen People idea is just as hypomanic.

Being "chosen" is not enough, however: one hypomanic idea fosters another. The thought that one will be tested and if found to be good one will live forever in an idyllic place, whether a mortal "City on a Hill" or an immortal Heaven, with one's loved ones again, is very manic and wishful thinking. Heaven is a manic idea, and mania can be like being in Heaven.

Again, however, as with xenophobia, the idea is not entirely negative. The idea of living forever may be individually - and species-adaptive in that it protects us from morbid ideation and fosters optimism, which in turn improves one's chances of survival, Oasis song "Live forever." There is mania in the idea that we can pray to God, who knows what we think and will protect us if we please him, but again there is advantage here in that we are encouraged by the feeling of Divine help - if God is with us, who can stand against us? This manic delusion feeds into the xenophobic delusion.

Allied to faith in God is fear of evil, a paranoid stance that no less feeds into the xenophobic delusion. In every war the enemy is demonised, and presented as the epitome of evil and the enemy of all that is good - and therefore of God - making it easier to justify killing them. Siegfried Sassoon speaks of the First World War as a time "When Murder wore the mask of Law", and in these years the Germans were indeed demonised.

Yet one needs to be careful in being too "enlightened" in this matter at any rate. *Schreckleitkeit*, roughly translated as "frightfulness", was official German policy at this time, and the infamous Rape of Belgium, and of parts of France and Russian Poland, saw thousands of civilians murdered and state-endorsed vandalism, notably the destruction of Louvain. This policy was, ironically, founded on a doctrine, endorsed by the military scholar Carl von Clausewitz, that terrorising citizens would deprive the enemy of popular support and therefore shorten any war, to the long-term benefit of both victor and vanquished.

Likewise, in the Second World War, the Nazis were objectively different morally to the Allies, as were the Japanese - whose bastardised Bushido code made them even crueller than the Germans. Though atrocities are committed in every war, it is foolish to pretend that Allied xenophobia was not well-founded.

At the same time, painting Germans (and Japanese) as "other", undoubtedly made it easier for individual soldiers to depersonify the enemy and shoot at a target rather than at a fellow-human being. Patton preached to his men that the secret of successful war was not dying for your country, but making the other poor son of a bitch die for his.

The notion of predestination - that one is chosen with the few to go to heaven after Jesus has come for a second time - appeals to our vanity and insecurity. The Second Coming (the Resurrection) is an even more manic ideal than heaven itself, perhaps, but other religions have equally unlikely scenarios: the Jews, who do not see Jesus as the Messiah but as a prophet, are very happy to have male sons because thus they might be parents to the "real" Messiah, who will lead them to the ultimate promised land - heaven on earth.

The whole idea, of course, has been used for thousands of years as part of a system of social control, the sweet carrot that entices on the masses, hell being the stick that drives them in the direction their elders, rabbis, priests, mullahs want them to go. The vision of heaven depends on societal beliefs. The Pope says that there is sex in heaven, and Muslim suicide bombers fighting Jihad are promised sex with 72 virgins in heaven. This perhaps more than anything indicates that Heaven is a figment of the imagination, a product of wishful thinking. Neil Young spoke of seeing "silver space ships flying in the yellow haze of the sun," a drug-induced vision of a New Age Heaven, with apparent endorsement of reincarnation: "flying Mother Nature's silver seeds to a new home in the sun."

JEWS

The 14 million Jews in the world comprise 0.2 percent of the world population but make up 25-30 percent of the Nobel laureates and Olympic medal winners. The 6 million Jews killed by the Nazi made up one third of the Jewish population in the world at that time. In 1948 the U.N. recognised the Jewish state of Israel.

Jewish success against the odds might suggest a certain manic activity and self-belief. It seems a bit manic to think that your son might be the messiah, as religious Jews do. For this reason, baby boys are more welcome then baby girls in most Jewish families. Jesus was a Jew, but is not recognised as the Son of God by the Jews. Does the fact that Christians believe he is - from the same hypomanic impulse as the Jews, presumably - indicate that Judaism affected its successor religions with its own particular manic delusion, or that such manic delusion is common to all people? In part rivalry between messiahs explains the hostility under which the Jews have had to operate through almost all of the Christian era.

During the Second World War the Germans saw Jews as being at the level of vermin. Six million Jews were exterminated with homosexuals, itinerants, mentally retarded people and foreigners who were not seen as part of the Aryan super race resulting in another 6 million being exterminated. In WW2 10 million Germans died and 40 million Nazi enemies died. China 15m, Japan 3m, USSR 20m, UK. 0.5m, Dutch East Indies 3m, India 1.5m

Thou shall not marry us
Thou shall not live with us
Thou shall not live

—thus Simon Wiesenthal summarised the way in which anti-Semitism was implemented in Germany.

But it would seem that Jews have always been outsiders. Anti-Semitism is as old as Judaism itself, the Old Testament detailing the persecutions inflicted by the Egyptians, the Assyrians, the Persians, the Philistines and others up to the Romans. In part this persecution stemmed from the Jews' own refusal to belong to another group, and especially from their jealousy of their own god, and hostility to those of other people (the same offence for which Christians were later persecuted in Rome). This persecution, culminating in the sack of Jerusalem by the Romans in 63 AD, led to the Jews becoming the wandering tribe of genius, specialising in work that travelled, should they have to flee from another pogrom - e.g. clothes, money and jewellery.

However, acquisition of a modern homeland has drawn out other hypomanic aspects in them: the mania of narcissistic nationalism has changed many of them into fanatics. Modern day Zionists are in the paranoid position, killing without guilt their Arab neighbours. The Palestinians live in primitive conditions, many in foreign ghettos, and their response to their persecution has been as hypomanic as belief in a messiah who would deliver the Jews from their earthly oppressors. The promise of heaven and unearthly virgins drives their martyrs to the ultimate sacrifice. The whole notion of a suicide bomber is almost outside our cultural understanding. Like what was found in the Northern Ireland "Hunger Strikers."

Israel is very much the loner in the Middle East and it needs help from Europe and America, an ironic reversal of much of the Christian era when the Jews were persecuted.

CHRISTIANITY

People need something to believe in, some higher power /idea. The Greeks and Romans had various Gods that satisfied the manic archetypes, notably Dionysus and Bacchus. The Greeks developed democracy; comedy, satire and the first joke book all signs of mania. Christianity, on the other hand, is a rather simple religion in that it postulates one God only, and an ultimately black-and-white set of rules for acceptable behaviour.

Nowadays, it may not be interesting enough to engage the intellectual soul-searcher, the human brain having been over-stimulated by advertising and the other excesses of a hypomanic age. Christianity does not have enough to appease the spiritual needs of many who number themselves Christian; it does not satisfy the psyche of all people at all times of stress.

Though religion may console and strengthen some people, the human spirit demands more than that which Christianity offers. The Gods in the mind need a more complex, imaginative, intriguing hypothesis.

Jesus' ideas were manic and attracted manic minds. Manic ideas make manic people more manic and lead them deeper into mania. This spiral of thought, emotion and experience leads to chaos.

To read, objectively, the gospel account of the preparations for the triumphal entry to Jerusalem on Palm Sunday is to see at least the possibility of passwords and plots. Reading of the actual entry in a similar way one may see a rebellion in the making, and Christ's crucifixion as a Roman felon goes a long way to convince an objective reader that Christ's mania overtook his common sense and he raised rebellion against the Roman authorities. Such an interpretation also accounts for such otherwise puzzling lines as "I come not to bring peace but a sword." Simon Peter's attack on the servant of one of those who came to arrest Jesus in Gethsemane adds evidence of armed rebellion, as does the fact that 500 soldiers (a cohort) were involved in this operation, and Peter's later denial of Jesus. Later still, of course, he and Paul both travelled to Rome and preached there, in defiance of Roman law, and died for their pains.

Christianity loves the poor and the meek - but was this Christ's original message? Or all of it? The New Testament is more hypomanic than the vengeance-centred Old Testament, with its dysphoric elation - though the Old Testament, with its graphic scenes of killing and rapine, does perhaps cater to the demands of the id. Is it coincidence that the Bible Belt, whose Christianity is strongly influenced by the Old Testament, has traditionally been the most violent part of America, a distinction it retains? The New Testament emphasises its charismatic leader and love; it appeals more to the super-ego and the ego than the id. Christians therefore have the ideal to live up to and the paranoia of both the devil and the wrathful Old Testament god to fear. (Christian churches traditionally have exercised control by putting people in fear of Hell.) (James Joyce, Portrait of an Artist)

RELIGION

"It's harder to get into heaven than it is to get a camel through the eye of a needle." Traditionally this, along with Christ's humble (mortal) origins, has been interpreted as meaning that wealth is the enemy of sanctity. Today, however, there is a new breed of celebrity minister that champions the gospel of "prosperity theology".[31] These preachers live in opulent mansions, enjoy the company of beautiful women, drive flash sports cars, proudly display their chunky gold jewellery and tattoos and revel in their celebrity status.

This doctrine, an offshoot of Pentecostalism and one of the fastest growing religions in the U.S., holds that financial wealth and physical health are the blessings of God, a material reward in this life for a faith that alleviates the curse of poverty and sickness. At least six preachers have "mega-churches" with congregations of more than 2,000 people a week; one, Noel Jones, a brother of Grace Jones, model cum singer, has 15,000 in his congregation.

People need something to believe in, some higher power - or at least many people do. Which churches are getting the crowds in? The manic evangelical churches promise forgiveness and supreme manic life everlasting. The Catholic Church, and organised Christianity in general, is losing out in the popularity polls. More and more religious beliefs are fragmenting and new religions are being developed all the time. Alternative religions - New Age, alternative medicine - are getting more followers. People are turning to Paganism, Druidism and Celtic Mythology.

There is disagreement over the interpretation of near death experience (NDE) such as seeing a tunnel or a bright light. That gorgeous blissful tunnel of light? That apparently is probably caused by a lack of oxygen to the retina. People are transformed in a positive way - becoming more altruistic and

---

[31] Philip Sherwell, *The Sunday Telegraph*, 27 October 2013.

having no fear of death.[32] Peter Fenwick a neuropsychiatrist and NDE expert talks about a study in the Lancet of 344 heart patients resuscitated after cardiac attest. All had been clinically dead at some point during their treatment; 62 reported near death experiences, while 41 described out-of body experiences, feeling of ecstasy, seeing dead relatives or tunnels going towards light. Paul Robertsons book Soundscapes: A Musician's Journey Through Life and Death. Interviewed by Christina Patterson. Sunday Times News Review 7th August 2016. Forward by Peter Fenwick.

With reincarnation people may not be focused or impelled to do better, as they might be under the terror of hellfire. They "know" they merely will be coming back to discharge their karma and for some this provides no impetus to improve in this life - perhaps partly the reason the early Christian belief in reincarnation was declared anathema at the Council of Constantinople. The idea of reincarnation is that you improve through each life until your build-up of positive karma makes you perfect and you enter Nirvana. Thus the main idea of karma is to love people more and do good deeds. Unfortunately if you love yourself, friends, family and country and other people you might get to the paranoid position and kill without guilt. Too much manic love is associated with the paranoid position. Love cannot be thrown around as it was in the Hippy-Dippy Sixties; it needs to be focused.

Belief in God may be an evolved adaptive trait, and there is evidence, albeit controversial, that people who pray and go to church are happier and have a higher chance of getting over cancer. Cultures such as Sweden that have turned toward atheism (no God) and agnosticism (some God) have a higher rate of suicide. This, however, may be a cultural meme or the consequence of Seasonal Affective Disorder rather than anything else. Dr Dermot Walsh, a previous Inspector of Mental Hospitals, suggested in a lecture that a blip in suicide at the age of thirty-three is due to an association with the age of the death of Jesus and copycat suicides.

The Catholic religion is almost stereotypically synonymous with guilt; it has a depressive view of Christianity and a fixation on sexual matters. So shameful is sex that Catholicism teaches that not merely Jesus, but Mary too, was conceived "without sin". Sinners will suffer damnation. On the other

---

[32] See Dick Teresi interview with Sam Parnia, *New Scientist*, 9 March 2013.

hand the Catholic Church offers a female deity – effectively - in Mary, Jesus' mother, and indeed an entire pantheon of neo-gods. Prayers are said to Mary and the saints and each saint has a particular cause, such as St. Jude for hopeless cases, much as old pagan gods did.

Parthenogenesis may occur in about 1 in a 50,000 births where sperm comes off the hands or sheets for example, without breaking the hymen. Aarathi Prasad describes how virgin women might give birth.[33] Could Mary have been the result of a fusion of male and female twin embryos, and thus have had XX (female) as well as XY (male) chromosomes? One in 1,000 people do. Could she have had ovotestes, gonads that are part ovary and part testes? One in 83,000 people have such organs today.

Other examples of "virgin" conception can be found in Germany, where a man sued his wife after she gave birth to a black baby, the couple both being white. The wife, who had not slept with anyone else, hired an investigator who found that her husband had gone to a prostitute who had just slept with a black man; the husband sucked up some of the black man's sperm into his penis and put it into his wife.

A South African who was shot in the womb became pregnant because the bullet had just gone through a man's testicle.

People sing less in the Catholic Church than in the Protestant churches. Singing is a bonding activity and makes people happier. When you sing you share emotion with the congregation as you do when you are being saved, talking in tongues and other aspects of emotion found in e.g. Baptist and Pentecostalism services. The Catholic Church controls the manic features of religion such as singing and making your own mind up about the scriptures; until recently, at least, it pivoted on a dysphoric Hell, not on the manic Protestant Heaven.

In Northern Ireland 3.000 reformist Presbyterians only sing the psalms. Martin Luther (1483-1546) had three sacraments, baptism, Eucharist and penance. He translated the bible into German. He believed in faith alone, the importance of scripture and the priesthood of all believers. He was musical and told people to sing in their own language. From the nailing of the thesis

---

[33] *Like a Virgin: How Science is Redesigning the Rules of Sex.*

to the door of the church from 1517 to 1522 he published 60 pamphlets and became the most published author in the world.

Though it is a sweeping statement, and a generalisation that does not apply to all, it may yet be said that there is little in Catholicism that makes people high. It is controlling and is largely driven by guilt and, in some instances, paranoia - the belief-system tends to make people manic, and paranoia may accompany this mania. Catholicism uses fear and guilt as part of its controlling procedures, the fear of the Devil and Hell. But religion cannot manifest itself independently of other cultural inputs. Thus Presbyterianism in Northern Ireland reflects the siege mentality of the Protestant community there, and differs hugely from the more enlightened brand of Presbyterianism, Methodism, Evangelical, Protestant mania found in distant cousins in the confident, more liberal USA. The Muslims of Bosnia were, at least until the genocide campaign against them in the 1990s, liberal, enlightened, and non-fundamentalist, unlike those in, say, Iran or Afghanistan.

Catholicism includes as part of its cultural input belief in the power of the Pope, and this imparts certain uniformity independent of the cultural composition of any individual Catholic community - at least much more so than would be possible in a Protestant faith. This central, reactionary control tends to make Catholicism a depressive faith. There is no manic high as in Presbyterianism whose adherents believe in predestination, or Congregationalism where hymns and chanting and rhythmic exhortation by a preacher often induces a religious ecstasy or frenzy - the ultimate religious hypomania may be the snake-handling cults of the Appalachians.

Historically, it was perceived that Catholics do not do very well in a democratic scientific culture. Though it was a Catholic country that gave modern democracy to Europe, France's revolution quickly gave way to the Terror, and the imperial hypomania of Napoleon. Ex-Catholics often gravitate toward socialism to satisfy a high intellectual non-scientific need and a crossover substitute of the universal brotherhood of the proletariat for the universal brotherhood in Christ which they have left; but Catholics historically make indifferent socialists as they do not have the scientific training and hence the scientific mind that would enable them to critically question the political legitimacy of the movement they embrace, or its leaders' credentials. Thus the Catholics of Italy adopted ex-Catholic

Mussolini's Fascism, as the Catholics of Bavaria were the first to champion National Socialism in Germany (a movement led by an Austrian Catholic).

Pius XI (1922-39) by 1937 had decided that Nazism was a greater threat to Christian society than communism. The Lateran Agreements of February 1929 recognised the Vatican State as a territory solely governed by the Pope in exchange for Italian recognition. But in 1938 Mussolini drafted anti-Jewish legislation; in response Pius XI secretly commissioned a draft encyclical opposing racism but he died the day before its publication, the same day he had planned to speak out against fascist violation of the Lateran Agreements on its tenth anniversary - 11 February 1939. Pius XII destroyed the speech and returned the encyclical and he took the initiative to improve relations with Hitler's Germany, to which he had been papal nuncio.[34]

In post-war Italy, support for the socialists and the communists was higher than in any country outside the Communist Bloc, but political stability was the worst in the Western world. Perhaps this is further evidence that Catholics do not do well in a democratic scientific culture and would prefer the tight control of their lives that both Fascism and Communism impose.

Catholicism believes more in nurture than nature, and depends on control, as one might expect of probably the last institution left in the Western world that accepts autocracy (that of the Pope). Catholic teaching denounces the contraceptive pill, condoms, the Morning-After Pill, and abortion. These procedures are accepted in most countries but condemned by the Pope. In a survey of attitudes in Boston toward condoms and abortion it was found that Catholics would have an abortion instead of, e.g., using ten condoms because they were sinning more often by repeatedly using condoms.

Traditionally, obedience to the pope meant that Catholics rejected the Enlightenment, and the subsequent shortage of scientific thought in Catholicism led to the accusation of simplicity in its approach to nature and nurture. Protestants believe in science that tends to undermine traditional belief in God and lead to a liberal democracy whereas, in post-Fascist times, Catholics tend to become socialist, a political substitute for God or organised religion.

---

[34] David Kertzer, *The Pope and Mussolini*.

Secularised Catholicism tends to lead to socialism. Europe is largely Catholic and socialist-oriented whereas the USA is predominantly Protestant and follows a liberal democracy agenda. Europeans often do not like the USA while the Irish media has an anti-US anti-Jewish agenda, perhaps a residue of its Catholic tradition.

In the North of Ireland, Protestant schools tend to emphasise science and technology whereas Catholic Church schools traditionally tended to focus on the arts, perhaps a consequence of a Classical Education having been required of their priests.

There are fewer jobs in the arts than in the scientific area. Though no one would attempt to deny the influence of political discrimination in the employment record of Northern Ireland, the Protestant artisan tradition, and the traditional Catholic leaning toward the arts may account, in part, for the differences in employment figures between the two religious communities.

Irish Catholics traditionally have been perceived as very nationalistic and the mix with socialism can be quite corrupting. The paranoid nationalist, and perhaps the paranoid socialist, requires an enemy and may murder without guilt, as happened with National Socialists and Marxist socialists; religious fervour facilitated the same in earlier centuries, with Islam being spread by the sword and the reactive Crusades.[35]

In the paranoid state hatred of the enemy is the manic high. When mixed with nationalism this is very dangerous. Eamon de Valera, famously - or infamously - nationalistic and puritan, was more responsible than any other person for the Irish Civil War and the economically devastating Trade War of the 1930s, as well as facilitating the creation of, in effect, a Catholic theocracy during most of his political lifetime. Yet perhaps the de Valera years had something of social value?

---

[35] The Irish, isolated by their monastic organisation from the diocesan European Church, took no part in the Crusades but the Oscar statue is a knight with a Crusader sword designed by an Irishman Cedric Gibbons who won 11 Oscars design.

2nd January 1921

Letter from the G.O.C. British Forces, Dublin.
SECRET & URGENT

The G.O.C. directs that the instructions with regard to no interference with De Valera be again impressed on all Officers that may be in charge of raiding parties, patrols, escorts or other parties.

Major, General Staff, Dublin Dist.

Diarmaid Ferriter UCD Professor Modern Irish History

"What their thinking is De Valera is more a moderate than the diehards who are driving for this campaign and if there's to be peace, "we need to have De Valera. "

It is said that Churchill wanted to thank De Valera for telling his men to phone the British Admiralty on a direct line when U Boats were sighted off the Irish coast. De Valera said that a thank you from Churchill would dam his support in Eire and this is why Churchill gave a speech that was against De Valera. The coast of Ireland was marked out by numbers made of stone and this helped U.K. pilots to know where they were.

    Winston Churchill
    Win- positive. Ton- weight
    Church-spiritual (left hand)
    Hill-spatial organisation (left hand)

As religious belief lessens there will be a change in culture. Within its remit, Catholicism has tended to control the mania that is latent in all our cultures. Maybe one day we will rue its demise, as this control, once lifted, makes way for increased anarchy in an increasingly hypomanic world. Was the grim, xenophobic suspicion of the de Valera years really worse than the ugly pornography and violence that increasingly is a feature of Irish life now?

Though individual priests might be reluctant to speak out against terrorism, might even actively support it, the Catholic Church provided a moderating influence on extremist movements and behaviour up until recently. But this was in a time when public - rather than private, as today - manifestation of hypomania was all but acceptable (in certain "respectable" circumstances). Now the grip of religion has declined markedly and Catholicism has taken a fearful beating over the many cases of child abuse by priests, so it lacks the moral authority it had, and is no longer the force for moderation that it was.

Richard Dawkins makes a good case for social controls being "memes," socially formed and determined and passed on through socialisation, not in the blood. But he also makes a good case for certain forms of behaviour, which we might call socially restrictive, being genetically adaptive in that subscription by the masses to these ideas better ensures the preservation of the genes of every individual. Seven of the Ten Commandments are concerned with ensuring the sort of social order in which all members may thrive; the other three are concerned with honouring the tribal god that keeps society in line. It is no accident that the Commandments were handed down after the Exodus from Egypt, where the Jews would have had to obey the laws of the Pharaohs - which would not have been very different from their own. All societies have to have regulations if they are not to collapse.

Another change in religion in Ireland is that many people who nominally profess Catholicism also accept what appear to be Protestant beliefs driven by mania and social change such as married priests, contraception, abortion, female clergy, and divorce, and same sex marriages and no belief in transubstantiation. Other social changes driven by mania and wealth in the past are one person one vote, abolition of slavery, no child labour, and feminism, NATO, EU, UN, and the International Court of Human Rights in The Hague.

It is easy to think the world is bleak, but poverty, malnutrition, illiteracy, child labour and infant mortality are falling faster than at any other time in history, argues Johan Norberg in his new book Progress: Ten Reasons to Look Forward to the Future. 11th Sept 2016. Sunday Times News Review.

A girl born 200 years ago could be taken away by tuberculosis, cholera, influenza, polio, plague, Black Death, smallpox, or measles or starvation.

We will need to distinguish between good and bad dirt. Dr. Blaser foresees an "antibiotic winter" in which we have no defences against new plagues to match the Black Death or the great flu pandemic of 1918-1919, which killed tens of millions. Covid was like the great flu. Blaser's (Missing Microbes: How the overuse of Antibiotics Is Fuelling Our Modern Plagues) belief that antibiotics are the most crucial factor in the destruction of our microbiomes is not universally shared, though no one doubts its importance. At birth 200 yrs ago she could not have expected to live longer than around 30 years, and often died in child birth.

Such changes began to manifest in the early-mid nineteenth century. Child care improved and legislation curtailed child labour and, for instance, outlawed child chimney-sweeps (who often died of testicular cancer due to soot around their testes). Soot is a carcinogenic which can cause cancer. Compulsory education saw children sent to school rather than sent down the mines - those under 10 years at first. Homes sprung up for children living rough and child prostitution was made illegal. In what may be construed as a benevolently manic way, people such as Dr Barnardo worked to make children be seen in an innocent way and in early-middle Victorian times Children, for the first time, ceased to be regarded as small adults.

The 1960s was a decade of major social reform in Europe and the USA, and one can discern a hypomanic edge to what went on. In Britain Roy Jenkins, Labour Home Secretary from 1965 to 1967, promoted reform of the divorce, homosexuality, abortion and censorship laws. He worked in the treasury and then in Europe as the President of the European Commission in the late 1970s. At the beginning of 1982, with the SDP ahead in the polls he was within touching distance of the ultimate prize, Prime Minister. But then Argentina invaded the Falklands, Thatcher won and the illusion was over. Jenkins is often cited as one of the best prime ministers Britain never had. He did not know how to change a light bulb, let alone boil an egg.[36]

AA Gill describes his - and Jenkins' - generation during the 1970s and the 1980s. Despite being past middle age by then, "we were the generation that were relentlessly for civil rights, gay rights, disability rights, human rights, equality, and fairness. We were implacably against racism and censorship.

---

[36] See *Roy Jenkins: A Well-Rounded Life* by John Campbell.

We defended freedom of speech, religion and expression. We will leave the world better fed and better off than when we arrived in it.

"Britain is a far happier, richer and fairer place than it was 60 years ago. And if you think that's wishful self- promotion, you have no idea how grim and threadbare Britain in the Fifties was. You weren't there, you don't remember."[37]

Ireland was more conservative and the change came later. Ireland has always been seen as an easy-going bucolic place, its people laid-back to the point of laziness, but this has changed radically. Irish people's belief that sex before marriage is always wrong in 1973-74 was 71 percent; by 2004-05 this was down to 6 percent. Many also do not any longer believe in Papal infallibility. Protestant services and beliefs exhibit some hypomanic qualities and, at least more so than Catholicism, attract hypomanic people - the image of Ian Paisley on full song illustrates this point - so is this tentative swelling of sympathy for Protestant ideas indicative of increasing hypomania? Every day alarm is expressed at the rise in selfishness, greed and violence in what was once a poor but sharing people.

---

[37] Quoted by AA Gill, *The Sunday Times*, 29 June 2014.

PROTESTANTISM

Catholic belief is controlling; Protestantism places more importance on individual faith and belief. Crawford Gribben's review Irish Times 25 th February 2017. The division of Western Christendom by the Reformation contributed to, or perhaps even created, the cultures of modernity: the rise of individualism, democracy, secularism and science. MARTIN LUTHER Renegade and Prophet by Lyndal Roper Sunday Times 22nd May 2016 reviewed by John Carey. Martin Luther's behaviour, in say nailing his 95 Theses up on the door of Wittenberg church in Latin the academic language of the church in1517 in public defiance, might indicate mania, or hypomania as salvation by faith alone(belief in Jesus and acceptance of sexuality as being natural and rejected celibate clergy he married a ex-nun. In January 1521 he was excommunicated by Pope Leo 10. Luther is concedes Roper a difficult hero. He was coarse, vulgar minded, bigoted and dogmatic. Anger and hatred were his commonest motives a dysphoric (irritable) mania. Mania was also reflected in his sexual disihibition. These Theses sought to discredit the Catholic Church's sale of "indulgences" which were to grant remission from periods of time in purgatory the money going to rebuilding St. Peter's Basilica in Rome. Within weeks Martin's ideas had spread by pamphlets, broadsheets and woodcuts throughout Germany, Europe, England and Scotland with religious zeal especially in Northern Europe smashing the power and unity of the Catholic Church and brought on the Protestant Reformation, with two main movements Lutheranism and the reformed tradition that began in Geneva under John Calvin. His paranoia might be reflected in his anti-Semitism He believed in free will, an outrageous idea in an autocratic age and therefore suggestive of mania, and placed Jesus, who also manifested manic qualities, above Mary, in Catholic thinking still the sympathetic, more human figure who is often asked, in various prayers, to "intercede" with her son on the supplicant's behalf. (Luther's attitude here might reflect his well-known misogyny, itself suggestive of depression/paranoia).

What we seem to be seeing now, with Catholics becoming more critical of their Church in Ireland and elsewhere - becoming "a la carte Catholics" - is a move toward Protestant-style belief: of taking responsibility for their own beliefs rather than having these dictated to them by a temporal power. The

Protestant and especially the Presbyterian Church offer the manic promise of life everlasting. In the sixteenth century Calvin in Geneva and John Knox in Scotland preached predestination and nominalism, 16th Century) the manic love of God for the chosen ones.

Presbyterianism is a manic religion but it is controlled and obsessive and cold. It did not allow graven images and smashed the stain glassed rose windows in churches. The Baptists offer joy and laughter and praise in their prayers. If Protestantism really is more hypomanic than Catholicism, than we seem to be seeing yet another aspect of how society in general is becoming hypomanic with the increase in evangelising in recent years. Africa is seeing a notable increase in this type of missionary, funding coming largely from the USA, where "televangelism" has become a huge phenomenon, generating billions from broadcast appeals by charismatic individuals like Reverend Jim Bakker.

Televangelism shows how the modern media can be used to exacerbate an already arguably-manic phenomenon. Believers can be "saved by Jesus" by putting their hands on the television screen. Preachers like Bakker become fabulously wealthy from donations extorted, one could say in one case, by the preacher tearfully telling his audience that Jesus will "call him home" if so much money is not given by such a date. Those who subscribe to such chicanery are as manic as the conmen, if in a different way.

Bakker - and others - have also used their charisma to their advantage in other ways. Bakker infamously was exposed as a philanderer, using his "God-given" authority to seduce star-struck women. (Perhaps significantly, Bakker is first cousin to another hypomanic, hyper-sexualised charmer, Jerry Lee Lewis, who bought him his first car in which to "spread the word" before the age of televangelism.)

Are Messianic delusions (thinking that one is Jesus, or that someone else, like Bakker, has messianic power) and the Ten Commandments hot wired into the brain? The Messianic delusion is common in manic depression and in people found G.B.I. (Guilty but Insane) of violent crimes (nowadays Not Guilty by reason of Insanity). In the Central Mental Hospital, out of 20 such murderers, approximately eight have had this delusion.

Jesus was an archetypal manic-depressive in his message of universal love and his belief that he was the literal Son of God, and his delusional teachings suited the new Christian religions. Jesus had a unique selling point: resurrection in love; he was the original thinker of the liberal utopia. "Love your neighbour as yourself."

The suggestion might be that not the delusion itself, but the capacity for the delusion, may be hard-wired, and is made manifest under the paranoid position. But if this is so, why would such a delusional capacity be hard-wired - i.e. adaptively selected for in nature? Maybe to be sacrificed as found in the royal bog bodies - *Eucharist* originally mean a feast to make such self-sacrifice, sometimes a cannibalistic one, something that finds echo in the Catholic belief that the Eucharist is literally the body and blood of Christ. Perhaps it is related to the sort of blind unquenchable faith in oneself that made millionaires of the likes of J.P. Morgan. As long as one's mental processes remain "normal," the capacity remains adaptive; in the event of breakdown its potential to exacerbate the delusional perspective may lead to tragedy i.e. killing a family member or loved one of whom the sufferer develops a paranoid belief that the other is the devil or some such enemy.

Protestanism in the USA would lead to the United States Declaration of Independence in 1776. Overtime, it would even influence the 1948 UN Declaration of Human Rights.

Capitalist belief in greed, and the concomitant fear that may be subtly encouraged in order to safeguard one's possessions, is associated in particular, nowadays, with the USA. This is not as predominantly Protestant as it was, but the Protestant ideas that made it materially great are still largely embedded there. Max Weber, a German in the early 1900s, coined the term "The Protestant Work Ethic", after visiting the St. Louis exhibition in 1904 and said it was the driving force behind north European and American prosperity. Capitalism certainly is likely to lead to material prosperity, even in Lutheran Germany today and the Puritan tenet that the Elect of God were favoured materially on earth would have tended to make the accumulation of wealth respectable and indeed virtuous. Weber argued that the growth of capitalism was helped by particular Protestant values. Ireland had little involvement in the Reformation and no part in the Renaissance or the Industrial Revolution and stood out as a sole Catholic Celtic country in

Northern Europe. Furthermore, Antinomian belief, popular in Puritan New England, held that moral law was not binding on Christians (a development of the doctrine of Holy Lying, subscribed to by, among others, Martin Luther). Perhaps this is a manifestation of the manic archetype Charisma, with its associated messianic delusion. Antinomian ideas may be discerned in America's vision of itself as not merely the City on a Hill but the self-appointed policeman, judge and jury of the world. One does not have to be anti-American to see Antinomianism in President Bush's rejection of the Kyoto Accord and his proposals to drill for oil in virgin Alaska wilderness, or to perceive messianic delusion in his invasions of Afghanistan and Iraq. Whether he was guilty of "holy lying" in claiming that there were weapons of mass-destruction in Iraq is still unclear, but his predecessor, Johnson, seems to have had no crisis of conscience in inventing the Gulf of Tonkin Incident to justify invasion of Vietnam.

Since September 11, 2001 paranoia has been added to the national mixture. Paranoia can be elicited in most individuals of all cultures, and may lead to the kill-without-guilt syndrome, developed to its - so far - climactic horror by the Nazis and Isis. Like Charisma, Paranoia is a basic manic archetype. With Christians' sense of a loving god there is also the paranoia of doing something to offend this god who, though loving, is also jealous and capable of impressive feats of wrath. But traditionally it has been possible to project this wrongdoing: onto the devil. The new god of the increasingly godless West is not one to be feared but one who loves, understands, forgives; a more manic Liberal Protestant god. Yet this manic god is possibly obsessive and paranoid as well, and the superimposition of this more complex god onto the wrathful, vengeful, terrible god of the Old Testament is often along a discordant boundary. (Heavy Metal music) The dissonance produced may invoke further hypomanic attempts by the new believers at rationalisation. The manic aspects of religious belief, as seen at, say, Baptist meetings, are shown by singing, dancing, chanting, preaching, witnessing and by believers' joyful faith that they are chosen ones (pop music); yet these aspects of celebration are embedded in an Old Testament matrix of paranoid fear.

Rationalisation must form a large part of any believer's psychological makeup. Broadly speaking, we may say that, like creativity and pattern-perception, faith is a right-brain (left hand) activity, rationality a function of the left-brain (right hand). Over the centuries science has explained, rationally, what used to be explicable only by religion. The consequence has been a severe curtailment of the domain of religion, and the rise of science as a virtual religion itself. Reflected in Right Brain, Left Hand Faith; rise of Left Brain, Right Hand and Science; Seeking Truth (analysis), another manic archetype, may now be a far more complex and stressful activity, given this other sort of dissonance: the inconsistency between, say, the Genesis account of creation and evolution. Astonishingly, over half the people in the USA still believe, literally, in the Genesis account.

Here we see an apparent contradiction: the Protestant mindset traditionally holds with rationalism and personal responsibility, yet the Protestant USA rejects rational explanations, the more fundamentalist warning, "Watch your intellect, lest it deceive you and lose you your soul."

One of the foremost members of a minority church on this island was poet and Church of Ireland member (Protestant) WB Yeats. On 11 June 1925 Yeats attacked the direction the new State was taking in a speech in the Senate. The new Cumann na nGaedheal (forerunner of Fine Gael) government was attempting to ban divorce, then allowed under the new Free State constitution. Yeats lost his virginity at thirty but made up for it in later life. He consummated his relationship with Maude Gonne on a few occasions and asked both her and her daughter Iseult to marry him. When he was 50 he married George, aged 23, who was into Automatic Writing and he got ideas from her. He had affairs in his sixties and famously had a vasectomy - a "monkey glands" operation - to improve his libido.

Yeats said *"I think it is tragic that within three years of this country gaining its independence in 1922 we should be discussing a measure which a minority of this nation considers to be grossly oppressive.*

"I am proud to consider myself a typical man of the minority. We against whom you have done this thing are no petty people. We are one of the great stocks of Europe.

"We are the people of Burke; we are the people of Grattan; we are the people of Swift, the people of Emmet, the people of Parnell. We have created the most of the modern literature of this country. We have created the best of its political intelligence."

In earlier centuries we also had Goldsmith, Sheridan, Farquhar, Berkeley and Sterne. In pre-1960 we had Shaw, O'Casey, Beckett, Wilde, Joyce and Synge.

Despite Yeats' best efforts, divorce was banned in 1924 as was the selling of artificial means of contraception. In 1937 a new Constitution recognised the special position of the Catholic Church as the denomination of the majority of the Irish people. It too banned divorce. In 1944 the Archbishop of Dublin John Charles McQuaid reinforced the 1875 ban on Catholics attending Trinity College Dublin under pain of excommunication. In 1970 this ban on Catholics attending where Beckett had studied and taught, was lifted by Archbishop McQuaid.

In 1992 a referendum amended the Constitution to specify that the prohibition of abortion would not limit freedom of travel into and out of the state or the right to distribute information about abortion services in foreign countries. In 1996 the ban on divorce was removed from the Constitution. In 2010 it emerged that in 1975 the Catholic primate Cardinal Sean Brady swore to secrecy two young people abused by Fr Brendan Smyth who had been abusing children since 1965 for years that was covered up.[38]

FUNDAMENTALISM

Several centuries before the Reformation a radically different meme had emerged: a new religion, Islam. Christian fundamentalists and Muslim fundamentalists share a paranoid dislike of alcohol, make-up, sexy dressing (Muslim fundamentalist women have veils), sexuality as expressed in rock 'n roll and other western modes of expressions. Both Christian and Muslim fundamentalists believe in heaven and that they are the chosen people and they do not believe in evolution. Both are very emotional about their beliefs. The Koran draws on its inspiration from the Judaic teachings and shows that Christian and Muslim fundamentalists share a good deal of common belief. Muslims detest alcohol and in the Protestant USA most states have over-21 drinking laws. Some Southern counties are dry and some do not allow cold beer to be sold.

---

[38] The *Irish Times*, 22 July 2011.

All fundamentalists too often lean toward hypomanic self-belief, which can turn to paranoid hatred of other people. Their obsessive quality needs direction and "a clean way of living" if their obsessiveness is to be channelled constructively: control of the psychotic position by obsessive action (super ego) over the paranoid (id) may prevent emergence of this hatred. Tragically, in Islam honour killings would seem to indicate the triumph of the id.

Can Liberal Capitalism survive without a manic leader like JFK (amphetamines), Clinton (sexual indiscretions) and Bush (a heavy drinker until he started out in politics. This trait can be seen in his nieces who have got into trouble over drink).

Differences in Protestant and Catholic can be seen in the way they support their football teams. The Protestant Swiss sit quietly in their seats and ignore the camera whereas the Catholic South Americans supporters are very emotional and vocal; they stand and dance and wave their flags. Protestants for some reason seem to fear individual emotional expression even though this is contradicted by someone like Van Morrison and Baptists.

Right now America seems to be on the cusp of a conservative wave that began to swell with Reagan. But the ambivalence and pragmatism that Americans have toward their leaders is illustrated by the sexual peccadilloes of Clinton which were forgiven with the famous expression that "It's the economy, stupid!" that's the important matter, yet implacably condemned by fundamentalists, who did their best, throughout Clinton's two terms, to bring him down. George W Bush, a Christian fundamentalist from the Bible belt, who nevertheless was a heavy drinker until he started out in politics, was very quickly forgiven this sin once he begged forgiveness. (Bush's history is reflected in the position of the dry alcoholic who sees things in black and white terms: his ultimatum in the aftermath of September 11, those not "with him" were "against him," illustrates this.

Perhaps a clue to voters' positions may be found in the Christian fundamentalist meme. There is something extremely puzzling for any outsider in what seems to be downright dishonesty at a certain level here. Bush won the presidential election in very unusual circumstances, whole sections of the electorate in Florida - of which his brother, Jeb, was governor - being disenfranchised, and clearly losing the popular vote. He is clearly not a very intelligent person, and it can seem terrifying that he was the most powerful individual in the world. Yet Americans, at least until recent reversals in Iraq, are not too worried about all this. It seems that as long as one believes unquestioningly in the bible as the literal word of God one can be forgiven anything else; certainly some fundamentalists at least subscribe to the doctrine of Holy Lying, and they would rather have one of their own in power, even under undemocratic circumstances, than a liberal. Also, traditional American suspicion of intellectualism would play to Bush's favour.

Is fundamentalism, therefore, another manifestation of hypomania? The rise in fundamentalism, political and religious, can be traced to the 1980s and two individuals who dominated that decade: Margaret Thatcher and Ronald Reagan. It was in part a response to the austerity that followed on the oil crises of the 1970s, mass unemployment and stagflation, 25 percent interest rate, top rate of tax of 98 percent in part, perhaps, a reaction against the - equally hypomanic - spirit of the Sixties.

The two leaders of the movement, however, clearly exhibited hypomanic qualities. Reagan was the only man who believed that it was possible to actually beat the Soviet bloc, and was prepared to risk Mutually Assured Destruction to do so. A devout Protestant, he nevertheless consulted horoscopes and may have been influenced by them in his decision making. Thatcher was a latter-day Boadicea who went to war to cover up a major security lapse, and who slept four hours a night or less, such was her energy level. Both, however, seem to have had the ability to bypass their rationalisation process and go with their convictions: hatred of Communism and faith, not so much in God, as in God being on their side.

Conservative Americans are absorbed by their perception of America as a biblical Promised Land and by their own sense of destiny. They salute the flag every morning as Muslims pray to Mecca. Three-quarters believe in Revelations and half do not believe in evolution, and perhaps a quarter of those in the southern states believe that Jesus will come back in their lifetime. There still prevails (with them) the nineteenth-century idea of Manifest Destiny. These fundamentalist Christians may make Americans susceptible to emotional and intellectual manipulation by politicians and the media by stimulation of the manic archetypes.

Why are these factors so? It would appear that the education of Americans in general is not very good and lacks emphasis on the scientific method. But this really is no answer, merely a restating of the question. Some psychologists (Hans Eysenck most notoriously, in his treatment of McNamara's paper on Irish measured IQ levels), have argued that America was the recipient of the genetic heritage of the most adventurous, brilliant and energetic blood of the Old World; and determinist theorisers aside, there is no evidence that Americans are statistically more stupid than other people, merely less well educated than people in some countries. Even in this regard, though quality ranges from the awful to the excellent, American universities do try to ensure a broad-based education in Freshman year, to make up for any shortcomings in their students' schooling - Composition 101, a foundation requirement, is as much about clear thinking as good writing.

Yet there persists a worrisome dichotomy even in science and technology schools: graduates remember the scientific principles that will enable them to pass exams and go on to make careers and money, but they seem to reject taking on board *scientific thinking*: up to a quarter of Americans with a higher degree believe in the literal truth of the bible. Is there a meme key to this phenomenon?

Consider American self-perception. Cocaine and the American dream are pervasive in the states. Life starts at 60. The dream is never lost. We're the best. Yet the great American archetype is the pioneer, the self-reliant, hands-on determiner of his own life and his own fate. This archetype was described "scientifically" by Frederick Jackson Turner in his 1893 treatise *The Frontier in American History*; in art it was portrayed by Frederic Remington and Charlie Russell, in literature by Owen Wiston (*The Virginian*) and Stephen Vincent Bénet ("The Ballad of William Sycamore"), among many others.

The extreme manifestation of this archetype is the cowboy, a frequent subject for Remington and Russell in particular, personified on the screen by John Wayne. In the classic American morality tale the hero stands alone against a plethora of enemies and shoots them down, sometimes at great personal sacrifice, as in Jack Schaeffer's eponymous *Shane*. Traditionally the bad guys have been the big ranchers, the good guys the homesteaders, but among these enemies are not the more insidious evil that is personified by wily bankers and businessmen, and educated Eastern dudes who despise the uneducated cowboy and his rough nobility. In the classic tale, of course, the good guy wins, and usually material wealth, or at least success, is his reward - along with the girl, of course, so he can spread his genes and his memes. He learns from his experience, and greater knowledge or even wisdom is an additional reward. But his essential nature remains unspoiled.

Even when this classic tale is wrenched to prove a subtler, even vaguely subversive point, as in *High Noon*, or *The Man Who Shot Liberty Valence*, the hero never becomes in any way intellectual. Gary Cooper rides off, rejecting the cheap adulation of the townsfolk, his only reward the love of a good woman for a good man. The real hero of Liberty Valence is not the James Stewart character, who goes on to political and financial reward, but John Wayne, who stays behind, despised by newcomers to the town, increasingly forgotten and ignored, until he dies a pauper. In *Heaven's Gate* corruption extends as far as government, but the "good" guys are grimy, illiterate East Europeans, perforce rustlers and prostitutes in a desperate hard land.

There is a huge irony in the notion that the frontier still is perceived as the defining American experience, 120 years after Frederick Jackson Turner presented his historic paper to a convention in Chicago, ironic because the reality of the frontier was almost the opposite of popular perception. The American West was always primarily an urban, not a rural, place. Though cattle-ranching was important, mining was far more so, and employed far more than did ranching - mostly those whose dream of getting rich had failed, for hard-rock mining was highly technological, and very, very few got rich with a shovel and pan off placer deposits. Though the pioneer was an icon of the West, even in his own time, he was also the victim of unscrupulous entrepreneurs, who foisted on him everything from the promise of paradise in a dusty back-of-beyond shack, to the absurd "scientific proof" that dry-farming methods actually change the climate - "rain follows the plough." In the classic American tale, the West was the place where everyone's dreams came true; in fact, it was predominantly a place of failure, where only the very strongest and most unscrupulous and ruthless survived, on the broken dreams and backs of others.

The appearance of the Dust Bowls in the 1930s was physical proof of failure of the dream and the lies. But that failure came barely a generation after one of the richest ecosystems in the world had been broken down by the very American Dream itself. For millennia the Great Plains had supported an impressively rich biodiversity in what was really a marginal zone. Rainfall was low, yet there was a deceptively fertile cover of native grasses, buffalo, gramma and bluestem, on which lived at least 20 million bison - "buffalo" - a keystone species that kept the entire ecosystem in good health for over ten millennia.

In this instance we see how the American Dream became a self-perpetuating myth that suborned everything from Christian well-wishers to professional scientists in order to serve its own interests. Driving everything, in this, the Gilded Age, was money and America's new/old god, Mammon, in a hypomanic rush to create a new kingdom of prosperity on earth. The wealth of the North American continent, even after centuries of exploitation, immeasurable, and the capitalists who followed Appomattox wanted all of it. If the Great Plains could support such life, why not replace the wild buffalo with the "spotted cattle" as General Phil Sheridan put it?

Getting rid of the buffalo, besides, would force "wild Indians" onto reservations or else starve them to death. With the Indians gone, the land could be settled by white people. The new railroad companies were persuaded to join the hypomanic dream by offering them land on each side of the tracks which they could sell to would-be settlers. Though land farther away from the tracks could be had for claiming title and making some minimum improvements, under the Homestead Act, the railroads would find buyers because proximity to the tracks added better access to markets and thereby commercial value to any land. Meanwhile, they could make money shipping back east the hides of the slaughtered buffalo for curing by the expanding Industrial Revolution, and selling the finished products - mostly for upholstery, military webbing and machinery drive-belts - to further Gild the Age.

Meanwhile, the railroad companies had to sell their land allocation, so they targeted potential immigrants in Europe. Here was cheap land and easy access to the American Dream! they proclaimed. Objections that the land was too dry to support farming were met by quasi-scientific gibberish: "Rain follows the plough", a restatement of the adage that God helps those who help themselves, for more sophisticated, sceptical folk of the nineteenth century. Those sceptics who turned hypomanic discovered the claim to be true - for a while. Rainfall actually did increase for more than a decade, but after 1910 it reverted to its post-Atlantean mean of 10-20 inches.

Crops failed so the pet scientists were wound up and rolled out again with "dry-farming" advice. A fine tilth given to soil by repeated ploughing and harrowing did indeed absorb more of the dew and such scarce rain as did fall. But it also left the land in danger from wind erosion when the rain did not fall. Besides, breaking the virgin sod also broke the established ecosystem which saw the deep-rooted native grasses both hold the soil together and pull up nutrients and water from deep down. Ultimately, "… you can't grow any grain if you ain't got any rain", the consequences for thousands of poor dirt farmers being the utter loss of their livelihoods and lives' work: "My Oklahome Home it blowed away".[39] Whole families packed everything into old Tin Lizzies and set out for a precarious and uncertain new life as fruit pickers and canning factory operative in California; three thousand miles away the skies of the Atlantic seaboard were darkened by the dust of the Great Plains.

The consequence of all these failures and disappointments is that rural Americans have good reason to suspect scientists' promises. In the 1980s, when the Popper husband and wife team proposed regenerating the Dust Bowl and returning traditional fertility to the Great Plains by creating a "Buffalo Commons", they received death threats.[40] The point is almost less that the American dream is false as that the American archetype is never intellectual, and that Americans at best distrust a paranoia, and at worst despise, intellectualism - however their civilisation is founded on wealth that is produced by, at some point in the conversion of ore to dollars, intellectual effort.

Perhaps this is a necessary deception: having accepted the myth for so long, to accept the fact now might be to fatally shake national confidence and self-

---

[39] Cis Cunningham, "My Oklahoma Home"; see Bruce Springsteen, *The Seeger Sessions*.
[40] A proposal for a Federal reserve of over 100 contiguous counties extending from Texas to Montana, across which the buffalo could migrate in accordance with their instincts, with culverts for animal traffic.

belief. So Americans persist in their dream, and their archetypes remain unchallenged. John Wayne believed in the bible, not in Darwin. He believed in American democracy - but if slopes and dinks threaten actual Americans, and their concept of democracy, nuke 'em! Bomb 'em into accepting democracy, or else back to the Stone Age. Examination of the complexities of freedom is an intellectual exercise and not to be contemplated. As one who clearly buys into the American archetype and the John Wayne myth, George W Bush unambiguously expressed it: the rest of the world is either with us or against us. Such an electorate is unlikely to question too deeply whether the Gulf of Tonkin incident was staged, or whether Sadam really was involved with Al Qaeda.

This national anti-intellectualism is in marked contrast to the Old World, where heroes include musicians, philosophers, writers and artists - hypomanic manifestations of a different sort. Ireland, a thousand years after the monastic age, still prides itself on being the Island of Saints and Scholars. An English mechanic, though he might never have read a word of the Bard, takes pride in the fact that Shakespeare was an Englishman. A German Nazi might have prided himself on killing the enemies of the state, but his eye might moisten at the strains of Wagner or Beethoven. Though Thomas Jefferson was an educated and cultured man, as an American icon he is best remembered for his Louisiana Purchase, and for sponsoring Lewis and Clarke's great expedition through the new American wilderness - as a quaint sort of frontiersman.

Whatever truth there ever was in the myth, it's all but hilarious nowadays to try to see a connection between Daniel Boone, Mike Fink, Davy Crockett, Jim Bowie, Wyatt Earp and Wild Bill Hickok on the one hand, and on the other the sort of hopeless fatties who binge in front of wide screen TVs all day long, venturing outdoors into the dangerous shopping malls only to stock up on soft drinks, chips and candy. The fatties may be very different from the Hickoks and the Earps, yet in this regard they are a hypomanic manifestation too. A truculent distrust of the rest of the world, to the point of paranoia, provides the connection.

Yet "trailer trash" fatties and "slackers" are inheritors of the American meme, too. The long-since noble cowboy was despised in his heyday as a looser, and today we have Beck's song "I'm a looser babe so why don't you kill me." Violence and poor image is now found in the trailer-park rather than the bunkhouse. Eminem, a famous white working class hero rapper, comes from a broken trailer park home - real name Marshall Mathers. Another working class coloured rapper is Jay-Z, a multi-millionaire a friend of his Notorius who was shot dead in New York. Another two rapper's Dr. Dre and Snoop Doggs friend Tupac was shot dead in Los Angele's. Snoop was a pimp had misogynist lyrics and was tried for murder when his bodyguard shot someone from a car Snoop was driving. He was acquitted from murder. Radiohead's singer Tom York sings "I wish I was special but I'm a creep". As the cowboy was likely to cheer Roosevelt's Rough Riders up San Juan Hill, so today's rappers are far more likely than not to cheer George Bush's gung-ho escapades across the world.

Perhaps in all this we can find the key to American fundamentalism - or at least for the scale of fundamentalism in America. (For the phenomenon is also found in Britain, Australia and elsewhere - certainly in Northern Ireland - just not so widespread.) If the American myth, the American archetype, the American Dream, is so at odds with the historic and current reality, then swallowing a lie may have become, at a very deep level, all but a patriotic duty. Factor in the unpalatable truth that the myth was founded on the literal genocide of native peoples makes the lie even more attractive - all but necessary to swallow for the patient's health. Finally, underpin this complex psychological mess with the tradition of Holy Lying, and one may approach understanding of the fundamentalist meme.

The keystone of the whole meme-arch is religious faith: the belief that God created the world according to the Genesis account, literally, 6,000-10,000 years ago. This belief is so at odds with all the evidence that it seems a joke that any even half-educated person, far less one with an advanced degree, could believe it. But fundamentalists have a perpetual get-out-of-jail card: anything is possible to God, and the "evidence" that things are other than they really are (in their eyes), is proof of the wiles of the devil, and therefore additional evidence that the bible is right. Perhaps subtly encouraged by a national myth that flies in the face of historical fact, they are able to really believe what they say; and because they "know" that what they are saying is the "real" truth, they feel certain that anything they do to advance their cause cannot be wrong in the eyes of God - hence the validation of Holy Lying.

This discordance with scientific evidence would be merely absurd were it not for the power that these people wield. One of them, George W Bush, has the power to literally destroy the world.

The doctrine of Holy Lying, in the cause of God, goes back at least to Pope Eusebius of the fourth century, and was championed by Martin Luther and other Protestant figures of the Reformation. In the same way that others of us might feel justified in using a "White Lie" to protect a child from getting harmed, if the truth was beyond his intellectual capacity to understand, some fundamentalists might feel justified in telling Holy Lies to bring the rest of us to see God's true path for us - once on this path, i.e. "saved," we will not only understand the necessity for this lie but be grateful for its delivering us from Satan. But while White Lies may be, to a point okay, telling them tends to make one colour-blind.

That some of these people absolutely do coldly tell lies is illustrated by the case of Duane Gish, of the Scientific Creationist movement. On his lecture tours Gish was in the habit of quoting a Canadian anthropologist, Sir Solly Zuckerman, to "prove" that the remains of the anthropoid, Lucy, were not humanoid, and thereby to strike against evolution. Some years ago Gish was challenged from the audience by a co-worker of Zuckerman, who conclusively proved that what Gish was saying was wrong. After a heated argument and with ill grace, Gish withdrew his point - but the very next night, on the next stage of his lecture tour, he was making that point again. He knew now, if not before, that it was not correct, so unambiguously he was lying; but presumably his thinking was that the seriousness of his case, the overall truth of his message, excused the departure from strict truth.

The very term "Scientific Creationism" is an oxymoron - a contradiction in terms - because the scientific method implies, and indeed demands, both testability and the possibility of being refuted by experimentation; "scientific" always implies "provisional" truth. Creation clearly must have been a one-off event, is utterly beyond testability, and its truth is so compelling that it is blasphemous to even question it. Perhaps the adoption of the adjective *scientific* shows how fundamentalists are quite prepared to press-gang anything that will confer perceived respectability on their cause, without feeling bound to the truth of what *scientific* means. Given this fundamentalist meme, what would happen if turmoil in the Middle East spins into international war there, with severe recession in the US due to the potentially high cost of oil as a result? The conservative religious right might come to the fore as people turned to religion to compensate for the financial and psychological setback. A leader who then said that Americans were the best/special/nationistic in the world would find his words strike a chord in the national psyche, evoking the national archetype as Hitler did in Germany, and tapping into American hypomania. He then well might come to power at the head of a metaphorical Seventh Cavalry and be able to manipulate the already hypomanic state found in the US.

Pre-Trump era

Generally the positive consumer index in the USA ignores the lack of real education - by international standards; though every once in a while an article such as "Why Johnny can't read" stirs unease - and relatively low GNP with high borrowings. Because of this positivism and national self-confidence people are blind to the large deficit (trillions) that exists in the USA economy, to which must now be added a further billion a week maintaining US presence in Iraq. With this sort of positivism a paranoid position can develop if the US itself is challenged, or even its values questioned. Such a paranoid position makes other people the enemy and provokes negative expression of the id. Their own country consumes Americans and few travel and know much about Europe or other parts of the world.

Due to 9/11 a lot of shrilly defensive nationalism already has come out in America, people being prepared to do whatever was necessary to protect their country. A lot of basic human rights were ignored and Muslims who were suspects were arrested and imprisoned without trial. Some people talked about the civil rights of these people but nationalist paranoia prevailed.

Again, we can account for this in terms of memes. Though imperialism is associated with the "decadent" Old World, nowhere was its evil better manifested than in the USA, which expanded at the expense of the Native Americans right up to the end of the frontier in 1890. Every single treaty ever made by the USA with native peoples was broken, the last in 1966 - ironically one of the first, and signed by none less than George Washington. The perception that governed such behaviour was that the native peoples, not being either Christian or white, were really not quite human. This belief was not confined to Americans, of course; it was used to justify slavery, sport-shooting of San Bushmen, the extermination of native Tasmanians, and other atrocities; but it was in America that it attained its greatest single congregation of believers. Genocide came to be seen as not merely a pragmatic necessity to realisation of the American Dream, to attainment of the Promised Land, but something that was blessed by science - rather the new, chilling pseudo-sciences of phrenology, eugenics and Social Darwinism - and even by the Old Testament. No longer respectable to acknowledge, this meme nevertheless survives, at none too deep a level in the American psyche - though also, and in an even more violent, fanatical fashion, and under different expression, in rival movements, notably Isis. Clearly Arabs now fill the diabolical role formerly allocated to the Native Americans.

Add to the national meme national hypomania. Generally, the positive consumer index (a reflection of the underlying cultural hypomania) in the USA ignores the lack of development and low GNP with high borrowings. Because of this positivism people are blind to the large deficit (32 Trillions) that exists in the USA economy and spend blithely, consumption in itself being a significant factor in the American economy.

But there is also a feedback loop at work: positivism generates hypomanic consumption, which increases positivism, which increases hypomania. For example, bright colours make people happy and when they are happy they spend more and this leads to them spending even more. Conor Pope Irish Times 18 May 2015, but hypomania may lead to a paranoid position that makes other people - Arabs, right now - the enemy if they threaten the source of the consumption - oil in this case. Consequent expression of the id may lead to war, as it has already in the case of Iraq.

Some people would say that American culture is probably the most hypomanic in the West and also dominates the West, from *Robocop* to *Friends*. Money is God in the USA. You can buy your way into the White House, if you can't act it. Yet is money bad? Some people say money is the root of all evil, but the saying is that the "love of money is the root of all evil." You may be rich and not love money and on the other hand you may be poor and love money and this may lead to robbery, fraud and distress.

For all the danger posed by hypomanic consumerism, maybe the fact that money is their God protects Americans from extreme fundamentalist Christians. Maybe money is the best God. Hollywood, which may have created the Western myth with *My Darling Clementine*, has become the modern day frontier of creativity in music, film and money. Some people say that Hollywood makes films for teenagers and that Europeans make film for adults i.e. culture and art. If the fundamentalists ever did get into real power - as opposed to "mere" political power - they would shut down Hollywood (as well as every university press and most museums in the country). The real moguls, the money moguls, would never allow this to happen.

THE "MODERATES"

Even traditional religion may have hypomanic input. Though there is little core difference between e.g. Catholics and Protestant, and even similarities between the beliefs of Muslims, Jews and Christians, these small differences are the focuses of great cultural conflict. In Ireland some say the differences are tribal, disguised as religious. Catholicism and Protestantism are almost the same theologically but they reflect different emotional backgrounds. Like all religions, they reflect emotional attachments, not intellectual ones. They incorporate attachments to parental, communal and peer groups, and perhaps most important of all, to tradition. Tribal attachment is emotional and beyond intellectual consideration; but the tribal attachment can itself be considered intellectually.

It would seem that, in Ireland at least, Protestants would appear to tend toward mania and Catholics toward depression. Catholics fear God and are depressive; Protestants love God and are manic - an oversimplification, certainly, but one that illustrates different and deeply-seated emotional states.

However, with the elevated mood of mania comes paranoia, with suspicion and fear of the perceived threat from the other culture and the development of an inward-looking tribal culture. The Protestant fear of being sequestered into a Catholic Irish state, whether real or otherwise, dominates their thought, ever since the early seventeenth century when dissenting Presbyterians, who had already suffered religious discrimination, went from Scotland to Ulster, with royal endorsement, after the Tudor wars had broken the power of the

Gael and the Old English. Massacres in the rebellion of 1641, when the displaced native Irish tried to reclaim their land, instilled a cultural fear of Catholics that might be described as manic in many cases. Reciprocally, Catholics feared and hated these tribal invaders. It is interesting to speculate to what extent tribal defiance was the reason why Ireland, almost uniquely in Northern Europe, remained staunchly Catholic and Celtic in the path of St. Patrick.

How religious control of wider affairs can feed into the tribal conflict was shown by the Ne Temere papal decree of 1908, a Roman Catholic Church law that said that when a Roman Catholic married a Protestant the Roman Catholic partner would swear an oath to bring the children up Roman Catholic. In 1920 there were 250,000 Protestants in the Free State and in 1990 there were only 90,000. The increase by 2002 to 115,000 was probably due in large part to immigration. A population normally doubles in 50 years so in theory there should now be 500,000 Protestants, and the decline of the Protestant population of the Republic is part of the basis of the Northern Protestant tribal paranoia. Since the Home Rule campaign of the nineteenth century, Ulster Protestants have looked on a United Ireland as a Catholic State, in which they feel that their belief system would cease to exist over time. But the fact the much of the decline was due to migration out of the "Catholic South" shows how tribal prophecies can be made self-fulfilling, thereby reinforcing tribal myths.

We may, indeed, consider religion itself as a hypomanic phenomenon. Broadly, religion is an organised system of interaction between humanity and spiritual powers, though no single definition will suffice to encompass the varied sects of tradition, practise, and ideas, which constitute different religions. Some religions involve the belief in and worship of a God or Gods, but this is not true of all, e.g. Buddhism. Some writers argue that Marxism is in important respects a religion, with the state or even the proletariat ideal as God.

It clearly would not be accurate to regard such a ubiquitous phenomenon as hypomanic in itself, but there are hypomanic aspects to religion, and the practise can evoke hypomania in its practitioners. Ian Paisley's high-profile performances have been alluded to already as a striking example, but even praying for divine intervention may be hypomanic in its expectation that an all-powerful deity would, to all intents and purposes - and to paraphrase Ambrose Bierce - set aside the laws of the universe to gratify an avowedly unworthy importunate. The near-epidemic of moving statues in Ireland in the 1980s testifies to the power of mass delusion and hysteria.

Protestants believe in the authority of the scriptures, justification by faith alone, and the priesthood of all believers, but the authority they claim to be divine comes through an unknown number of human agents: the anonymous writers of the books of the Old Testament; the evangelists and apostles of the New; but also the various early church fathers who selected the four evangelist gospels from the eighty-odd Gnostic gospels as being, unlike the others, inspired by God. Extreme fundamentalists, challenged to say whether God meant, say "Peace on earth, good will to all men," or "Peace on earth to all men of good will" - each an equally valid translation from the Greek, but with vast if subtle differences in meaning - refer the questioner to the King James version as always correct, therefore including seventeenth century Anglican churchmen, and the lay-polymath, Sir Francis Bacon, in the long chain of human agents inspired by God.

While one must always respect people's religious views, it remains legitimate to ask how they can allow themselves to unquestioningly overlook such logical conundrums, not the least being how God could entrust an eternal and enduring message to humanity through the medium of human language, which changes not merely in translation, but over time. One can ask even more legitimately how they can kill each other in the name of a God of love, and indeed invoke God's blessing on the slaughter.

Yet surely there must be something adaptive in religion; otherwise it must have resulted in extinction of believers. There may be something in the statement: if God did not exist, man would have had to invent him. Perhaps hypomanic men did?

If life is to have real substance, if it is to lead to something worthwhile—be that merely the passing on of our genes successfully—it has to offer more than endless and aimless pursuit of luxuries and indulgences. The fact that Americans, the wealthiest people in the history of the world, have ongoing relationships with their psychotherapists that have become a standing joke, might support this old idea. Civilisation means more than mere freedom;

without discipline, freedom degenerates into chaos, which destroys freedom. As Alexander Pope wrote, "Order is Heaven's First Law". Freedom must operate within framework institutions that demand obedience, or at least within a culture that encourages obedience.

Through the twentieth century the West went from a society in which all were conscious of their duty to one in which most seem narrowly focused on their "rights," one in which "society" must be held responsible even for personal carelessness. Crazy claims for compensation when such carelessness leads to loss or injury threaten the moral, and even the financial foundations of society.

The other potential danger in Western "freedom" is that when the manifestation of this freedom - say in the form of revealing dress - offends the religious sensibilities of other cultures, it invites hostility and retribution. When this "freedom" is allied to the Western totems of Liberty, Equality and Fraternity in such a way as to make capitalist laissez faire doctrine all but sacrosanct, it creates the perfect atmosphere for twenty-first century imperialism. This Western capitalist-imperialist dream, perhaps itself in part the creation of the hypomanic mind, is driven by consumption, which in turn is driven by advertising, which is designed to engender a certain hypomanic spending pattern.

But imperialism always comes at the cost of loss of freedom to someone, and leads to resistance movements that threaten the lives of innocent parties as far away from the "colonies" as the Twin Towers. Hence this potential danger of Western "freedom": religion can no longer dictate to the "free" peoples of the West on moral duty, and their own "freedom," and their focus on their rights to the exclusion of their responsibilities, prevents these people policing their own behaviour.

Freedom in fifteenth century Bohemia ended in chaos, when the Catholic Church's burning at the stake of proto-Protestant Reverend John Huss (1369-1415) resulted in the Hussite Wars that lasted until the mid fifteenth century. This may have been a bad decision by the Church in hindsight, but the Catholic Church was well aware that freedom without authority leads to chaos, in which their own privileged position comes under threat; hence their persecution of John Wycliffe and execution of William Tyndale for translating the bible into vulgate English. Though the Reformation created a critical mass of "heretics" that proved too great to put down, centuries of pogroms, inquisitions and crusades testify to the seriousness with which the Church regarded the threat from personal freedom. Something of the same could be seen in America during the McCarthy era, and perhaps right now at Guantanamo Bay (costs approx $1billion per prisoner) and in the crackdown on illegal immigrants.

The other thing that religion provided in the past was knowledge or at least certitude. The need to know is a driving force. We seem to have been aware always that knowledge is power - hence, perhaps, human curiosity. One of the ways we add to our knowledge, the scientific method, is to formulate a hypothesis, and then test it until the test results advocate acceptance or rejection. So primitive man did with the god hypothesis. The results seemed to confirm a force outside mankind that was sometimes capricious and vindictive, and that needed to be mollified with gifts - sacrifices. But we may see how such a fearsome, powerful being was actually of enormous value in preserving the wider community, because it became something of an endorsement for co-operation - in offering obeisance and in other fields - and for charitable and self-sacrificial works. It enforced a sense of duty, and even a loss of sight, to some extent, of one's "rights." Thus we should not covet our neighbour's wife or goods because this powerful, wrathful deity might strike us dead for disobeying his will.

Really, of course, the adaptive value of not coveting our neighbour's wife or goods is preservation of social harmony, which, for social beings, whose very survival may depend on successful co-operation, is essential; but for a society without a great capacity to understand logical and philosophical niceties, the wrathful god was a good policeman. Today, with almost all of God's powers accounted for by science, which most people now accept is and perhaps ought to be amoral, the question must be asked: can religion survive in the long term and if not, how do we replace its directives and its penalties?

To the extent that keeping them is species-adaptive, and the fact that the moral code they frame is universal, the commandments are probably hot-wired in the brain, older than mankind. However, with a rise in rationality we may assume that individuals began to see the personal advantage of breaking these commandments. Successfully doing so might confer a short-term advantage to the individual and enhance his opportunities to pass on his genes; but in the long term such behaviour is maladaptive. Hence the need for rational reasons to obey our deeper instincts: a formal code, rigidly applied, and strictly enforced, i.e. religion. It is surely significant that the Ten Commandments appeared immediately after the Israelites left Egypt, and were no longer subject to Egyptian law. Any wise man that went up the mountain would have come down with the same commandments as Moses. This is for the simple reason that morality, in a general sense, is innate and species adaptive - a meme, as Richard Dawkins claims - and commandments, or laws, formulate this morality.

However, it seems reasonable to suppose that it would take a person of unusual qualities to impose these laws on a desperate rabble. Moses perhaps was not so much wise as hypomanic: he had the energy and conviction to demand of the most powerful man in the world that he "Let my people go," and then lead them, against the reservations of many, surely, into the desert. He clearly had auditory hallucinations if he heard the voice of God speaking to him from a bush - or else he was clever enough to disguise his common sense commandments in a form that would over-awe his followers into accepting them. But his hypomania may not have been entirely benevolent: if he took forty years to lead a group of people across a stretch of land maybe 200 miles wide, with no more direction needed than to keep walking into the rising sun, Moses may have been delusional rather than simply incompetent. Yet for him to hold his people together behind him, despite this, indicates a huge amount of energy and self-confidence - hypomanic qualities.

While Protestantism looks to the scriptures for answers to unanswerable questions, seeking truth for all truth seekers and promising the ultimate reward in order to maintain social control, the Catholic Church has looked instead to impose authority from above. It controls its adherents by quasi-divine fief, claiming legitimacy of divine descent from the "Petrine passage" in Matthew (16: 16-19), and becoming more and more autocratic over the centuries as accretions of secular power were added to the original sacred office. One can distinguish elements of hypomania in some of these characters from history, notably in the warrior-popes like Julius II and the Renaissance popes who built St Peter's at massive expense. Some of these popes, like the Borgias, were as decadent and ruthless as Roman emperors, but they were temporally very successful men.

MUSLIMS

Fundamentalist Muslims, like fundamentalist Christians, take their sacred scripture literally; they believe it is the word of God and they are very strict (obsessive) about following the laws. Though their Arab ancestors safeguarded classical science and literature through the European Dark Ages, nowadays Muslims are often backward in or even hostile toward science, reluctant to credit it as it undermines God, in their view. While Billy Graham, the American evangelist, had columns in newspapers, the biggest Christian magazine, radio shows, T.V. programmes and preached all over the world, fundamentalist Muslims hold that any literary discussion of the Koran is blasphemy; like fundamentalist Christians in this and other matters, they leave no room for discussion or analysis. Their religious leaders must not be questioned and may never be wrong. Even moderate Muslims have to be much disciplined, pray to Mecca four times a day, and every year observe Ramadan, a month-long fast throughout daylight hours. It is a tenet of Muslim faith to aspire to sharia law, and most moderates so aspire. This sense of discipline can be led into manic avenues, all the way to self-slaughter in the cause of Allah.

Fundamentalist Muslims have a medieval world-view that can lead to apostasy being punishable by death (notably in Saudi Arabia, criticised by bin Laden for not having a sufficiently strict Muslim legal code). Stark, simplistic belief can satisfy the unsophisticated mind, as their quite similar belief does Christian fundamentalists. Sometimes people like to be told what to do with their lives; the imposed order gives them certitude and solace, especially if they are told that they will be saved as Chosen Ones by God and go to heaven. As discussed under Christianity, the idea of being chosen by God is arguably manic, but the jihad warriors believe in addition that 72 virgins will greet them in heaven, a notion that seems bizarre at best. Very extreme and vicious forms of Islam have emerged in recent decades, notably wahabbism, and such Muslims are willing to murder or die in a suicide bomb for their God.

The rise of Muslim extremism may well be due to the certitude and solace of an imposed order in an often chaotic world, and the promise of eternal bliss after this unbearable life; but it is helped by the narcissistic nature of their beliefs and the love of their fellow men. This love, however, is restricted to fellow-Muslims, and narcissism leads to paranoia, which perceives an enemy; the paranoid partners, Israel and the USA, fill the role of heathen devil. Manic love, paradoxically, leads to the most passionate hatred. But this is something seen throughout Judeo-Christian history too, from the genocidal excesses of some of the dysphoric Old Testament leaders to the Christian crusades to the destruction of the Twin Towers.

Extreme Muslims pose a threat to the stability of the west - and even moderates aspire toward a sharia legal system. Muslims in America therefore will be seen as a danger within the States, an enemy in their own country. However, by educating Muslims in America the USA might be able to influence Muslims in the Middle East, by expanding their understanding of western culture.

Apart from educating individuals, how can we pacify these Muslims powers and terrorists? Do we ameliorate their condition with aid, so that the resentment felt by often desperately poor countries may be tempered? But capitalism would look to claw back some of this aid by advocating consumption, and more coke, cigarettes, coffee, might serve to increase Muslim hypomania, thereby exacerbating the problem. The agent provocateur, i.e. the USA, stimulates mania and hatred; and a response to American aid might focus the terrorists' attention on a different enemy, i.e. Israel. But in the eyes of extremists, though individually they may hate Jews more than any other, Israel is no more than an out-station of American imperialism, so aid may do no good in reducing fundamentalism. However adaptive it may be in certain aspects, hypomania ultimately tends toward mania, which is madness - and how does one deal with a madman?

Most extremism emanates from wahabbism, which developed in what is now Saudi Arabia in the nineteenth century. Muslims in the Far East seldom feature in atrocity stories; usually it is those who draw their cultural, as opposed to strictly religious, influence from the Middle East.

Experiments indicate that whether one emerges from a farming or herding culture determines to a very great extent one's sense of honour.[41] Farmers are cooperative, depending on each other, while herders need to be more self-reliant and pro-active in seeing off predators and rustlers alike. Herders therefore are more prickly and aggressive, farmers more back-biting but tolerant. However, because herders may spend long periods alone, visitors are very welcome and usually treated with extravagant hospitality - after the herder has been satisfied that the visitor is no threat. The American Deep South was populated by "Scotch-Irish", who brought their border-reiving cultural identity with them; the North was populated more by Irish, English and North European farmers.

As a consequence, the South is justly famous for its hospitality, more so than the North - but it also is infamously far more violent. This is after centuries away from the milieu that created the culture. Wahabbism emerged from Arabian herders in recent times, and the grandfathers and even the fathers of today's Muslim extremists, even the extremists themselves, may have been actual herders.

By contrast, Indonesian Muslims come from a farming culture, so do not tend toward manic extremism. The problem may not be Islam, but the prickly aggressive honour code of goat- and camel-herders.

The relationship of Muslims to alcohol and sex may bear examination. Muslims are not allowed to depict the human body in art. Even when they live in hot climates they cover their bodies and this is taken to the extreme when women's faces must be covered by veils and even their whole bodies by chadors. There is no sense of sexuality in their dress. Devout Muslims do not drink alcohol, and therefore they would not tend toward sexual and intellectual disinhibition and be less inclined toward hypomania, in this regard, than would the West. They would not have the mania of a hangover, but mania of prayer and belief, to say nothing of genocidal impulses, would contradict the idea that they would, overall, be less vulnerable to hypomania.

"In Muslim countries women experience marital rape that is legal, honour killings, violence against women, stoning, public floggings, child marriage which is o.k. after their first period, forced marriages and female genital

---

[41] Malcolm Gladwell, *Outliers* (New York: Little, Brown & Co, 2008), pp. 166-75.

mutilation. Homosexuals face public flogging, imprisonment and in ten Islamic states [homosexuality] is punishable by death. For converting religion or becoming an atheist one can be sentenced to death. Women get half the inheritance of the male sibling. A man can have four wives and give one up with notice. Iraq gets a lot of coverage but Sudan, Somalia, Nigeria, Syria and Iran are ignored."[42] Women walk behind their men. Suicide bombers are rewarded with 74 virgins in heaven. Taken in total, these beliefs and attitudes suggest widespread hypomania.

A Channel 4 survey in 2015 showed that in Britain a quarter of Muslims wanted sharia law, 5 percent supported stoning for adultery, a third supported polygamy, two fifths thought that wives should always obey their husbands and more than half thought homosexuality should be illegal. Half of British Muslims were born outside of Britain.

In Islamic culture there is grandiose belief in men with a superiority complex and paranoia/morbid jealousy along with sexual control of women that is partially done by the forced wearing of a burka that covers the body and a hijab that covers the head and the face. Genital mutilation is a more extreme form of control, removing physical pleasure from women's experience of sex.

Most Moslems, those of the Middle East in particular, grow beards. This is touted as religiously-mandated, but it also allows them to cover up their facial emotional expression i.e. fear, love and hatred.

Isis are fundamentalists who are vicious and deliberately cruel, cutting people's heads off or shooting them in groups. They destroy artefacts in museums going back to the year zero, as their fellow-travellers, the Taliban, vandalised the Buddha statues in Bamian in 2002. They rape girls young and old and sell them to each other. They are very much anti-Kurd and anti-Christian. They are the ultimate id (Freudian) machine with grandiosity, paranoia and psychopathology driving them.

The male Islamic sexual drive needs to be questioned and examined, along with the Islamic world view. Negativity, fear and hatred are characteristic of Moslem men. They display fear of homosexuality; they deny freedom of thought; they have powerfully-developed id and ego but low self esteem.

---

[42] Carol Hunt, *Sunday Independent*, 3 August 2014.

They tend to have a binary world view, and addictive, paranoid personalities. They are anti-Zionist, anti-Jewish, anti-American and anti-capitalism. Shari law, a body of doctrine that governs Muslims, is very severe; for example, you lose a hand for stealing.

Islamic Terrorism in Europe a history by Peter Nesser reviewed in the Sunday Times 24 Jan 2016 by Christina Lamb. "Al–Qaeda tend to be poor and troubled, others highly intelligent, a sign of MDI falling from upper S.E class to lower S.E. class. Teachers are Jihadi veterans or radical preachers who are politically or ideological driven.ie (MDI) They groom "drifters" in search of communities or (MDI) "misfits" with personal grievances' /paranoia like Hitler and Jihadi John who thought the police were after him before he went to Syria" Just because your paranoid doesn't mean they're not after you.

Mohammad was the founder of the Islamic religion. Born in Mecca in 570 AD, in 595 he married a rich widow. At 40 he had a vision of the Archangel Gabriel calling him to preach the word of God, which he did in 613. In 620 his wife Khadija died, but he took eight more wives. He had many enemies and fled to Yathrib, now Medina, city of the Prophet, from where he returned to pagan Mecca as the avenging agent of Allah, and smashed the idols of the three main goddesses of the local pagan tribes. He died in 632 AD. His teachings were recorded in the Koran, the sacred book of Islam, as revelations from God.

Islam had been called, with much historic justification, as a religion of the sword. Unlike Judaism, from which it developed, it is a proselytising religion, with a long tradition of forced conversion. It is not the only religion based on manic paranoia. St. John had visions which he recorded in Revelations, of Satan in the form of the Dragon. In addition to manic paranoia, fanatics of these religions are dopaminergic, and the elevated levels of neuro-transmitters can give vivid hallucinations. Convinced that their actions are endorsed and even mandated by God, they can become addicted to violence, and this can reinforce the paranoid position of killers who think that people are against them.

HELL

Christian churches traditionally have exercised control by putting people in fear of Hell. Hell is the depressive superego, appealing, in a perverse way, to the sinner. He thinks he is the worst, and that nobody is as bad as he. This is reversed self-confidence yet a definite form of egotism. The acceptance of the fantastic vision, the farfetched notion of eternal torment as punishment for such victimless sins as say, sexual ones often are, suggests hypomania: the hypomanic believes that he is actually bad enough to deserve this fate.

The paranoiac factor may be at work here too. The Christian believes that an omnipotent being is personally watching him, every moment, and all his life long. Such misplaced importance again reflects the whimsical egotism of the person who imagines he deserves hell for his sheer badness. But this egotism may quickly turn to paranoia, especially when the person thinks of the omnipotent being not as a guardian angel character, but a busybody clerk noting every transgression in order to enter it into some sort of balance sheet at the end of one's life, the "final figure" determining whether one goes to hell or to heaven.

The fact that the result must be either/or reflects intolerance for anything but the perfect, exact formula for living. Such a formula is usually based on a worldview that incorporates non-rational explanations involving gods, angels, and the superimposition of the supernatural world - "miracles." Miracles account for creation, but for other things too, any that may be necessary to reinforce whatever message the religion is trying to impart. Both subscriptions to non-rational explanations, and intolerance for anything outside the religion's explanations, may reasonably be deemed non-rational behaviour. From there to hypomania may be a small step.

SATAN

Fear can lead to low self-esteem and people with low self-esteem think they're evil and deserve to die. Evil is the manic opposite to high self-esteem and God. Is Satan a paranoid manic archetype, a depressive archetype or a dysphoric archetype? If we have a God in the manic ideal we also need to have the opposite and Satan satisfies this need in a paranoid world: fear of hell, of the bogey man, of dirt and germs and madness; also the fear of foreigners and of authority, whether the church or the state.

Psychiatrists believe that people with religious delusions are schizophrenic but this is not necessarily true. The religious high (identification with Jesus) and low (with Satan) are part of mood disorders such as manic depression (bipolar affective disorder) or depression. People who have a dysphoric elation (irritable and poor mood) are more likely to get into Satan. They are often manic and need to be put on mood stabilisers such as Lithium, Tegretol etc.

Jesus' sacrifice in the New Testament famously was anticipated by Isaac in the Old Testament, and he brought it to the ultimate point of laying down his life for, not just his friends, but the world, as Christians see it. His followers believe they are eating the body and blood of Christ at communion (Catholics literally, Protestants figuratively so), a cannibalistic rite that can be traced back to primitive societies where the sacred king was sacrificed and his body eaten by his followers, in order to partake of his divinity and satisfy the gods at whose whim the people lived.

Cannibalism is an extreme form of disinhibition, and cannibals like Jeffrey Dahmer are reviled as evil monsters and satanic; even the cannibalism that was resorted to after the plane crash in the Andes in South America was regarded with revulsion. But Christians are not condemned for their cannibalistic rite.

The devil can be identified with earlier pagan gods, notably Pan, the god of the woodlands - the original pagans, the *pagani*, were simply those people who lived outside Rome, in the "wilderness." The perceived evil nature of Pan may be traced to the first commandment of Moses: "Thou shall not have strange gods before me." Thus the gods of the *pagani*, epitomised in Pan, were necessarily evil and in total opposition to God. Might this mutual exclusivity, which has been narrowed through history to intra-Christian and sectarian levels, account for the sort of isolation, sense of siege and eventual dissonance that may lead to breakdown in a no longer homogenous society?

This may be an especially moot point today, with enormous numbers of Moslems coming to Europe. Islam is essentially a medieval religion, with a penal code long abandoned by the West, and a world view at odds with

Enlightenment values. All the evidence suggests that Moslems resist assimilation, and all but flaunt their otherness. This inflames xenophobia in others, and reinforces social heterogeny. Many Moslems hold the same views of Christians as early Christians did the *pagani*; America is "the great Satan"; who are the "little Satans"? Certainly some Enlightenment values are among them.

ALIENS AND ASTROLOGY

For those who cannot see salvation in traditional religion - and even for some of those who can, like Reagan - there is astrology. Looking at the stars is therapeutic and a source of wonder. We are literally looking back across billions of years when we look at a distant star; on another but parallel level, we are looking at eternity. The sense of distance, space and scale can induce in the most sober person a feeling of awe and perhaps incredulous delight, or even religious import.

Any apparently mystical connotations of this experience may be explained by the necessary involvement of the right brain's spatial discernment and perception of non-linear connections in merely looking at a star-filled heaven above. Perhaps men are more likely to report such feelings, because men usually have a better sense of direction and the heavens are the ultimate orientation system.

Fascination with the stars, however, may also indicate mania or hypomania. *Lunacy* comes from the Latin for moon, and in Irish *gealach* is the word for moon and *gealtach* that for madness, but it is hardly fanciful to imagine that, in some cases anyway, mania may be induced by the mystery of the stars and space, rather than the moon.

We have looked to the stars since prehistory, so it is hardly surprising that they have worked their way into our subconscious. Joseph Campbell discusses the development of gods from stars to nature to man himself - man as god. Some people believe that they are aliens, often coming from the Dog Star, Sirius (brightest star) in the constellation Orion; others, less hypomanic, may believe that the ancestors of the race came from this star.

Aliens are mentioned in Revelations, in an ambiguous context,[43] but in such a way that might support those who believe in aliens in a post-1947 way. If imagining oneself to be Jesus is indicative of mania, belief in aliens, especially that one is an alien, is rather similar.

The popular fascination with aliens can be dated to the years immediately following the Second World War, notably an incident in Roswell, New Mexico, in 1947. Ever since then, popular interest has waxed and waned, perhaps driving or being driven by such films as *Close Encounters of the Third Kind. Star Wars* has consistently got high ratings since its release, and was recently voted the best film ever by Channel Four. The TV series *X-Files* is one of the most popular on the air; like *Star Trek* before it, it has cult status with many people. Along with the films have been books, some of them simply silly, some, like Von Daniken's series claiming to offer spurious scientific proof for their claims.

Does this increase in popularity of the manic idea of aliens indicate that people as wholes are becoming more hypomanic? More credulous? It is interesting that the spread of belief in alien origins has been at a time when human evolution has been mapped in finer and finer detail, and each discovery brings yet more ancient ancestors. But perhaps the sense of despair at the end of an appalling war, and the threat of literal destruction of the world with the onset of the nuclear-armed Cold War, might have driven people to look beyond the human species and the world itself, for salvation?

"In 1914 God died," wrote Virginia Woolf, so many people, unable to look skywards for salvation from this source, and in the scientific spirit of the day, transferred their hopes onto a more tangible, if equally unlikely, saviour.

A popular haunt for aliens is supposed to be "the Bermuda Triangle" in the western North Atlantic. Also called the Devil's Triangle, it is alleged to be everything from some sort of teleport to another dimension to a place in which magnetic anomalies may more reasonably account for losses of air- and water-craft. The more fanciful point out that the Sargasso Sea, to which eels are drawn over thousands of miles to breed, is found in this area (as though this somehow offers support for the "special" quality of the area).

---

[43] For instance, "a star fallen from heaven to the earth" - 9:1.

The reality may be far more prosaic. This area lies off Florida, a popular tourist resort, and north of Cuba, for over half a century a country from which refugees leave in unseaworthy craft. It is perhaps not surprising that so many disappearances occur in the Bermuda triangle. The American sense of confidence and adventure exacerbates the problem: in the mid-1970s the Coast Guard rescued a senior citizen who was, apparently, on her way to Cuba, alone, to make perhaps a protest, perhaps a symbolic invasion of Castro's domain. She was navigating with a school atlas.

Perhaps it's a question of a little knowledge being a dangerous thing. The increasing speculation that life may indeed have "come from the stars" - in the form of organic "seeding" - adds spurious "scientific proof" to the hypomanic claims that the first humans came from Sirius. This may be merely a quaint notion, like belief in fairies. But when people believe in such unsustainable notions, or in creationism, to the exclusion of scorning real science, it points to a potentially serious failure in society. Either the education system has failed, or something else has.

Some people, at least, resent or even reject science. Given that science, or at least its child, technology, gave us two disastrous world wars and threatens us with nuclear extinction, such rejection makes emotional sense, especially if the "alternative" is all-providing access to immediate gratification and over-indulgence. At the same time science has robbed us of the therapeutic belief in God. Perhaps it is not surprising that the prospect of aliens offers, some at least, a substitute: redemption from a rotten world by men from space.

But it is rational nonsense. Science also drives the hypomanic engine, in everything from the creation of surplus wealth where 1 percent of the population own 33 percent of the wealth in the U.S.A. to the internet where e-mail was started by Ray Tomlinson in 1971 and in 2010 there was 247 billion hits on the internet or 2 million a second - all for no charge. In Davos 2017 (The Guardian 18th January 17) the eight wealthiest people in the world (mainly technology companies) own more than the poorest 50 percent of the world population. But it is estimated that 80 percent of internet traffic is based on humour, music and porn, all manic archetypes.

The power and capacity of all 1950s computers in the world would fit on to one mobile phone today; what landed men on the moon would fit onto a single iPod and a £100 pounds would now buy a memory of 20 million pages. Internet speed and traffic, as well as text messages, Twitter, Facebook, with attached files and photography communications, are getting faster, leading to or possibly indicative of mania. You Tube had 1 trillion views last year, 3 billion a day, equivalent to 140 views for each person in the world. This was up 30 percent in eight months; You Tube, like everything else in the virtual world, is getting faster and faster getting more manic leading to overload and the potential for chaos. As for internet culture, we are bombarded, frustrated, addicted, disrupted, interrupted and strung out.

Dr. Mary Aiken cyber psychologist based in Dublin reviewed by Barry Egan in the Sunday Independent 23 October 2016, talking about the issues that modern society is facing online said; "As a society we are facing a tsunami of criminality coming down the line...online, from hacking to malware production, identity theft, online fraud, child abuse material/solicitation, cyber stalking, IP theft/ software piracy, data breaches, organised cybercrime, ransomware, extortion and cyber-attacks - therefore it is critical that we understand the dynamic nature of cyberspace as an environment- and ongoing criminal behavioural evolution in this domain" Mary also pointed out earlier this year in June, NATO officially recognised cyberspace as a new frontier in defence. "That is, NATO formally acknowledged that modern battles could be waged not only on land, sea and air, but also on computer networks-this new recognition of cyberspace as a potential conflict zone presents important challenges to society in term of international jurisdictional issues and cyber ethics."

In terms of future threats Dr Aiken pointed out; "At the Europol Cybercrime Centre we are very concerned about the evolution of "Crime-as-a–Service" online-that is procurement services for criminal activity from rentals of botnets, to denial-of services-attacks, malware development, data theft, and password cracking.

The internet also offers the potential for central control. *Smurfing* allows the CIA to turn on and off smart phones and listen in without the owner knowing.[44] The purpose of such technology is national security, and the fears

---

[44] *Panorama*, BBC2, 6 October 2015.

of being eavesdropped upon by voyeurs are baseless, but there is certainly Orwellian potential in the system.

This increase in computer speed and power may not indicate hypomania, merely a careless approach to reality, no worse than an uncritical acceptance of traditional religious belief, or perhaps indulgence in wishful thinking that all will work out for the best. But when people deliberately reject rationality, in favour of the wishful thought, something more ominous may be suggested. The rash of crop circles that was a feature of the 1980s was taken by some as "proof" that aliens were visiting; when the men who had actually made these circles not merely admitted doing so but described in detail how they had done it, they were either disbelieved or, it was claimed, there were other circles that were not hoaxes. Even before this, the lines scored on the ground at Nasca, in the Atacama Desert, were taken as proof that aliens had visited earth in ancient times, the rationale being that as the patterns could only be discerned from high up, earth-bound people could not have drawn them. This is the same as saying that ground plans of large buildings could not be conceived or drawn except by spacemen. Such an attitude may indicate nothing worse than an uncritical approach, but the determination to cling to a fanciful explanation, in the face of common sense, shows a quite remarkably pig-headed approach to reality, determination to see what is not there, an emotional labiality that suggests a hypomanic archetype.

END OF THE WORLD

People think about various scenarios when in a manic frame of mind. These scenarios range from the horribly absurd to the idealistic. People think that their time in the world is the most important time of all, but some take this perception to extremes. All of us find it difficult to imagine the world without us; some postulate our continuing on a different dimension, but others conceive of the world as ending with, or shortly after, their own death.

At the end of the nineteenth century millenialists felt that something would happen to destroy the world; toward the end of the twentieth this fear was even greater, as the event marked the end of a millennium rather than a mere century, and the alleged Y2K bug added spurious scientific proof that world order would collapse, after which the Kingdom of God would come. Notably in America, unscrupulous profiteers cashed in on these fears by supplying everything from guns to K-rations to the greatly increased number of survivalists. Charlatans, street preachers and evangelists have always attempted, in extroverted modes of behaviour, to convey to a passive public that "The end is nigh," often for cynical reasons of their own. Writers and movie-makers find a strong demand for such fare too - for example the 1980's post-apocalyptic films *Mad Max* and the virulently anti-Soviet *Red Dawn*, and the many others that were released coming up toward the millennium, such as the fatuous *Waterworld*.

The world will not end but will change. Conflicts will continue to spring up and ecological deterioration may continue; perhaps the global economy will indeed implode when "the credit is called in," or some rogue nation may cause catastrophe with atomic weapons; but the world will continue as it did after the dinosaurs.[45] The concern of the prophets of doom reflects an anthropocentricity that often has as its foundation a religious belief system, usually Christian (understandable, given that it was the Christian calendar that created the millennium and its alleged accompanying doom).

One can sense from some of the prophets of the last century an excitement at the prospect of the world ending, even an impatience for it. Those who would welcome such an event would see themselves as "the elect" who would be saved from the collapsing world and brought to heaven, either permanently or in order to wait for the establishment of the reign of Christ on earth. Such a belief suggests manic delusion, but given the near hysteria in the latter part of the 1990s in certain quarters, notably in fundamentalist circles of America, it suggests that culture is dictated by manic delusions - at least in part. American culture is also sustained by fear and paranoia of the devil, onto which may be projected mortal enemies like Osama bin Laden or Saddam Hussein.

Nor is the Religious Right the only group to suffer thus: the so-called New Age also emerged, in part, as a response to a perceived imminent shift in the world order, and prophets of this also perpetrated manic acts of recklessness, notably the cult that committed mass-suicide in order to ease their members'

---

[45] A possible exception, outlined by James Lovelock in *The Gaia Hypothesis*, would be caused by biological mutation of plants which would overcome the earth's capacity.

translocation to the spaceship that they claimed accompanied Halley's Comet. As early as 1971 Neil Young had anticipated such a belief in *After the Gold Rush*: "Well I dreamed I saw the silver spaceships flying /... /... The loading had begun / Flying Mother Nature's silver seeds to a new home in the sun." Young, however, acknowledged that a drugged dream had inspired his vision; the self-martyrs of Jones' comet-spaceship clearly were suffering from delusions of some kind.

TRIBE AND NATION

Such delusions may be found in tribal attachment, which can be, and often is, emotional and beyond intellectual or logical justification. People talk of the emotion-laden Mother tongue, Motherland (or *Vaterland*) and Homeland, and the Faith of Our Fathers, and the Biblical exhortation to Honour thy father and they mother may reinforce such emotional, non-logical thinking. In modern Western society, tribalism manifests as nationalism, religion and politics - which often incorporate aspects of the first two.

Nationalism is a crucial meme: a collection of people who have cultural similarities such as language, history and religion. It is often integrated with religion, which, like nationalism, is an emotional attachment based on female vowels, not an intellectual one based on male consonants. The two are attachments to parental, communal and peer group loyalties and are suffused with emotion and express subsidiary memes.

But nationalism at least is also a manic archetype, an extension of the ego, and as shown by the Nazis can be used to manipulate people's self esteem, thinking and behaviour - to manipulate the memes themselves. Politics almost always has a nationalist, pan-nationalist, underpinning, and sometimes more grandiose delusions, imperialist or universal socialist beliefs, and frequently a religious one as well. Like other memes, it is often "inherited."

What makes a child follow tribal influences, and "inherit" the tribal meme? The Jesuits say, *"Give me the boy and I'll give you a man."* First impressions are important, and they reverberate at various levels of the psyche: i.e., in an interview, the mind is made up in 12 seconds.

- ❖ Our church: Super Ego
- ❖ Our parents: Super Ego
- ❖ Our tradition: Super Ego
- ❖ Our school: Ego
- ❖ Our peers: Id

The emotional and psychological connection is important and tends to develop in teenage years. Even as we question and challenge the views we inherited and grew up with we grow deeper into an appreciation of them, a sometimes complex but always more emotional depth of appreciation - or else we reject them, an even more emotional experience. Though today there is greater cultural expression of intellectual, emotional and spiritual ideas, we still like things to stay the same: like father like son; the same enemies and friends.

The Irish meme is in a state of flux today, therefore. In fact, it is now more accurate to speak of several Irish memes (though there always was more than one). In any society there are likely to be profound political and social differences between working class and middle class ideas, working class ideas tending to be more rigid and less sophisticated. Working class people are also likely to lack the manic gene that is well documented in socio-economic classes 1 and 2, and its immediate and genetic input. Memes will vary from Catholic to Protestant communities, but working class Protestant memes are different to those of middle class Protestants.

Factor into the meme the elevated mood of mania that nationalistic fervour imparts and we get paranoia, with suspicion and fear and perceived threat from the other culture being heightened; this reinforces development of one's own inward-looking tribal culture. Though the manic gene is primarily a middle- and upper-class inheritance, in the case of Ulster Protestants paranoia is as likely to be a working-class phenomenon, because of the "Revival" tradition and the annual commemorations of various events in the glorious Protestant past, when they were in genuine danger of being eliminated by their displaced Catholic neighbours. Thus the mania of either being "saved" by God in the present, or of memory of being "saved" from Popery in the past may degenerate into paranoiac fear of their neighbours.

Presbyterians in the North of Ireland are perceived as being dour, stubborn and lacking in emotion and creativity, but this does not imply a lack of cultural mania. Their belief in being God's chosen ones is contradicted by and not reflected in their dour expression. It was manic Ulster Scots Presbyterians who wrote the American Constitution, with its rigid separation of church and state, and became the first presidents in the USA, and the Protestant fear of being sequestered into a Catholic Irish state dominates their thought to this day.

Cultural bonding can be encouraged by artistic portrayal of cultural icons or mythology, such as the image of King Billy on his white horse (it was probably brown) and upraised sword painted on walls in Protestant areas of Belfast. On the other side of the cultural divide, the Celtic resurgence of the late nineteenth century, led by Yeats and Lady Gregory, set the stage for revolution, as Yeats admitted in his poem "1916." But such cultural bonding may not be entirely positive: artistic representation of the revolutionary years 1916-22 in song and story, and such paintings as *Men of the South*, set the stage for de Valera's repressive Ireland of the 1930s-1960s, in which huge sections of reality were denied, such as the deaths of 60,000 Irishmen in the Great War, fighting for the British Empire, while the revolution supposedly raged. Such denial clearly has pathological components to it. On a strictly manic level, we have Yeats' description of the post-war/post-revolutionary/post-modern world:

"The best lack all conviction, while the worst / Are full of passionate intensity" ("The Second Coming"). The *passionate intensity* is the dysphoric mania.

NATIONALISM

Love of one's country as an extension of self (ego), compared with love for other people, is a manic archetype. An enemy is needed by this archetype: the British in the case of the Irish; Tamil Tigers, PLO, ETA, all have their own enemies. Every individual thinks he's special and every nation thinks it's better than any other. The strength of the myth and the dangers of the idea are seen in manipulation of the Germans during Hitler's reign; they are also evident in the mobilising of public opinion against him on the Allied side, in the American myth of Manifest Destiny and the British myth of the White Man's Burden in the nineteenth century.

Nations are collections of people who share a common language, culture and territory. Their culture binds them - at least to an extent. But the idea of a United Country is a manic delusion, an ideal. The difficulties of a new nation state may be seen in Afghanistan, where various tribes are in conflict over just what nationalism means for them; their competing perceptions reveal the difficulties. Indeed, it is questionable whether nationalism can flourish or even exist in Moslem countries, where manic energy is directed rather toward a world caliphate, in which nationalism would have no place and would even be anathema.

The rise of European nationalism in the eighteenth and nineteenth centuries set off wars between empires and subject peoples, and between empires and republics, but it did not lead to peace in Europe, and the most ambitious attempt to implement "legitimate" nationalist feelings, the Versailles settlement of 1919, led directly to the most destructive war in history. "The war that ended peace", as Margaret MacMillian describes the First World War, came at the age of peace movements, disarmament talks and international friendship societies. The naval race between the Germans and the British effectively had ended two years previously, Britain had just acceded to German plans to complete the Berlin-Baghdad Railway, even though this accession had angered her ally Russia and could potentially endanger Britain's own security in the Persian Gulf, and even communications with India. So rosy did the future seem that Europeans were preparing for the next Hague conference, scheduled for 1915.

Inbuilt into the idea of nationalism is the problem of where to draw the boundaries, geographical, linguistic, and cultural, as well as political. This was made very apparent in 1919 in Europe, when plebiscites that favoured inclusion of, say, West Prussia and Posen in the new German republic were ignored in favour of giving the reconstituted Poland access to the Baltic, while those areas that favoured opting out of Weimar - as in Schleswig and Eupen-Malmedy - were readily acted upon. But even on an island scale our own small country (Ireland) shows the difficulties of drawing nationalist lines.

In the 1890s came the Irish cultural revival, under Yeats, Lady Gregory, Douglas Hyde, and others. This revival developed a culture and mythology that was expressed in writing, painting and drama, but its influence did not end there. In the rabid rhetoric of *The Leader*, a propagandistic Irish journal of the early twentieth century, D. P. Moran claimed that Irishness required a Catholic and Celtic tradition, and that Protestant Irish were really "West Britons," despite the ironic fact that the leading lights of the cultural revival were almost all Anglo-Irish Protestants. Ultimately the cultural revival led to insurrection in 1916 and Yeats's "terrible beauty" being born.

Irish cultural nationalism led to a republic - of sorts - for a country that had been in subjection for 800 years. But the attendant creation of the artificial statelet, Northern Ireland, with two rival nationalities and cultures, led to one of the most intractable civil struggles of the twentieth century. Competing egos led to an expression of the id in terms of mutual exclusion and violence of the darkest sort. People fought for the aspiration of a united Ireland; others fought against them to preserve the British link. A measure of the manic delusion of both is that, increasingly, Northern Ireland is not particularly wanted by either the Irish Republic or Britain.

EMPIRES

Imperialism is little more than nationalism writ large. Certain efficiencies of scale - and comparative administrative and military advantage - may improve the conditions of even subject peoples: thus in the age of Pax Romana it was said that a woman could walk the length and breadth of the Roman Empire without fear of insult, and Pax Britannica went a great way to eradicating slavery and famine in Africa and India.

However, as empires get more manic they get more chaotic. Material security leads to complacency, and boredom leads to the search for sensual outlets. Public expression of sexuality becomes more acceptable and widespread. People go to spectacles and see people being injured and even killed in the name of sport. Leaders get manic and think they're gods or the next thing to that (though as yet none of the modern era has matched Caligula in making his horse a senator). Money systems overheat and there is credit for all. Then the backbone breaks and the economy collapses or else stronger more primitive cultures win the wars or take over the empire.[46]

Ancient empires like the Sumerian, Macedonian, Assyrian, Egyptian, Greek, Roman, Persian, and more recent European powers, British, Dutch, Spanish, Portuguese, French and now the Americans, all show how nationalism grows into imperialism and how the process ends in different ways, usually chaotically. In more modern times capitalism, driven by hypomanic advertising, leads to over-consumption, chaos and eventually the end of empire. Lehman Brothers went bust in 2008 due to subprime lending as did Fanny Mack and Fanny Mae mortgage brokers went broke.

A Samarian clay tablet from 2,000B.C. in the Chester Beatty Library (Dublin) describes the payment for education of an out of control teenager, proving that juvenile delinquency did not first appear with rock ' n 'roll as Marlon Brando in. "Rebel without a cause"

Initially the empire provides both raw materials and markets, to the great advantage of the motherland. Thus much of Britain's greatness and wealth came from the riches of its colonies, notably India. The culture speeds up as more wealth comes in, people see their prosperity as proof of the benefits of the system or even of their being chosen by God to rule the world (certainly in the case of the British, and, latterly, the Americans), and the process of imperialism becomes self-generating. Thus after the Suez Canal opened Britain established a protectorate over Egypt in order to secure her sea-lanes to India, and later took over the Sudan in order to safeguard Egypt. The logical end of the process was Cecil Rhodes' ambition to have a red streak all the way down Africa, a dream that was almost realised before the entire colonial system collapsed in the mid-twentieth century.

The sun, it was said, never set on the British Empire. The idea of such an empire is quite manic, implying world presence and dominion. But the notion of the sun never setting on the Empire can have another connotation. People think they're better than other people and this gives them some sort of right to do anything from making other people the butt of jokes to subjugating them. Imperialists feel they're cultured, grandiose, superior and sophisticated

---

[46] Ian Morris describes the triumph of these cultures as "counter-productive war" in *War: What is it Good For?*

- manic ideas. The reality is that it was insufferable arrogance more than anything else that turned Indians against the Empire.

Colonialism is a development of **nationalism, the archetype of self-love**. The opposite archetype **(socialism), the love of others**, emerges to fight colonialism - as early as the turn of the twentieth century the historian Hobson was arguing that wage increases that would create more domestic spending power would be better than imperialism both for British industry and British society. **However, when socialism joins nationalism, as it did in Nazi Germany, it evokes the paranoia archetype, and people in that delusional situation can kill without guilt**. Thus two conflicting spirals, imperialism and its reactive system, may develop. Culture speeds up and becomes more manic, and this inherently leads to a paranoid position that may lead to unstoppable chaos and cultural collapse.

Gandhi and Martin Luther King took the manic non-aggressive approach. Their manic love of man defeated colonialism in India and helped remove the worst excesses of the Jim Crow laws in the USA. **Pacifism without nationalism is a good anti-imperialism position**. The sense of being a person in the world deflects nationalism; but unfortunately the larger and more manic society grows the more difficult it becomes to really feel like an individual. Certainly the United Nations has become a quasi-manic organisation, akin to the European empires that dictated to subject peoples. To argue that the UN is ultimately a democratic organisation seems fatuous when Saudi Arabia can have a place on the UN Human Rights Council, something she gained through secret dealing with Britain.[47]

Sometimes, as empires become very wealthy, cultured elements within them become pacifist and try to tone down the empire's war exploits. Perhaps the current power of political correctness in academe is evidence of this. Thus the utterly unsupported notion of Afrocentrism, which claims that all European civilisation came out of Africa, has a certain cachet in American universities, and there seems a marked reluctance to raise objections to it, just as there often is to reject the more extreme ideas of feminism and postmodernism. At least one history department back-pedals on the hard fact

---

[47] Owen Bowcott, "UK and Saudi Arabia 'in secret deal' over human rights council place", in *The Guardian*, 29 September 2015.

that it would have been impossible for Aristotle to have gained his knowledge from the library of Alexandria (700,000 books), as the Afro centrists claim, because he died in the year the library was started (if not before). Afro centrists and militant feminists seem to combine hypomania with obsessive-compulsion, which enables them to plant the seeds of intellectual nonsense even in universities, and thus revise the history of their civilisations.[48]

Language can be misused toward propagating such fashionable nonsense. Language possibly emerged about 250,000 years ago and became more subtle and nuanced as it developed. It also enabled the development of ideas, and this in turn affected how language further developed. For instance, people can exchange goods or services across language barriers - the rudimentary sign language of the American frontier, or the pidgin English of the Pacific islands and elsewhere, is adequate - but it takes language-proper to make possible discussion of abstract ideas. The Phoenicians of 1,000 B.C. (named after the purple dye they made from rare shells) had few vowels in their alphabet, but the Greeks had 20 consonants and five vowels which made their language more expressive and gave us the great works of Classical times. The *Iliad* and the *Odyssey* were pre-literate, and whether anyone called Homer ever wrote them down is debatable, but they are the oldest recorded stories and it was the Greek language that recorded them. When the Golden Age (which developed a manic democracy among the culture of the aristocrats with love and paranoia at its apex) was destroyed by the more primitive Roman culture, the soldiers of the conquerors said, "Leave the Greeks their libraries for with libraries they will not raise up against us." This apocryphal remark contains a good deal of truth.

The Golden Age belonged to the Bronze Age, and the Iron Age of better tools and weapons that succeeded it was succeeded by a cultural Dark Age in which hypomanic religious fanatics deliberately destroyed the great works of the Golden Age. The poetry of Sappho is the best example, Sappho having been not merely a woman - bad enough in the misogynistic religion of St Paul and St Augustine - but she also was lesbian and wrote lyrically of sexual love.

---

[48] Mary Lefkowitz, *Not out of Africa: How Afrocentricism Became an Excuse to Teach Myth as History*.

The same sort of destructiveness can be seen in what the Taliban did to the Buddhist statues of Bamian and what Isis is doing now to archaeological treasures of the Levant. But language can be targeted more subtly by ideologues in mainstream Western culture. After its political defeat in 1990, Marxism took refuge in universities and other corporate homes and we may see in Bryn Mawr's hosting of an Afrocentrist lecturer perhaps evidence of Marxist "revolutionary defeatism". Another manifestation is "sensitivity training" workshops in British civil service and local council departments, such workshops being a continuation of the tradition of "re-education camps" for enemies of the regime.

HYPOMANIC AMERICA FOREIGN POLICY

"No matter how selflessly America perceives its aims, an explicit insistence on predominance would gradually unite the world against the United States".

— Henry Kissinger

America believes in itself. The American Dream is a belief in the self, the belief of a Protestant country against that of a predominantly Catholic Old Europe. What's missing, Henry Kissinger argues, is "vision", accompanied by "enlightened leadership." America needs "an unapologetic concept of enlightened national interest" that nonetheless acknowledges the concerns of other nations. "America's ultimate challenge is to transform its power into moral consciousness, promoting its values not by imposition but by their [i.e. other countries'] willing acceptance" of American values.

This reads like Kissinger looks for the USA to become a "globocop", a stern but benevolent policeman of the world, keeping the peace to the benefit of all. Britain fulfilled this role in the nineteenth century, but the cost of the two world wars, and the loss of her empire, left her unable to do so after 1945 - even compromised her power after 1918. However, unlike Britain, the USA was never an unchallenged global power, and in more recent years the emergence of asymmetrical warfare has made the very possibility of a globocop unlikely.

Such an aspiration suggests hypomania, and Victorian hypomania drove the British Empire into becoming one on which the sun never set and allowed an army that was little more than a colonial gendarmerie to become the best, if one of the smallest, in the world, and to dictate to other countries. The British largely eradicated slavery, even in Moslem lands, where slavery was, and indeed still is, regarded as divinely ordained.

Similar hypomania drives the USA, and always has. Fourteen men, eleven of whom were Ulster Scot Presbyterian, a religion that leans toward hypomania, the chosen ones, wrote the US constitution. The constitution is very wide ranging in the freedom it offers the individual person, especially by the standards of the eighteenth century. People had genuine rights that must be respected and after the Fifth Amendment was passed did not have to speak if it compromises their sacrosanct individuality (grandiosity).

Here we see the archetype of the free man; man above nature (in that in nature freedom is often the freedom to kill or starve); the American belief in the individual above all else: man is the elite in nature and above the law of nature.

In the USA everybody, in theory, is part of the elite, power coming from the people and vested temporarily in one who is primus inter pares, not permanently in power like any king or emperor. In part because of justifiable pride in their democratic system, in part because their country is large enough to be self-sufficient, Americans are often self-centred and self-concerned and relatively few of them know much about the world outside. They have the biggest of everything but often have the irrational belief that if something is good, then more of it must be better.

Similarly, their placing of man above nature easily can translate into placing Americans above other nationalities. The ideal warriors that save the world and makes people feel safer emerged mainly in the U.S, in Dell Comics super-heroes like Superman, who indeed acts rather like a globocop, as the USA sees itself as being. Thus the constitution that set out to establish the sacrosanctity of the individual human being becomes the lofty excuse for American imperialism.

Cultural imperialism is an important factor, to an extent that it was not in the days of earlier empires. The European Union and countries on the periphery are scared of the all-encompassing American culture. Not all of this is cheap or negative; along with McDonald's and Walmart is enormous confidence. There is little guilt in American culture and few excuses. Everybody can make it. Only I am to blame if I don't. Shame on me, not guilt, if I don't, and there is very real shame in the USA if one is on welfare, unlike in socialist Europe.

But with globalisation, itself a manifestation of trans-national hypomania, national differences are unavoidably expressed, and the most powerful country will export elements of its culture. The danger then becomes that the lowest common denominator - American consumerism - dictates cultural norms to all. English is becoming the global language long after the end of the British Empire because English is the language of the USA.

Riverdance, a strictly Irish cultural phenomenon, met with widespread, enthusiastic acceptance in the USA, but this is insignificant - almost a patronising indulgence - when set against how the entire American cultural-value system has been imposed elsewhere. Riverdance sexualised Irish dancing.

Cultural icons reflect the cultures out of which they arose. Batman, Spiderman, Superman, the Invisible Man, Superwoman and the Incredible Hulk emerged out of the culture of America from the Depression to the Cold War mainly reflecting mania/grandiosity and paranoia. They are larger-than-life characters with the reassuring power to save whole cities and even the planet from gangsters and global "empires of evil", to borrow from Reagan. But they also reflect their creators, who were somewhat outsiders, often the children of Jewish immigrants. Stan Lee, who still writes for Marvel Comics, developed Spiderman; Iron Man, X Men and the Incredible Hulk. The Dell and Marvel heroes emerged from a remarkable meeting of an old European storytelling culture and an immigrant's sense of alienation as he was tossed by the ferocious energy of the American dream.[49]

In computers Europe is only represented by Spotify , the music-streaming service out of Stockholm whereas the USA boasts Apple, Google, Facebook, Amazon, Instagram, Uber, AirBnb and Twitter, whose combined value is greater than the GDP of many European economies.

Look at the contrast with British comic-book "heroes" from DC Thompson. There is nothing remotely *super* about any of these except Desperate Dan,

---

[49] Review by John Harlow and Josh Glancy in *The Sunday Times*, 22 November 2015.

and he's a parody of the Western Frontier hero and the Dell and Marvel Superhero, a man who dresses as a cowboy but lives in a working-class terrace house of an industrial English city and never draws his gun. Dan's heroic attributes extend no further than eating cow-pies, shaving with a blow-lamp and smoking dustbins (before Health and Safety and other concerns obliged him to give up smoking). Other DC Thomson heroes are heroic only in their mischievousness - Denis the Menace, Beryl the Peril, Korky the Cat - or even stupidity - the Bash Street Kids.

An added factor is American superheroes' dress. There may be little sense, as has been observed, in wearing one's underpants on the outside, but Superman is much more sartorial than Desperate Dan despite that. It's as if the British refuse to take themselves too seriously, whereas the Americans do the opposite. It was famously remarked that the British acquired their empire "in a fit of absence of mind",[50] but the Americans take their globocop responsibilities very sternly and seriously indeed.

For better or worse, the American Dream can be translated into the World Dream; culture can expand from a national base to a universal one. People want to sing; dance and act (Michael Jackson) but often are too wary or even scared to do so. Thus on the very day the Taliban was driven out of Kabul cheering crowds greeted the "godless" liberators, women raised the hems of their burkhas, and men lined up before barbers to have their first shaves in six years. The next day newly reopened music shops catered to long queues. Mindsets can be tuned into similar wavelengths so that people get on through shared cultural values and appreciation. Muslim hatred of the US can be reversed if cultural openings can be found between the two traditions.

It is heartening that this was the very approach taken after the Twin Towers attack: the American president cautioned against reprisals against individual Muslims and took care to build a coalition against the Taliban, a coalition of Muslim and non-Muslim nations all sharing a cultural rejection of terrorism. "Fate has propelled a nation convinced of the universal applicability of a single set of maxims into a world characterised by the multiplicity of historical evolutions requiring selective strategies" (Kissinger).

---

[50] John Robert Seeley, *The Expansion of England.*

On the other hand, to one extent or other culture depends on and is driven by paranoia. The problem is that with love of others who share our cultural values there has to be an enemy, something or someone we can compare ourselves favourably with and focus the blame on when things go wrong. This enemy may be America, terrorism, drugs, death, nature, global warming, illness, and pollution. We may trace Riverdance back a century and more to the Celtic Revival of the 1890s, a cultural resurgence that gave the Irish back a sense of identity and national pride, but that also contributed greatly to the blood-letting of 1916 and what followed - i.e. success of this cultural phenomenon, for all its enthusiastic reception by the Anglo-Saxon Americans, was built on hatred of the erstwhile cousins and grandfathers of its latest enthusiasts.

We need to love each other and ourselves without being nationalist (American) or socialist (European). We need to love the differences - as the Coca-Cola ad put it: "I'd like to teach the world to sing / In perfect harmony." But when the masses like one thing, the creative leaders another, the creative leaders lead, simply by virtue of marketing budgets, more money spent on Coca-Cola, a relatively new factor in cultural promotion. Merchandising is a huge part of marketing all products for much of the twentieth century. Films sometimes earn more money through merchandise than in box-office returns. Such merchandising techniques are often used to promote cultural values, and - more significantly - denigrate the cultural values of the enemy.

Propaganda has been a significant part of the war effort through modern times, and it often concentrates on painting the enemy in a sub-human light (paranoia), the "home side" as superhuman. Thus in the Great War the Kaiser was represented by the Allies as a mad dog, the Germans as simian Huns; the Germans portrayed themselves as the noble defenders of civilisation, holding Europe against the marauding Asiatic hordes and their Entente allies.

In large part through advertising and merchandising, Coke and Marlboro are among the biggest sellers of any product in history, each worth some fifteen billion dollars a year. The album *Bad* by Michael Jackson, *E.T.* and the film *Star Wars* are colossal cultural milestones that have exported American culture into all parts of the world.

COLD WAR

Pitted one against the other, the Superpowers had to keep doing one better: nuclear warheads, ships, spies and planes. In this manic environment, in which a nation threatened was a world threatened, there was a lot of paranoia. The Cuban crisis was a very manic time, people praying for a political resolution or, if that failed, favourable winds that would spare us the evils of fallout. We may have been closer to nuclear catastrophe than anyone realised: JFK was on medication for chronic pain, steroids and speed/amphetamine that could have made him manic and paranoid. The paranoid position meant that both sides could kill without guilt.

Josef Stalin murdered at least 15 million of his own people (some estimates go as high as 40 million) as he tried to enforce Communism, an unnatural political entity.[51] To his admirers - Ché Guevara Lynch being one (Irish Times, Letters Page 12 October 2017, Gerard Casey, Guevara wrote "Hatred is the central element of our struggle! Hatred that is intransigent ...hatred so violent that it propels a human being beyond his natural limitations, making him a violent and cold blooded killing machine...We reject any peaceful approach. Violence is inevitable. To establish socialism rivers of blood must flow!") Saddam Hussein another - he was a faithful student of the teachings of Karl Marx; to his enemies, he seemed the devil incarnate. The "fundamental fact" about him is not that he was a monster: it is that he was a Marxist and ideologue. Lenin, the thinker and orator, driven by emotion as much as by ideology and the drive of anger and hatred. "You have to hit them over the head, without any mercy." Both Stalin and Lenin were equally the creators of the Soviet terror system. In his quest for power, Lenin promised people anything and everything. He lied unashamedly. Winning meant everything; the ends justified the means". The whole Soviet system was base on a lie. Lenin and Trotsky, were messianic Marxists, Stalin the journalist and organiser, but all saw the deployment of state terror in the cause of Communism as perfectly legitimate. This way of thinking is what any ideologue risks falling into. The ideology, however admirable, takes over the ideologue, which will literally kill in its cause. Thus the Irish Revolution

---

[51] See, for instance, *Stalin: Paradoxes of Power*, by Stephen Kitkin; *Koba the Dread: Laughter and the Twenty Million*, by Martin Amis; *Stalin: The Court of the Red Tsar*, by Simon Sebag Montefiore.

began with the idealistic Pat Pearse and ended with the ruthless Dan Breen. The French Revolution quickly went from *liberté, égalité, fraternite* to the famously "incorruptible" Robespierre, who declared, "Pity is treason".

However, Mutually Assured Destruction - the apt acronym MAD - lead to a mutual understanding between the KGB and the CIA that there would not be a nuclear first strike by either side. It was a stand-off position between **Communism (love of others, paranoia) and liberal democracy (truth seeking and spending**, both manic archetypes). MAD and detente eventually gave way to more a confrontational stance taken by Ronald Reagan against the "evil empire" of the Soviet Union, and trying to meet and match the manic concept of "Star Wars" (a CIA invention) broke the Soviet economy and ended the Cold War with the fall of the Berlin Wall in 1989.

Engels wrote that the greatest position in nature was for two people to fall in love above money and religion, which is not true. It is for access to love their children that they fight in divorce courts, and most people believe in money, capitalism, tradition and religion that is the opposite to the teachings of Marx's. Mao believed in Marx. The feel-good factor of grandiosity in the USA and the paranoia of the Cold War era allowed those in control to foster popular belief that nuclear war would meant the end - or End Times, for some. When a secret deal between the KGB and the CIA had been agreed that they would not attack each other (After Dark) Channel 4 Tony Benn. This was a crude form of thought control. "I never knew?" said Tony Benn. "You never asked," replied CIA.

I used to talk about nuclear war and the paranoia that goes with it to people but when they had the same ideas I found it boring and changed the topic. My other obsession was God and that religious delusions i.e. messianic are found in Schizophrenia and Mania.

It was not coincidence that a popular uprising which also contributed to the downfall of Communism started in Poland. The Vatican was anticommunist and the appointment of a Polish pope threw a holy spanner into the Cold War works. Stalin's sneer, "How many divisions has the pope?" developed a hollow ring. The Holy See, however, had Protestant allies in Washington and London; years later Lech Walensa thanked Margaret Thatcher for giving Solidarity £5 million which was a lot of money at the time.

Now the Cold War is over, but people need to have an enemy onto which to project their paranoid archetype; there has to be someone to hate in the same way there has to be someone to love. It used to be the Reds; now it's terrorism, climate change, Islam and drugs, drugs at least being as artificial a threat as any the CIA previously fabricated.

But fabrication of causes is not restricted to the political right. Wives talk of control of husbands. Hatred of others and love of self brings out the paranoia on both sides. Those in control, and those who aspire to control, may manipulate this need toward their own ends. Thus climate change, drug culture and terrorism are seen by socialists as a way of attacking capitalism. "Revolutionary defeatism" calls for Marxists to use whatever comes to hand to bring down the capitalist system and replace it with the Workers' Utopia. That just about every Marxist state has failed is beside the point: "Marxism has never been tried" is the answer to this obvious objection, i.e., they never killed enough!

Despite the end of Communism, there is still a pre-socialist agenda in some western countries, including Ireland where there is an intellectual anti-American bias in the media that is filled with sleeping Trotskyites. Fellow travellers have infiltrated the print media and TV journalists and third level academia. The frantic pace demanded of journalists means that many are hypomanic and derive a great solace from ideas that are dialectical and require intellectual rigour and argument. Journalists and academics kneel at the foot of left wing icons associated with alcohol (Bacchus) and cocaine, and they tend to be hypomanic and follow the liberal left wing agenda. Journalists boast a disproportionate number of what are called socialists, according to at least one of their number, the maverick John Waters,[52] though many are "champagne socialists". They live and think the manic dream of breaking the big story such as the Watergate scandal. They see their duty as seeking the all-powerful truth. Of course there is no objective truth, and only the seeking after it can provide a fulfilling life, not the defence of any dogmatic "truth".

I once went up to Trotskyite Paddy Smyth - son of Jennifer Johnston and latterly an *Irish Times* journalist - as he held a Trotskyite poster at a student

---

[52] See, for instance, the *Irish Times*, 22 January 2010.

march and I showed an interest. I told him to call up to my rooms in TCD where I was staying that year. Soon afterward a friend came up with a bottle of champagne and eggs, bread and milk for French toast as promised. While we were drinking and eating Paddy came in and I said "Not today Old Boy".

In Cuba, which is one of the few communist countries left, a waiter in a hotel can make $33 a night on tips, the wage of a doctor for a week. This inconsistency can only last for so long. Castro is seen as a God to socialist fellow travellers, despite the oppressiveness of his regime. Recently the relationship between the USA and Cuba has opened up.

Persuaded away from one manic ideology, Russians have embraced another: they have embraced with enthusiasm liberal capitalism. However, Vladimir Putin is a self-admitted admirer of Stalin, and Russia lurches from one crisis to another, with nuclear-powered submarines threatening to rust away and perhaps unleash ecological catastrophe of global proportions. Such a threat may well elicit the sort of manic response that Stalin unleashed on the kulaks. Putin is a manic paranoid and small (aggressive)

NATIONAL SOCIALISM

Nationalism is a manic archetype i.e. love of self, and it reflects the ego. Socialism is another manic archetype i.e. love of others, and it reflects the super ego (control by peers, parents and police). Under German National Socialism, however, "others" was strictly confined to the German people, and of a particular type: the Aryan. The notion of racial purity inherently excluded those who did not belong, notably the Jews. This love of self and a restricted group of others necessarily led to suspicion of all outside the group, especially when these were blamed for Germany's degradation after the Great War: the former Allies but even more so "the November criminals" - Jews and Bolsheviks - within the state.

Suspicion developed into paranoia as a consequence of Germany's neighbours' understandable alarm at the rapid rise of her old enemy (which would again make war "after an interval of twenty years for a change of moustache"),[53] and the paranoid position became established. Paranoia is a

---

[53] David Low, *Europe at War: A History in Sixty Cartoons with a Narrative Text.*

manic archetype and it reflects the id (basic instincts). The paranoid position allows people to express the id in acts such as murder, rape and incest, killing without guilt, as happened infamously in the death camps.

In Ireland we have the National Socialist-type party Sinn Fein which has emerged from a terrorist foundation and which, like the Nazis, incorporates both nationalist and socialist ideals and maintains a private army. It claims descent from the true republican nationalist party of 1916 and denies that either Fianna Fail, the self-styled Republican Party, or Fine Gael, political descendants of the "Free Staters" of the Civil War, have any right to make such a claim. Sinn Fein attracts 20 percent of voters, mainly young adults. Like the Nazis, they have an enemy onto which to project all evil, initially the Protestant Unionists but latterly any opponents in the Republic. Significantly, when Martin McGuinness was asked, during his presidential campaign, about criticisms made about him, he dismissed these contemptuously as coming from "West Brits", Britain being the traditional and indeed racial enemy, as the Jews were the Aryans'; such dismissal solidifies Sinn Fein belief in a National Socialist Ireland.

Like the Nationalist Socialist party in pre-World War II Germany, a mythical vision of a Celtic race is being sold by Sinn Fein. Sinn Fein may well be increasing their vote but unlike Germany in the 1930s we do not have high unemployment but inflation is rising and we do not need a messiah like Hitler or Adams to save us.

COMMUNISM

Of course, any ideology may subscribe to lies in order to serve itself. Stalin's use of the airbrush to officially remove former allies, later enemies, from the record is infamous. The former Italian communist, Italo Calvino, once frankly acknowledged that any idealist, faced with a choice between ideology and truth, will always pick ideology and even today, two and a half decades on from the fall of communism, the system has its apologists. Universities rightly decry "Holocaust deniers" and none would give such a denier academic status; yet Marxism flourishes in both history and English University departments, TV, radio, print journalism and politics.

Why do people, especially those in academia and perhaps in the media, focus on the National Socialism of Hitler as the worst regime in history, one that caused maybe 65 million deaths in World War II, whereas Marxist regimes of the 20th century resulted in perhaps twice that many deaths? Marx said "no great movement has been formed without the shedding of blood". The French historian Stephane Courtois's devastating book *Black Book of Communism* is left on the shelf and rarely referred to by media and academics, many of whom have a rose tinted view of communism as the grandiose viewpoint of being better than the rest, as opposed to the paranoid view of the right wing. Political correctness (another meme, perhaps), is in part responsible, but is more likely to exist symbiotically alongside communism rather than account for its continued existence.

In the modern rock and roll poseur fashion, the Manic Street Preachers talk of going to Cuba, where doctors are paid £15 a month, as being cool. The name *Manic Street Preachers* is probably one of the best names in Rock and Roll encapsulating how a manic depressive person would act. Another good name is U2, a number and a double vowel (balancing the left and right brain so the whole brain is involved) and Dexy's Midnight Runners (*Dexy* being Dexedrine - amphetamines or speed).

Again, perhaps there is a meme that may account for this. Communism emerged from the rottenness that was finally exposed by the Great War but had been pointed out by writers and intellectuals from Charles Dickens' time and before. The "dark satanic mills," decried by Blake had developed out of the Industrial Revolution that had made capitalists unimaginably wealthy and their workers unimaginably miserable. When these same exploited workers went off in their tens of millions to be slaughtered in "a capitalists' war", as Lenin denounced it, the truth was brought home to the disillusioned public by the "trench poets" and other writers: Erich Mariah Remarque, Henri Barbusse, Ernest Hemmingway, Dalton Trumble, an illuminated state

When Remarque's *All Quiet on the Western Front* was released in 1930, the great acclaim it got worldwide seemed to signal agreement that there could be no going back to a situation where the masses could become cannon-fodder for the wealthy few. When the Nazis ritually burned the book and film, and exiled Remarque, it was a short and apparently logical step for those who espoused the new egalitarian society to claim that the end of the Great War had promised a swing toward the pendular opposite of Fascism: Communism. Thus through the 1930s many intellectuals, up to the Bloomsbury Set and the cynical, shrewd George Bernard Shaw, endorsed Stalin, and returned from Russia with glowing reports of the new workers' paradise. Even the infamous show trials of 1936-37 were excused by otherwise intelligent people: after all, if such dedicated communists as Zinoviev had denounced themselves, then the cause, Communism, must be greater than mortal and corruptible individuals.

In the years between the wars it became all but necessary for any intellectual, free thinker or liberal to be at least benevolently disposed toward Communism. The meme for this benevolent disposition may have evolved out of Christian precepts - Good will to all men, and Do unto others as you would have done unto you - and Enlightenment ideals, and it still is "inherited" by many intellectuals and radicals. The revelation of the true extent of Nazi evil, after the concentration camps were opened, seemed endorsement of the pro-Communist stance. Though rumours of Stalin's purges had been current from the 1930s, and Stalin himself joked at the Yalta conference that the kulaks had been harder to defeat than the Nazis, his apologists excused him on the same grounds that Padraig Pearse had said in 1913 "We may shoot a few people by mistake at the beginning."

It was only after Kruschev abolished the "cult of Stalin" that the full truth emerged, and then only over a period of many years. The lowest estimates are that 20 million kulaks and incidental peasants were starved to death and otherwise slaughtered in the collectivisation drive of the early 1930s (the best-agreed figure is 5 million families, and peasant families tend to be large). The full extent of the genocide of Mao's Cultural Revolution has yet to be determined but could be 65 million and some historians hint at up to 100 million. Hitler deliberately killed perhaps 10 million.

However, there is more to this matter than raw numbers. Himmler and many other Nazis were involved in the occult and astrology, and looked toward a pagan Teutonic future. The Aryan race consisted of tall, blond blue-eyed men who could grow family trees free of "inferior racial origin".

But even the Aryans might need artificial help, as their leader did long before the end. The invasion of Poland was led by 1,200 panzers, their crews taking chocolate amphetamines to keep them awake. Immediately afterward SS death squads descended on the country's elite determined to kill as many teachers, intellectuals, clergymen and politicians as was deemed necessary to ensure that the Polish nation would never rise again. Some 6 million Poles or 16 percent of the Polish population died in the Second World War; of these 2 million were Jews who died in the death camps. Pre-War Poland had more than 3.3 million Jews and now has 11,000 Jews. In one example in Jedwabne 1,600 Jews were rounded up into a barn and burnt alive by locals' in July 1941. Had the Nazis won the war they would have killed an estimated 11 million Jews in Europe and an unknown Slavic population.

The extremes of Fascist and Communist emotion share different sides of the same coin that leads to similar expressions of the id, notably the "paranoid position" that allows killing without guilt; but traditionally liberals have excused communists' "shooting a few people by mistake," while shrilly decrying anything fascist. **Communism and Fascism make up the opposite ends of a circle where they become the same**. Even contemporary liberals buy into the old meme that enabled their parents and grandparents to support Stalin.

Communism seems to be based on a paranoid view held by the proletariat of the educated as well as of the rich. This paranoia damns these and elevates the working class in a *folie à deux* grandiose delusion. The ongoing support of Communism by the educated becomes more baffling in face of the paranoid hostility that is often their reward in the Workers' Utopia. An irony often missed by Communism's intellectual apologists is that during the Cultural Revolution, and certainly in Pol Pot's Kampuchea, people with spectacles were often shot on sight - on the grounds that they were "obviously" intellectuals. Clearly, this meme has had a complex genesis.

However, quite aside from its survival in academia, it would seem that communist belief has not gone away - notably, it is still alive, if rather far from well, in Cuba and North Korea, and survives in name and totalitarian control in China. Though Communism as an "official" opposition to liberal democracy lost its place after the Velvet Revolution, how we confront it remains a problem, if only in academia. It is still there, trying to impose its vision on literature and history in particular, in universities, and on all aspects of society through political correctness. Though avowedly antireligious, it might well hide under the umbrella of Al Qaeda: if the latter can use drug-smuggling, oil and artefacts to finance and further their aims, they should be capable of forming a devil's pact with Communism with which they share an anti-western philosophy including denial of climate change.

Pol Pot, head of the Khmer Rouge, killed 2 million or 30 percent of the population of Cambodia between 1975 and 1979 through execution, malnutrition, disease, and overwork in the "killing fields" where he had tried to create an agrarian Communist utopia. The soft spoken, French educated Marxist ideologue who masterminded the revolution, died in 1998, almost 30 years after he was defeated by the Vietnamese - also Communist - and in 2011 two of his former ministers were tried for war crimes.

Collectivisation in Vietnam was stopped in 1986 because it was not working and individualism was developed as a form of farming. The ideology was discarded piecemeal, as in China. There are now billionaires in Vietnam who make their money from coffee.

The Vietnam War was hypomanic, as all wars need to be. Four times more bombs were dropped in the course of it than in the whole of World War Two. Four million Vietnamese and 58,000 U. S. soldiers died in the war, but more American soldiers died of suicide then and in the years that followed than were killed in combat.

HITLER

Of the 65 million people who died in World War II. 2.5 percent were British and 50 percent were Russian. Enoch Powell, hostile to the USSR, appreciated the sacrifice of the Russians late in his life. It was a different form of hypomania than Communism than enabled the Russians to make such sacrifices, however: they died for Mother Russia, a nationalist hypomanic archetype. The war is remembered in Russia as the Great Patriotic War.

Probably the ultimate manic trip of a manic era was that of Nero and his reign. Nero believed he was a god and that he had total control of his people. Agrippina Minor and Messalina were wives of Claudius, the former emperor, and Agrippina was the mother of Nero whom she crowned Emperor (and who ultimately murdered her, thinking he was a God and probably paranoid at the same time). Messalina was sister to Caligula and liked to go out at night dressed as a prostitute and see what she could earn when she got tired of the wild parties within the palace - a sign of manic lack of inhibition and of madness in the family.[54]

This was a time of manic chaos, the beginning of the end of an empire and its civilisation. Almost a hundred years of manic Caesars followed Augustus in 31 BC to 68 AD: Tiberius; Caligula; Claudius; and Nero. This was a genetic line of paranoid maniacs, immoral, murderous, cruel, sexual perverts who perversely ruled an essentially peaceful society. Today in the Western world we are speeding up and becoming more manic and paranoid and this may well end in similar chaos. Until recently we had Saddam Hussein and in the relatively recent past we had Stalin, Pol Pot, Hitler and Mao. But perhaps it was such strong men that maintained a certain peace, comparable to the Pax Romanus? It was the fall of Saddam and Ghadaffi, and the challenge to Assad, that precipitated the current unrest in the Middle East.

Hypomanic displays marked Western Europe for long before the Nuremberg Rallies, which now can easily seem to be evidence of National Socialist political mania whose belief system was based on semi-mythology and quasi-history. Such a belief was not new: pan-Germanic sentiments, and half-baked mythical notions of Teutonic archetypes and gods, had marked the last years of the Kaiser Reich. In Britain, public displays of near-hysteria marked the fall of Khartoum, the relief of Mafeking and, as all over Europe, the outbreak of the Great War. Rupert Brooke expressed it thus: "Now, God be thanked who has matched us with His hour".

Hitler was a failed artist as was Nero who acted in his own plays and ordered Seneca to commit suicide.[55] Hitler made himself his greatest creation, the messianic saviour of Germany, but he did so by offering the people of Germany striking symbols and displays of Teutonic might: the red black and white swastika of nationalism, a re-casting of the colours of Prussia and the Second Reich; the emotion instilled in the flag and the anthem; grandiose delusions - "we're the best"; exaggerated gestures, notably the goosestep

---

[54] See Annelise Freisenbruch, *The First Ladies of Rome: The Women Behind the Caesars*, Jonathan Cape, 2010.
[55] *Adolf Hitler: Leading Millions into the Abyss*; RTE 2 TV, 26 July 2014).

and the Nazi salute (borrowed from the British and the Roman Empires respectively); the majestic eagle staffs (from Rome and Prussia); the glorious, intimidating Nuremberg rallies, captured on film by Leni Riefenstahl for further propaganda purposes.

The Hitler Youth were indoctrinated from an early age to buy into all the glory and promises and went on to join the S.S., sinisterly uniformed, and effectively a state within a state. However, it's interesting to note that not more than 10 percent of the German people were ever in the Nazi Party, and when we consider that many joined for pragmatic or business reasons - John Rabe and Oskar Schindler, for example - that figure would likely be halved. Consider then how many members had grown up entirely hoodwinked by propaganda and Nazi "history" and "biology": in his last letter to his wife before his hanging concentration camp commandant Rudolf Höss wrote: "Based on my present knowledge I can see today clearly, severely and bitterly for me, that the entire ideology about the world in which I believed so firmly and unswervingly was based on completely wrong premises and had to absolutely collapse one day".[56]

Possibly as few as 2-3 percent of Germans were convinced, idealistic Nazis; the rest just went along or were forced to do so. The problem for the people of Germany was that the relatively few hypomanic Nazi ideologues were far more feared than the rest of the world lined up against them.

We may be seeing a modern reprise of Nazism in Daesh. The Lebanese prime minister, basing his estimates on figures from refugee camps, believes that about 2 percent of Syrian "refugees" are terrorists. This figure is probably close enough to the percentage of German who were committed Nazis in the Third Reich. Most Moslems, like most Germans in the 1930s and 1940s, are decent people; but how might their decency be sapped by fear of their own terroristic elements?

Another historic parallel may be in the demonising of the "politically incorrect" of those of today and those of the 1930s. Then, when appeasement was popular, those like Churchill who warned that appeasement would lead to war were called warmongers. Today, those who warn - quoting Daesh's

---

[56] Ivan Klima, *My Crazy Century*, p. 424.

own words - that the sort of untrammelled immigration Europe is witnessing will foment religious war are condemned as Islamophobes.

Notions of the perfect Aryan race with blond hair blue eyes contrast almost amusingly with the five foot four inch demagogue runt with the toothbrush moustache, the Great War corporal who would lead them to a new Germany with his spellbinding oratory with its thrilling infectiousness. But he had the inner self belief of a gambler, and his early victories were a gambler's. In 1936 he gambled that the French would not militarily contest his march into the Rhineland, demilitarised by the Treaty of Versailles. He had bet the farm on this, and later admitted that the 48 hours following the move were the worst of his life, for if the French and the British had chosen to fight, the German forces would have been defeated and Hitler would have been ousted.

A number of historians have observed that had Hitler died in 1936 he would be remembered as one of the greatest German leaders. In his three years of power up until then, he had done much to restore German well-being and prestige. In the next three he took further gambles, annexing Austria in 1938 and dismembering Czechoslovakia in 1938-39. Every time his generals argued caution, and Hitler's payoffs encouraged him to discount them - a sign of mania.

Hitler had suffered gas attacks and shellshock in the Great War and looked on his surviving these, and the later attempts on his life, like von Stauffenberg bomb plot, as evidence of his great destiny. The risks he took in his battle plans at the end of the war, which went against his generals' strategies, convinced him further but probably lost him the war. His payoffs also encouraged him to disregard Western political leaders, whose policy of appeasement had allowed him to make such territorial gains in Europe. Even after he over-stepped himself by invading Poland, he continued to take breathtaking risks and come out on top, further encouraging him to gamble more. But hubris led to over-confidence, and the nadir here was probably Stalingrad, where, against all his generals' urging, he insisted on no retreat. The entire Sixth Army, and its commander, General von Paulus, were forced to surrender in February 1943. From there on the Germans retreated all the way back to Berlin.

Nazi Germany was an almost classic hypomanic society: *"ein Reich, ein volk, ein fuehrer"*. There was no tolerance of difference; Nazism was the purest form of xenophobia. Hitler despised the weak, boasted that his people were better than others and had a paranoid hatred of the Jews. After a book burning he said that Jewish intellectualism was at an end. He was charismatic and had a long straining stare looking deep into your eyes, and was aware of the power of persuasion. When he was 30 he went to a course in propaganda and his Minister for Propaganda, Josef Goebbels, was the first ever to exploit the power of radio. Goebbels was skinny, mean-featured, club footed, failed playwright i.e. a failed artist like Hitler (and, to a lesser extent, Lenin). In his regular radio pronouncements he talked of a great rebirth of a nation that satisfied the common German's aspirations, but may also indicate subconscious compensation.

Hitler was obsessed about rebuilding Germany and a new 1,000-year Reich. Art, music and painting followed Aryan mythology and great gatherings such as the Munich Olympics and the Nuremberg Rallies were staged by Goebbels' propaganda machine. When Hitler took over Austria and saw it as the new Germany he had 99.9 percent approval rating in Germany - or so Goebbels' propaganda would have it.

Before he'd fought in the First World War, Hitler had gone through a period as a failed artist, which may go some way to explaining his bitterness and even paranoia, and his energy in creating something more impressive than a canvas - his canvas was to be the whole of Europe. In the paranoid position that Hitler was in, Fascism and Socialism are at one in expressing the id. **Left wing and right wing become the same at the extremes of the circle.**

Hitler said that if the war was not won then he would leave Germany in ruins. If he could not win the war then he would kill his child – Germany - as the Germans were unworthy of him and his Iron Cross. When the war in the east began to collapse, he notoriously remarked in November 1941: "On this point, too, I am icily cold. If one day the German nation is no longer sufficiently strong or sufficiently ready for sacrifice to stake its blood for its existence then let it perish and be annihilated by some other stronger power...I shall shed no tears for the German nation."[57] Such "icy"

---

[57] From the afterword of Martin Amis's novel, *The Zone of Interest*.

detachment suggests the psychopath as well as the hypomanic fanatic, but it may also hint at madness. After all Hitler's core notion, a Jewish world conspiracy, comes straight out of a primer on mental illness - it is the schizophrenic's first and most miserable cliché. In the street, then, gutter Judaeophobia (or at best the unnatural indifference adduced by Ian Kershaw), a fulminate nationalism, and herd docility punctuated by mass intoxication.

Hitler was not mad in the way that word is usually meant. He exhibited signs of mania, and his performances now may look mad but really he was a most effective demagogue. What is more terrifying than any real madness is the way in which this "madman" could have brought a whole country to share his manic vision and almost destroy civilisation. Is the madness in human nature?

Hitler was loved by his mother, and perhaps particularly because before him she had three male miscarriages. He was no less very close to her - her Jewish doctor attested in 1944 that he had never seen such grief in any man as in Hitler when his mother died. He no less feared and disliked, maybe hated, his father. Psychoanalysts have had much fun trying to account for Hitler, but all has to be speculation.

Was Hitler intrinsically evil or was his evil a consequence of his abusive upbringing, being knocked unconscious by his father once as a child, his artistic failure (mania), the displacement of affection for his brutal father onto an adopted Fatherland, and the enduring sense of shock and betrayal when that country was defeated - or, as he preferred to believe, "stabbed in the back" by "the November criminals"? To say nothing of his gassing and perhaps shellshock in the Great War.

Recent scholarship indicates that Hitler's blindness, which he suffered in a gas-attack toward the end of the war, was hysterical. In fact the attack that had "blinded" him was made using chlorine gas, not mustard.[58] Several were affected by the gas, but the others were all treated locally; Hitler alone was sent to Pasewalk Lazarett, a special hospital for shellshock victims north of Berlin. He was cured by a very harsh method, by which the physician "used

---

[58] David Lewis, *The Man Who Invented Hitler: The Making of the Führer*, p. 164.

his dominating personality essentially to bully the soldier better".[59]

This experience almost certainly affected Hitler's personality - it was the "crucible" through which all great leaders have to pass. Pasewalk's isolation was designed "to prevent the spread of hysterical symptoms", but such hysterical conditions were seen at the time as evidence that the sufferer was "to be branded as best weak-willed or feeble-minded and at worst a cowardly malingerer". This would have been anathema to Hitler, or to any Nazi, and to make matters worse, successful treatment was "a battle of wills between doctor and patient", one which recovery proved the patient must have lost. So sensitive was this matter that after Hitler took power it became "an offence punishable by imprisonment even to question the cause of Hitler's wartime blindness ... and to provide medical proof of hysteria was likely to invite an even harsher response".[60] Sinisterly, the doctor who had cured him, Edmund Forster, was probably murdered.[61]

This explanation may account for the strange transformation in Hitler from a courageous soldier who never sought leadership of even a platoon, to the most magnetic and forceful leader in the world. Fritz Wiedemann, his regimental adjutant in the First World War, later testified: "Hitler was an excellent soldier. A brave man, he was reliable, quiet and modest. But we could find no reason to promote him since he lacked the necessary qualities required to be a leader."[62]

Part of the difficulty of engaging clinically or even imaginatively with Hitler is that we still are all but forbidden to consider him as other than an inhuman monster; it's truly difficult to even imagine him as the human being that he was. One scholar, Claude Lanzmann, maker of *Shoah*, comes close to claiming that it is morally wrong to try to understand Hitler, on the grounds that to understand his humanity may carry with it the obligation to forgive his moral failings. One suspects self-serving elements in Lanzmann's reasoning, though, for he also claims that his film is the definitive account, and no one should try to add to or take from it.

---

[59] Ibid, p. 20.
[60] Ibid, pp. 138, 16, 148, 243.
[61] He was alleged to have committed suicide, but his family doubt this. See Lewis, op cit, p. 303.
[62] Ibid, p. 4.

Recently the balance of scholarship seems to emphasise the importance of nature as opposed to nurture in a person's makeup - therefore must we admit this as a mitigating factor in his case?[63] Ultimately, of course, one must be held accountable for one's actions, but in Hitler's case there was another factor, the collusion of the German people in his crimes. Can we blame Hitler alone for the atrocities of World War II when without the backing of the German nation he would have been but one crazed bitter anti-Semite out of millions?

This argument needs to be treated with caution, however, since never more than 10 percent of Germans were members of the Nazi party, and some German scholars hold that the ordinary people were more afraid of the party than of Allied bombers.[64]

Before the war, though, Hitler assuredly was beloved by many if not most his people in part because he exonerated them from defeat in the recent war. People's powers for self-delusion are impressive. Twenty years after the Battle of the Marne General Ludendorff claimed that it had been a German victory.[65]

Hitler's control of the Germans reinforced their sense of being a chosen people and gave them defined enemies against which to measure their distinction: the Jews, traditionally the Chosen People of God and the Communists, now filled in "the legend of an enemy, invisible, ever-present, and attacking the nation from within".[66] James Joyce once observed that a nation, like an individual, has an ego, and if so, why not an id? People tend to need an enemy in order to express their id, and a common enemy, a hatred shared, produces a group id. Though many have claimed that the Germans, in general, were ignorant of the Final Solution, in *Hitler's Willing Executioners* Daniel Goldhagen makes a case that the vast majority of ordinary Germans knew what was going on in the concentration camps. This claim is supported by the initial denials, followed by traumatic admission, by local community

---

[63] The nature-nurture argument has a political dimension, conservatives favouring nature, Marxists and neo-Marxists insisting, as they must, that nature can be trumped by nurture.
[64] WE Sebald, On the Natural History of Destruction, pp. 14-16.
[65] General Joffre was more subtle in his analysis. "I don't know who won the Battle of the Marne, but if it had been lost, I know who would have lost it."
[66] Sebald, op cit, p. 102.

leaders when they were brought to places like Dachau by the Allied liberators of the camps.

Even if Goldhagen overstates his case, as most historians would hold, it was only with the collusion of the German people that Hitler was able to direct a war that caused 60 million to die. Was an entire nation, therefore, complicit in another crime of monstrous proportion - the genocide campaign against the Jews and others - or were they too intimidated to protest? Those Germans old enough to remember the Third Reich claim angrily that the notion of public protest then is fatuous. Those few who dared to object to Nazi policies quickly vanished into the camps themselves, or were simply murdered.

To speak, therefore, of communal madness, more so, of communal evil, is simplistic. The fact has always been that one man with a gun can impose his individual will on a hundred unarmed men. Stanley Milgram's experiments prove that authority is itself a compulsive force; yet does this not suggest that the many defences advanced at Nuremberg - "I was simply following orders" - may have been valid? In 1963, in a climate of Cold War suspicion, not unlike the suspicious period in which Hitler came to power, the Milgram experiment had volunteers being told to ask questions of a man strapped into a chair, the volunteers being under the mistaken impression that they were inflicting physical pain (through electric shocks) to the point of endangering the "subject's" life. They were given orders by men in white coats. Sixty-five percent of volunteers were prepared to administer a potentially lethal dose. This shows how people may act when simply "under orders" - a defence put forward at about the same time by Adolph Eichmann in Jerusalem. Until 1944 it was a legitimate defence for Allied soldiers, and it is impossible to doubt that such a defence was changed to illegitimate in anticipation of it being deployed at post-bellum war crimes trials.

The Semitic-looking waif, Hitler, was seen and promoted as an Aryan icon by the Germans, the all-powerful leader of the blond super-race. This certainly suggests simplicity of intellect, an uncritical mindset, but it does not mean that the Germans were mad or stupid. Look at all the other inane notions that have been swallowed by people before and since, from the cynical revenue-gathering witch-hunts of the late Middle Ages to the "Satanic panic" of the 1980s and early 1990s, to the now-discredited yet still defended self-evidently dangerous theory of multiculturalism. What the Satanic panic suggests is that when someone is merely accused of a crime that is, for the moment, regarded as particularly abhorrent, society responds in a hysterical rather than a logical fashion. Other experiments, like Asch's on social conformity, prove that people will agree to what they clearly can see to be wrong, in order to reduce the dissonance of differing with others. Hence it would have been immensely difficult for anyone in Nazi Germany to speak out for the Jews, even without the threat of the Gestapo - look at the pillorying that people who murmur that even alleged child rapists deserve a fair trial may find themselves subject to in Ireland of the twenty-first century. Does this make society's member, society itself, mad?

Was Hitler that bad? He liked children and animals and could be charming even to his enemies - notably, the shrewd Lloyd George was beguiled by him. Though he never forgave Mussolini for forcing him to intervene in Italy's botched invasion of Greece (thereby deferring by a possibly fatal six weeks Hitler's own invasion of Russia), he found sympathy for the old dictator at the end and even treated him with affection, despite Mussolini's terrifying his fellow-dictator with aerobatics (Hitler was a nervous flier). His affection for children and animals proves that he was not the inhuman monster many would believe, but rather in ways as normal as the rest of us - like all hypomanics. His mother's Jewish doctor testified in 1944 that he had never witnessed a young man so grief-stricken as Hitler when his mother died, and his grief for his niece in later years also seems to have been genuine and long-lasting.

But some historians say that Hitler didn't have any close bonds with people and that he was very cold. Rumours have circulated for almost a century about sexual impediments like monorchidism and a micro-penis, as well as copraphilia and other perversions. His biographer, Ian Kershaw, dismisses these claims as being without objective evidence and likely to be politically motivated. But his niece, Geli Raubl, with whom Hitler is said to have had an affair, committed suicide, and his mistress and later wife Eva Braun made two suicide attempts in the 1930s. There seems to have been a darkness in his soul of which he probably was not unaware, as his nickname for himself, Wolfie, suggests, and the *gotterdammerung* of the last dark days in the bunker is well-captured in the film *Downfall*.

Perhaps he had to have an enemy to hate as he had Nazi Germany to love, and by the 19th century anti-Semitism was even more pronounced in Russia and Poland, and even France, than in Germany.

Hitler, however, was specific: he blamed the Jews for the defeat in 1918 and expressed his hatred, his negative id, in the killing of Jews, homosexuals, criminals, gypsies, Slavs and the handicapped. He was a charismatic speechmaker in the early days in beer halls where the atmosphere would have been hypomanic. He developed German hypomanic myths and manipulated the Germans to believe they were the best in the world: the strongest, the fastest, more sexual, more creative and intellectual than any other nation. But of course there was nothing amusing about Hitler. He and Stalin were in a full blown paranoid delusional state as they killed people. They and other dictators, notably Saddam Hussein, seem to have had in common **a manic belief, a paranoia - that fatal combination of the emotions of "anger and fear" - that leads to the "paranoid position" and results in killing without guilt**. Anger and jealousy are emotions that are related to paranoia and then mania and to a lesser extent, I believe, to schizophrenia and, sometimes, religious delusions.

Hitler was jealous of the Jews' wealth and financial power, real or imagined, and of the Allied victory in 1918; Stalin, having seized power himself by ruthless cunning and force, feared losing it in the same way. Hence his otherwise inexplicable purges of 1936-37, when all the Old Bolsheviks and most of his army generals were killed. (When he was visited by top generals and Party members after the German invasion in 1941, he was quietly expecting to be told he had been deposed and was about to be killed. Nothing happened). All three dictators sent their soldiers on what some generals considered suicide missions. All three had no sense of remorse. Saddam and Stalin killed where there was any possibility of threat or dissent including top political and military adversaries and in the case of Saddam his in-laws. Saddam's hero is said to have been Stalin and his favourite film *The Godfather*.

Hitler, Stalin and Saddam were cruel, using Gulags, concentration camps, chemical bombardment of Kurds, or the football stadia mass executions. All three had very efficient propaganda organisations and a personality cult with statues and large pictures of themselves in public and radio and TV programs dominated by their propaganda. All three went on building programs that reflected their egos, not unlike the Pharaohs who built pyramids and statues and went to wars that eventually bankrupted Egypt. Hitler through his propaganda minister Gobbels sold an ideal image of the blue eyed blond haired people singing, dancing, exercising and eating ice-cream like a Coca Cola add. Everything was filmed and speeches were broadcast on cheap radios daily in every house. Despite his nervousness at flying, Hitler canvassed in a way never before, going by plane to 21 cities in seven days.

Hitler exhibits many other characteristics of hypomania. He dabbled in art, perhaps itself indicative of the Creativity manic archetype, but was not a success at it, something that may have channelled his energy into other hypomanic areas. His grandiose ideas indicate the Charisma manic archetype of the messianic delusion and he had enormous plans for Berlin, keeping in regular contact with his architect Albert Speer and together designing and planning the new Germania. In fact, a quick check of the list of hypomanic traits will suggest that Hitler exhibited a large number of these. One was paranoia and barely a year after seizing power he killed Ernest Röhm the head of the S.A. and 100 of his followers who Hitler felt were plotting against him. The injections of amphetamines (speed) that he was given by his personal doctor Theodore Morrel during the Second World War would have led to higher self-esteem, greater energy and more loquacious, irritable and paranoid behaviour (to the extent that near the end he had fits where he would fall to the ground and chew the carpet). But for most of his public life Hitler was a spellbinding orator and an inspiring leader whose very wish was the command to many Germans.

The adaptive side of Hitler's hypomania is shown by his rise from failed artist and lowly trench corporal to become the most powerful man in the world, within a few short years. Extraordinary levels of energy and enthusiasm and a messianic delusion that gave him the faith to move mountains achieved this. Thus he took over the demilitarised Rhineland, in the teeth of not only international opposition, but that of his own generals - and with a tiny force of 25,000 men. Quite extraordinary. Similarly, he was willing to take enormous risk with the Manstein Plan, which successfully broke the Anglo-French forces in 1940, and ended the war in the west in a matter of six weeks. Again, this risk caused consternation among his own generals, and the creativity and daring of sending tanks and mechanised infantry through the broken country of the Ardennes took both friend and foe by surprise.

His great nemesis, Churchill, exhibited a few hypomanic traits of his own. Like Hitler, he dabbled in art. Churchill was famously dogged by depression all his life and was a heavy drinker. Yet he was able, by sheer energy and self-belief, to overcome his depression and, in the eyes of many, save western civilisation from Nazism. But for his inspirational leadership Britain would have capitulated in 1940 - the Foreign Secretary, Lord Halifax, favoured negotiation through Italy. Churchill utterly refused and instead, with the promise only of blood, sweat, tears and toil, he managed to rally a nation of shopkeepers, friendless and alone, to defy and eventually defeat an empire of warriors.

Churchill was uninhibited about changing his mind and his party, crossing the floor from the Conservative to the Liberal benches, and later back again. Nor was he inhibited by the unpopularity of his stance through the Thirties, when, virtually alone, he warned against the Nazi menace and Chamberlain's appeasement policy. As Prime Minister through the war, though in his late sixties, he travelled incessantly to meet Roosevelt and Stalin, and also at home, touring blitzed areas with his famous V-for-victory sign, a respectable version of the two fingers to Hitler. His energy was prodigious, for not only did he become the greatest Briton - in a recent poll - for his role in the war, but he wrote a quite amazing number of books, including multi-volume histories of the Great War and his ancestor, the Duke of Marlborough, and *History of the English Speaking Peoples*, winning the Nobel Prize for Literature. All the time drinking enormous amounts of alcohol. Again, a quick check of the list of manic archetypes will suggest that Churchill displayed several. Brendan Bracken was Churchill's best friend, a spin doctor, Tory MP, Privy councillor, Lord of the admiralty and Minister for information who set up the Financial Times and the Economist to pay Winston's bills and later in life, Winston's books and celebrity tours made him debt free and on death he was worth $7million.

SINN FEIN

Socialism, ostensibly the alternative to capitalism, is also a manic archetype. The socialist is therefore emotionally inclined to mania, and the enduring image of, say, Jim Larkin is one of a man speaking and gesturing with a passion that seems even more manic than Ian Paisley's. Socialism, though, is an emotional delusion, as its failure everywhere, total in the case of the USSR, partial in Britain and China, indicates.

Like nationalism, socialism is a manic archetype as well as a political meme, and is therefore emotionally inclined toward mania; it is an emotional delusion. Even though Gerry Adams denied being a socialist in an interview with *Playboy* (much as he continues to deny IRA membership) the raison d'être of the Provisional IRA is a "United Socialist Republic." This neo–National Socialism leads to the "Paranoid Position" and killing without guilt, as the Seventies and Eighties proved in Northern Ireland.

It is hardly unfair to call Sinn Fein a National Socialist party, given the Fascist characteristics that it displays: the Ireland irredenta fixation, with an appeal to nationalist myth and "the dead generations"; complete intolerance of dissent, and readiness to employ ruthless violence to enforce discipline, with a private army to do so; and the cult of the charismatic leader. While in its republican tradition Sinn Fein eschews anything like sectarianism, and has worked with the Democratic Unionists in Northern Ireland for years, nevertheless they retain a binary attitude: their opponents are ultimately "West Brits", as Martin McGuinness dismissed his critics in the recent presidential election - to criticise is to oppose, and to oppose is to be a tribal enemy. They never speak of "the Republic" in a 26-county sense but in the Republican ideal of an all-Ireland unit - *großireland*.

The aim of Sinn Fein's military wing, the Provisional IRA, is an All-Ireland Socialist Republic, a Nationalist Socialist state in which a quarter of the population would clearly be alienated. The tribal difference between Catholic and Protestant is reflected in the everyday rivalry between Rangers and Celtic, with the addition, in Northern Ireland, of bombs and bullets in the mix. Sinn Fein's aim is as much a manic ideal as was Hitler's ethnically cleansed Germany, and less dangerous than Nazism only because of its comparatively stunted scale but not for long. The political situation in the

Republic is again volatile with financial pressures and a divide between the struggling masses and wealthy bankers and property speculators, social disruption and high emigration - not unlike the scenario that Hitler found in Germany in the early Thirties.

The heightened danger occurs when a meme that lends itself to violence coincides with a manic gene. Paranoia feeds on itself, and the greater the levels of fear, whether generated by paranoia or genuine danger, the more paranoid the sufferer gets. Brendan Hughes, a Belfast IRA commander opposed to the Peace Process, felt that attacks like Loughgall might have been sabotage designed to remove hardliners that might have been against Gerry Adams (Belfast IRA commander) and Martin McGuinness (Derry IRA commander).

Memes, no more than genes, are not immutable. The appearance of the haemophilia gene in the line of Queen Victoria can be more-or-less dated, and it now seems to be dying out; similarly, it would seem that the Sinn Fein meme is being co-opted. Even though Adams and McGuinness have a past (McGuinness was chief of staff in the Derry brigade, Adams, despite denials, a major player in the Belfast IRA) they have been protected by the British establishment so that they can talk peace. The Bishops Gate bomb on 24 April 1993 cost £1 billion and The Canary Warf bomb on 9 Feb 1996 that threatened the city of London as a financial centre and cost £1billion (more than the total cost of all previous bombs during the Troubles) these together changed things fundamentally. After this the I.R.A. sent letters to all the top financial institutions and banks saying they would bomb them out of business in London (as a financial centre) and force them to move to New York, Japan and Frankfurt; this the City of London could not afford or permit. Both militarily and monetarily the IRA could not be beaten. Some people believe that it was the mortar bombing of Heathrow airport in 1993 that resulted in the threat of Lloyds to withdraw insurance cover from the City and also a Japanese bank threatened to withdraw. The bankers backed the Good Friday Agreement and peace became a business decision. The power of the pound ensured success, as it ensures the success or failure of an advertising campaign. The death of Army and RUC members did not matter. Thus everywhere hypomanic factors played a part in both the destruction and the settlement.

Early in Sinn Fein's life de Valera infamously remarked that "the majority has no right to do wrong," and Sinn Fein has always claimed, almost by divine revelation, to know what "right" is. In this it illustrates the parallel between political and religious memes. It would seem likely that, even as education and scientific enlightenment dismisses more and more of, say, the Old Testament, there always remains a hard-core rump of fundamentalists who will believe anything that's in the bible - literally. So, even as the Sinn Fein meme is bred out over the generations - out of Cumman na nGaedhael, Fianna Fail, the Workers' Party - it stubbornly survives, now in the Real and Continuity IRA. The hope may be that the gene pool in which it swims will dry up in the heat of enlightenment. Peter Brookes, a UK minister, gave a speech, a copy of which was given to the IRA beforehand. "We have no selfish strategic or economic interest in Northern Ireland." The go between people who were talking to the IRA for example, Father Duddy put words into IRA mouths that said; "The war is over but we need your help." (A white lie) This brought the UK government into the picture and started off the peace process. Gerry Adams said on TV, "John Hume was serious," "So am I."

RIGHTS AND DUTIES

It is almost trivial to ask if there is more to western civilisation than the endless and aimless pursuit of luxuries and indulgences. A more profound question centres on the concept of freedom, and especially the Western version of it. Perhaps the Chinese sage's Chou En Lai opinion of the impact of the French Revolution on western civilisation is hyperbolic ("It's too early to judge"),[67] but our concept of freedom is actually rather young. Universal male suffrage was granted in Britain as late as 1884 (in rural areas), and female suffrage only arrived in the West in 1919-30 for 30 years of age, and you could be a member of parliament in their twenties (in 1990 in one Swiss canton); blacks were enslaved in the USA until 1865, serfs in bondage in Russia until 1861, and until a few years earlier in parts of the Austrian

---

[67] A less flattering interpretation of this "profound" response is that Mr Chou was aware that any substantial answer to the question might be followed by another question, this one on the Chinese Revolution, and the answer to that might well see him end his days in a re-education camp.

Empire. Until the end of the Great War freedom was conceived as being tightly constrained by "Duty" (it was considered bad form at school, even a caning offence, to spell this word with a lower-case d). Freedom was more or less a by-product of the Enlightenment, and emerged organically and gradually out of it as civilisation itself developed. It was, perhaps, a reward for responsible, constructive behaviour, well expressed in the maxim, "The price of freedom is eternal vigilance."

But in recent decades the notion of freedom as intrinsically sacrosanct has emerged - of a quality so sacred that it is beyond price; even to question its value being a cause for denouncement. Is this a new meme, or an old one showing rapid mutation? In America in particular great lip service is attached to it - to the extent, as the cynical saw has it, that America is determined to give their freedom even to people who don't want it. Freedom is now viewed in a subtle but very different way than it was by our grandparents. Now it is not the reward for good behaviour, so to speak, but an entitlement open to all, and which all, somehow, must share - to the extent that we can often sound like spoiled brats crying for the moon.

Freedom indeed is a great and valuable resource; but as history shows, it is something that is the reward for those who pursue it and act responsibly in holding onto it. To try to "impose" it, as America is doing in Afghanistan and Iraq, is to misunderstand what freedom really is - if not a cynical subterfuge for imperial adventures. A civilisation that advertises and aggressively markets freedom of its own brand, to people of another culture, might be so far wide of the mark that its own destruction might seem inevitable. Not merely is freedom the reward for eternal vigilance against one's enemies - rather than something to propagate to those enemies - but the enemies' own brand of perceived freedom may compel them to fight against the imposition of another's. Particular manifestations of "sacrosanct" individual freedom, such as bare limbs flaunted in the face of religious prohibitions, is an assault on the piety and cultural freedom of another group of people, and one that invites retribution.

Here, de Valera's claim that no man has the right to do wrong in Ireland's cause may be relevant; he defied the democratic mandate for the Treaty on the grounds that it didn't accord enough freedom to the country - as he saw freedom measured - yet he later handed over much potential personal freedom to a de facto theocracy.

As well as being a meme, freedom is a manic archetype: love of the self and love of others. If America is more hypomanic than any other country of the West then one might expect to find the notion of freedom as a pure quality lauded there more than elsewhere. But, as in de Valera's case, the particular vision of freedom is what matters: it must conform to the "popular" vision of what "pure" freedom is: accept our freedom or we'll put you in jail or to death. And always there is a price to pay for our brand of freedom. A century ago this price was the duty to fight, and if necessary die, for King and Country, *Gott und Vaterland*. In Ireland's case the price was economic ruin, political and cultural division (or rather, further division), a heritage of bitterness, and domination by the Catholic Church for decades.

The reality of the Free State's freedom was questionable. It was, to some extent, a sham as nominal political independence was not under-written by economic independence. The new state remained in economic thrall to the British market and when de Valera tried to break this dependency he did so without first finding a substitute market, Britain remaining effectively the only outlet for virtually Ireland's only exports and foreign currency earners: agricultural produce, in particular, live cattle. De Valera tried to make the country self-sufficient, but this could only be done to a limited extent and behind high tariff walls, inside which shoddy products gave Irish manufacturers a bad name at home - there was no export markets for any of their products. Not until the mirage of self-sufficiency was abandoned in 1959 did the country begin to make progress, and only after joining the EEC in 1973 did it begin to prosper - and the price for this prosperity was the sacrifice of part of the country's sovereign freedom.

In the first fifty years at least the Free State, and later the Republic, was as much theocracy as democracy, yet for another country to invade and impose a more "pure" freedom would have been anathema to the notion of freedom itself: if we so desired, we were free to enslave ourselves, to the extent that we did, however that compromised the ideal of "pure" freedom. For an outside power to invade and refuse to leave until, say, the clergy had been removed from influence, would have been an unacceptable and unforgivable act of foreign aggression, however better off the country might have been without a semi-theocratic quasi-dictatorship. Our freedom to go to hell if we so wished was more important than our conforming to any "objective" vision of "pure" freedom.

Freedom, therefore, is an ideal and welcome by-product of civilisation, but a civilisation cannot be built on freedom alone, and especially one that is imposed from outside. Freedom alone may degenerate into chaos, which abolishes freedom. The idealists of 1916, in the name of freedom (and albeit with the unwitting connivance of General Maxwell), inflicted mob rule and anarchy on Ireland, compromising whatever chance a democratically mandated and perhaps more enduring freedom, Home Rule, might have had. Freedom has to exist within framework institutions that demand obedience, such as a constitution or the Ten Commandments, so that the freedom of both the individual and the broader society of which that individual is part is maximised. There has to be a culture therefore that encourages obedience.

Yet the encouragement of obedience may grade into totalitarianism, and to this day the self-appointed custodians of "freedom", "the spirit of 1916" and other such lofty claims, condemn their opponents as "West Brits", as has already been noted, Britain being "the enemy of freedom". For much of Ireland's history this was the case, but one could argue that in the 20th century Britain sought, in the Third Home Rule Bill of 1914 and the Government of Ireland Act of 1920, to give to the Irish people, Nationalist and Unionist, the optimum amount of freedom that was consistent with the mutual suspicions, even paranoia, of the two traditions, and the perceived need in Whitehall to have a secure "back door" against Continental enemies. The Council of Ireland, a component of the 1920 Act, was charged with coordinating governance of Northern and Southern Ireland and gradually seeking to integrate the two.

In this scenario the enemies of real freedom were the "freedom fighters" of 1916 and later years, for they sought to impose their version of freedom on 20 percent of the island's population, by force of arms and a putative appeal to the might of the Second Reich, which in victory would recognise the claims of "the men of 1916". In this we can see elements of revenge for centuries of Catholic oppression as well as pursuit of the ideal of freedom. The rebels' very commitment to a republic has been questioned. Jeremiah O'Donovan, one of the founders of the IRB, which led the Easter Rising, points out that originally this meant the Irish Revolutionary, not Republican, Brotherhood, and according to Desmond FitzGerald, after proclaiming a republic Pat Pearse and Joseph Plunkett discussed an Irish kingdom, offering the throne to the Kaiser's son Joachim. At this time the radical but still-constitutionalist Arthur Griffith was in favour of a dual monarchy, so the rebels' favouring a German prince over the King of Great Britain and Ireland as head of state is not too fantastic.

It is not difficult to see aspects of hypomanic nationalism in the Rising, but there is also hypomania of other kinds. There is a strange sort of fanaticism in the delicate weakling Joe Plunkett being appointed Director of Military Affairs - and in his accepting it. Plunkett was by all accounts a very brave man,[68] despite his debilitation, but courage does not make for a military strategist and according to William T Cosgrave, another IRB man who was "out" in 1916, the rebels' plans were close to "madness". Digging trenches in Stephens Green, where they were overlooked by several storeys, is a particularly striking case in point, and the Green had to be evacuated as soon as the British Army mounted a machinegun in the Shelbourne Hotel.

According to Ezra Pound Yeats had said before 1916 "that Pearse was half cracked and wanted to be hanged. He had Emmet delusions the same as other lunatics think they are Napoleon or God." The entire Pearse family could be said to have been rather strange. Patrick was proud of the fact that he and his siblings came from "widely remote traditions, English and Puritan and mechanic on the one hand, Gaelic and Catholic and peasant on the other", but this dichotomy may have created pressure in the family. [69] The father, James Pearse, was a Birmingham stone mason, a Unitarian turned freethinker and eventually atheist who settled in Dublin in the 1850s and died in 1900. His spiritual journey suggests hypomania - indeed Unitarianism, in its rejection of the Trinity and proto-Humanism, to say nothing of atheism, may be considered hypomanic for that devout time - and he was intellectual and creatively curious about history, politics, religion and philosophy. He was baptised a Catholic, but only to suit the clergy and obtain business as a monumental sculptor in his adopted country. His second wife was much

---

[68] James Connolly is said to have testified in the GPO that Plunkett had "more courage in his little finger" than most men have in their entire bodies.

[69] Cited by Ruth Dudley Edwards in "Patrick Pearse", *Sunday Independent*, 4 April 2016.

younger and a traditional Catholic - who can say what effect such a union, in a time and place when piety was all but ubiquitous, may have had on family dynamics and the moulding of young minds? Possibly immersing himself in Irish mythology, and the simplistic history tracts available at the time, became a distraction or displacement for the growing children.

None of James' second family married and there was an unusually tight bond holding them together. Patrick and Willie often conversed in a strange language they'd used in childhood (teenager language) Lypton Village (U2 group) and Willie was quite pathetically devoted to his big brother. Willie was an art student, and tried to maintain his father's business, but in hero-worshipping style he gave it up to help Patrick at St Enda's school.

It is credibly claimed that Patrick kissed pretty boys on the lips. His poem, "Little Lad of the Tricks", contains the disturbing line, "Raise your comely head/Till I kiss your mouth"; another poem begins, "Why are ye torturing me, O desire of my heart?" One could infer from this evidence that Pearse was a sublimated paedophile, and Thomas Mac Donagh and Joe Plunkett were concerned enough to caution him about such lines. His biographer Ruth Dudley Edwards suggests that Pearse was an "unconscious homosexual" and many historians believe, or suspect, that he died a virgin. It would take a certain innocence to publish such lines as those quoted, and they may have indicated affection and nothing more.

In addition to hypomanic nationalism, it is easy to perceive a distinctly elitist quality to the revolutionaries of that time. The Fenians' founding father, Jeremiah O'Donovan, having been persuaded that he was the descendant of the chieftains of Ross - as, likely, was everyone else in Ross - accorded himself the title *Rossa*. Similarly, a generation or so later, the decidedly wealthy Michael O'Rahilly decided that he was *The* O'Rahilly. Constance Markowitz traded on her husband's bogus claim and passed herself off as *Countess* Markowitz. Such grandiosity suggests hypomania, if not clinical derangement, when these self-appointed elite presume to act without mandate for the ordinary people of Ireland.

There is nothing amusing in their delusions of grandeur. When deluded or unbalanced people assume power the results are seldom pretty. French Revolutionary Terror reached its nadir under the famously-incorruptible

Robespierre, pitiless in his idealism: "Pity is treason". The Irish Citizen Army, ostensibly champions of the ordinary people, murdered in cold blood two unarmed policemen and two Dublin civilians, and their leader, James Connolly, handed over to Mick O'Rahilly a captured policeman with instructions to take the man outside and shoot him; to O'Rahilly's great credit, he let the policeman go. (Another rebel shot him as he was trying to make his escape, and he died of his wounds.)

Such delusions of grandeur and self-elitism survived the Rising. In January 1919 Dan Breen and Sean Treacy took it upon themselves to make war on behalf of the Irish Republic, as Breen later admitted; they had hardly more a mandate than the 1916 rebels, for the Sinn Fein "landslide" of December 1918 was based on just over half the Irish vote, and war had not been on the manifesto - it was to take more than two years for the Dáil to endorse the War of Independence, after murder and atrocity had resulted in the deployment of the Black and Tans and Auxiliary Cadets, and reprisals had become official British policy.

At the end of the War of Independence the Rising's only surviving garrison commander, Eamon de Valera, retained his delusions of grandeur and self-elitism. He denounced the democratic mandate for the Treaty, claiming that "the Irish people have no right to do wrong" - *wrong* being as he perceived it to be. Later, as President of the Free State, he claimed that he merely had to "look into his own heart" to know what was best for the Irish people, further evidence of grandiosity and hypomania.

Such people, when they attain power, may try to subvert other forces, and extend their power. *"L'état, c'est moi"*, famously said Louis XIV, the Sun King, who used his power to build the opulent Versailles and other Parisian palaces and emasculate the power of his nobles. He also made aggrandising war against much of the rest of Europe, as Napoleon would a century later. In Ireland such corruption was less grandiose but it was there. De Valera set up the *Irish Press* with funds he had gathered in the USA for the Irish Republic; one could defend such use if, as de Valera claimed, the paper was to be an organ for the "Republican party" - his own, Fianna Fáil - when others, the *Irish Independent* and *Irish Times*, respectively, were pro- Fine Gael and -Unionist respectively, but he made up the shortfall by selling shares, and ensuring that only 200 (the "B-shares") conferred executive power or paid dividends, while the actual funding was raised by useless "A-shares". National businesses controlled by Government include Bord na Mona, Sugar Beet, Erin Foods, Sweepstakes, New Ireland Insurance.

De Valera set an example for others. The PMPA insurance company was something of a Ponzi scheme that made its founder very wealthy but which the Irish insurance customer eventually had to bail out. The most blatant was the Irish Hospitals Sweepstakes, set up by IRA-man Joe McGrath, who used his gangster connections to sell the scheme abroad, notably in the USA and other countries where such a lottery was illegal. The Sweepstakes made McGrath and his cronies wealthy men.

Quite early in the revolutionary years, de Valera distanced himself from the Edwardian radicals, many of them feminists, Protestants and secularists, who had largely driven the extra-parliamentary independence movement. Alone of the 1916 commanders, he refused to have women in Boland's' Mills, and in government later he allied himself firmly with the Catholic Church. Effectively the Free State became a Catholic state let, not as viciously sectarian as Northern Ireland, but sectarian nevertheless. Divorce was banned in the 1937 constitution and condoms even earlier. They remained illegal in Ireland until the 1980s, and then only on prescription to married people; because the Catholic Church condemned artificial contraception, non-Catholics were compelled by the law of the land to conform to an alien religious doctrine. Likewise, divorce only became available again in 1996.

To an extent de Valera was making a virtue of a necessity: the War of Independence and - much more so - the Civil War brought ruin and destruction on the new state, which was glad to hand over responsibility for health and education to the Catholic nursing and teaching orders. These did sterling work for Ireland, but unsurprisingly there was a quid pro quo, and Ireland's political leaders had to toe the ecclesiastical line. The most telling example is Noel Browne's abandonment of his Mother and Child Scheme in the teeth of opposition by Dr John Charles McQuaid, Archbishop of Dublin. (Though it should be noted that before independence the Irish bishops had successfully opposed the extension of social insurance to Ireland on the same grounds as they opposed Noel Brown's measure: it might give single women unwelcome independence.)

Conservatism is characterised by convention and obedience, the foundation stone of Nazism and Communism alike, any deviation punished perhaps by death. Encouragement and if necessary enforcement of obedience is therefore essential. Whether Hegel actually claimed that Germans would prefer order to injustice is a moot point, but there is some truth in the claim, and this probably helped account for the rise of Nazism.

The Catholic Church's conservatism is of a different order than Nazism's or Communism's, but in the past it was little different - it was in Catholic Venice that the first Jewish ghetto was established in 1516. A core belief of Christianity is free will, but the doctrine that freedom without authority leads to chaos helped establish and sustain papal temporal power. With years of experience the papacy tried to control manic movements, denouncing them as "heresies". Examples range from the Gnostics and Cathars, Troubadours, Manicheans, Knights Templar, Illuminati, right down to the Freemasons, now at any rate a fraternal organisation but still proscribed by Rome - though there is said to be a Vatican lodge. Such political concerns were far from the spiritual ones with which the papacy was ostensibly concerned, and the Church inevitably became corrupt and even manic in its own way.

This corruption eventually was recognised and confronted, but why did the Reformation succeed when it did and not centuries before? The great voyages of discovery, and Marco Polo's adventures earlier, had both revealed to European eyes a wider world and developed new technology to access it, the caravel and galleon in particular. Wider horizons had prompted questioning of received wisdom and the resurrection of ideas of Ptolemy and other Ancient Greeks. The voyages to the Orient had brought back not merely tales of a wider world but also great wealth in the form of silks and spices, and mercantile trade created wealth and power in the Italian city states from whose ports trading missions departed and returned. Surplus wealth made possible sponsorship of artists, who drew on the wider imaginative world to create *objets d'art* of a sort not seen in over a thousand years.

The Renaissance proved not merely the rebirth of classical learning in the 14th and 15th centuries, it indirectly encouraged greater questioning and the emergence of new aesthetics. This in turn led to greater confidence, and the combination of all this with mercantile wealth fostered hypomania - certainly by comparison with the conformity and superstitious fear of the Middle

Ages. Confidence and nonconformity led Jan Huss and later Luther and Calvin to question papal authority, and the very authenticity of the "petrine passage" in the New Testament from which this authority allegedly derived. Hypomania also led to reading of the bible in the vernacular (self-improvement) and singing of hymns by the congregation.

By this time the Renaissance had spread from the Mediterranean to the emerging great naval powers, the Netherlands and England, and the greater distance of these from Rome's temporal authority allowed for greater independence of expression. The Reformation, by and large, had greater success farther from Rome, and in the late 17th and early 18th centuries it was in Protestant countries - France being an exception - that the Enlightenment developed, and this encouraged greater self-responsibility and more trust in science and empirical observation. Technology had been a factor in the Reformation, Gutenberg's printing press allowing for cheap copies of the Bible in the vernacular and rapid propagation of the new ideas, and at the time of the Enlightenment better education and further technological advances permitted even more rapid spread of new ideas.

In the late 19th century cheap paper and almost universal literacy (in Western Europe) led to the "yellow press", which quickly became an important propaganda tool. Bismarck was the first to see the potential and he bribed both German editors and foreign correspondents with the Guelph Fund, underpinned by reparations taken from Hanover after the Austro-Prussian War. Propaganda became increasingly important to Germany after Versailles, when the *Zenstralstelle für Erforschung der Kriegshuldfrage* was established to exonerate Germany of responsibility for the Great War. Later, Göbbels masterfully exploited the relatively new medium, domestic radio, to propagate the Nazi message, while Leni Riefenstahl created impressive, exciting films of German might at the Nuremberg Rallies and the 1936 Olympics. Things had moved a long way from the Vatican's Medieval attempts to control manic movements to twentieth century attempts to direct them toward different ends, and a case can be made that over the centuries hypomania had become more widespread.

It is likely that different but related factors, over the centuries, led to the evolution of a new meme that valued individualism and indeed made individual responsibility for Salvation a virtue. The older meme was one that valued above all prostration of individualism to the will of God as expressed through his high priesthood in Rome. Memes mutate, and sometimes the mutation is adaptive; as with genes, the fittest survive. But as the Nazi era illustrates, maybe the change is not that radical at all: the people obeyed the state now, not the pope, but still out of frenzied fear and faith and hope.

It must not be forgotten that frenzied faith remains a factor in the world today. The Ten Commandments may have ceased to be framework for Western institutions but in a mutated form they underlie the constitution of religious states, as Sharia is in some Muslim countries.

HYPOMANIC HEROES

As early as the late nineteenth century Buffalo Bill's and other travelling Wild West shows were very popular, perhaps proving both a universal capacity for self-delusion and the need for heroes. We still need the myth of heroes and icons to make the movies more interesting, commercial and better entertainment for the audience, and as far as the West is concerned, we have needed it for over a hundred years with criminal accounts expressing paranoia, as far back as Edgar Allen Poe at least.

When people are depressed they have depressing thoughts; when they are manic they have manic thoughts. Emotion dictates thought. Thus to the hypomanic, the cowboy who comes into town and changes things for the better, against the wishes and even the best efforts of the weak majority and/or authorities, is the ideal man.

Alternatively or as well, he may be a fighter, a card-player, or heavy drinker - Victor Mature's portrayal of Doc Holliday in *My Darling Clementine* is of a hard-drinking, fighting gambler who is a magnet to women but who treats these like easily disposable extras to his life. Such men are often sexualised with power to the point where they become dangerous even to their friends and have to leave - riding off into the sunset like Shane to preserve the marital honour of Marianne before his sexual power becomes irresistible. "Often such men, aware of the danger they present to society, may kill themselves to safeguard that society," according to Dr Aidan McGennis.[70] At

---

[70] Late Consultant of Admissions Unit, St Brendan's Hospital, Grangegorman.

times of war, however, they may see themselves as an asset to society—hence, perhaps, at least in part, the decline in the suicide rate during wartime. For example, the "hypomanic hero" of the desert war, T.E. Lawrence, may have committed covert suicide after almost two decades of stultifying peace.

Perhaps indicative of rise in hypomania is the Olympic Games, evolved from the Ancient Greek Games held at Mount Olympus, which go back at least to the eighth century BC. The Christian Emperor, Theodosius I, probably because of their pagan practices, which had manic aspects to them, banned them in AD 393. The games were revived in 1896, in the very middle of the "gay 'Nineties," a manic phase toward the end of the Victorian age.

The idea of representatives of different countries from around the world, playing competitive games, is a manic ideal. It is one that has worked for more than 100 years and survived two world wars. Athletes became heroes of the Cold War, with Russian and American vying to be the best in the world. Heroes in our hypomanic world are often athletes.

Sport cuts across nations class, colour and clan, and thus helps to erode racism. Jesse Owens exposed the bankruptcy of Nazi racial philosophy: a black man, not a blond, blue-eyed Aryan, was the best in the world, in one field at least. At the same time Joe Louis defeated the Aryan champion, Max Schmeling, greatly to Nazi embarrassment and anger.[71] After the war that followed the US armed forces was integrated, and blacks allowed to play professional sports together.

But sporting instincts can find an outing in mania of the most negative sort. Football is one of the biggest if not the biggest sport in the world. From the slums of Rio to the stadia of the World Cup, people are joined in a love of football. Manchester United fan club is believed to number 50 million worldwide.

However, soccer, especially English soccer, is all but synonymous with hooliganism. This hypomanic activity is not restricted to the working class supporters; many well-known hooligans are in middle-class professions, and their activity is often extremely well organised, with use made of the Internet and mobile phones.

---

[71] Schmeling was never a Nazi and in later years he befriended Louis, and even gave him money when Louis was impoverished.

Hypomanic concerns in the arena of sport are evident in the prevalence of advertising, drugs and sponsorship. In turn, this has led to enormous sums being paid to successful athletes, not merely for their achievements - Wayne Rooney earns £300,000 a week, for instance - but for their endorsement of anything from running shoes to razor blades to kitchenware. Some players get over $1 million a week now. Kylian Mbappe earns £1million per week playing for P.S.G.

The end result of commercialisation, paradoxically, may be the end of sport. Athletes are now professional, the Irish rugby team included; perhaps soon even those in the GAA will be as well. Professionalism may lead to the result being what counts, not how the game is played, so performance-enhancing drugs are almost inevitable especially in Russia and America. Such drugs, and the cruelly demanding training schedules, both driving up testosterone levels, lead to dreadful violence, off the field as well as on it, and may also contribute to young men dying of heart failure, a relatively commonplace occurrence now in Ireland alone.

Another hypomanic manifestation of sport is the aggressive defensiveness when there is a conflation with the manic archetype nationalism, i.e. when "our" athletes are accused of drug-taking, as happened in Ireland when Michelle Smyth was so challenged in 1996. Again, we may see here evidence for increased hypomania across society as a whole.

Despite their enormous success, financially and as popular heroes, athletes often prove failures. After scoring a goal in the World Cup in 2009, with his ego high, Cristiano Ronaldo met Paris Hilton but is said to have been too shy to talk, displaying low self-esteem, low self-image, low self-confidence despite his high ego. Alcoholics and addicts tend to have a high ego but a low self-esteem which seems contradictory but the pattern is well-established, Paul Gascoigne being probably the best example from recent times. Boxers are even worse: Joe Louis and Mike Tyson are well-known examples, for whom racial inferiority complex may have been a factor, but the white John L Sullivan, the first athlete to become a millionaire, died with less than ten dollars. The good-looking, glamorous George Best, too, fell victim to alcoholism and failure.

FEAR

Fear keeps people going: fear of loneliness, of debt, of poverty, of death, of standing out in a crowd; the unknown and the unknowable; straying from the beaten path and being forced to conform; separation and agoraphobia; authority and anarchy; doing wrong and being a wimp; paying taxes and not paying taxes. They fear bad Karma, fear fear, fear the feeling of fear (paranoia). They fear the parent and breaking the superego rules. Fear may lead a parent to "beat the child out of a person" through fear of being like a child. Ultimately such fear can breed "the lost adult," who perhaps repeats the cycle with her children.

The experience of overcoming one's fear can lead to the feelings of power and control that may be found in a psychopath. The fearless psychopath doesn't appear to feel pain in the way normal people do and this engenders similarities to the manic creative who along with schizophrenia have a higher pain threshold whereas depressives have a lower level. To such a person everything is possible. There are no rules. He's the best, the quickest, the funniest, the sexiest, the all-powerful God, the Superman, the mad genius, (Nietzsche). Harold Shipman might be a good example, though in ways he was untypical in being middle-class and professional. Many if not most psychopaths come from the working class or are poorly educated, the latter at least in part as a result of their cold detachment, which interferes with their engagement with intellectual matters.

It is also possible that with such acceptance by society of unrestrained sexuality, or perhaps deliberately outrageous behaviour, such as that of Marilyn Manson, may become commonplace, especially in the advertising culture where gimmickry has to get ever more outrageous to make a marketing impact. Eventually such deviant or quasi-deviant behaviour may become so commonplace that society collapses, bereft of any sense of acceptable behaviour, order or discipline, much as the decadent societies of ancient Greece and Rome did. Thus we see further evidence for hypomania: erosion of traditional cultural values and the restraints they formerly imposed, leading to manic-creative advertising in the interests of amoral capitalism, all perhaps leading to, ultimately, paranoia, perhaps, and certainly chaos.

In *The Cultural Revolution: A People's History 1962-1976*, Frank Dikötter describes this chaos, when young people, hypomanically infatuated with Chairman Mao, set out to defend the Communist Revolution, and ended up killing each other in the name of Marxist purity. Up to one in fifty Chinese died in this crazy period, and all were traumatised, to some extent or other.

As well as by this route, anxiety can develop from depression - perhaps at the loss of tradition and traditional values, such indeed as was the case in China after the Communist - as opposed to Cultural - Revolution. In such an unravelling society we may become understandably anxious. Anxiety becomes fear and fear becomes paranoia. Out of the depth of our darkness we become paralysed by fear. In the depressive phase we have anxiety, in the manic phase we have paranoia, but in either case we have fear, which may lead to individual and even social paralysis.

In the religious past fear of anything from societal change to the devil could be assuaged by the priest in confession, or a sympathetic vicar or rabbi (indeed you could buy your way into heaven with indulgences, and people's fears were hyped up to encourage them to do so, thereby increasing Catholic Church revenue), but now few people have that resource.

Fear and worry, though, up to the point at which it becomes debilitating, is natural and adaptive. Desmond Morris, anthropologist and author of *The Naked Ape*, says:

> *We all have the same capacity for worry hard-wired into us. We developed worry about the future thousands of years ago as a way of being prepared for potential threats so that we might overcome them. As cave dwellers, we worried about predators, finding food, tribal relations and the elements. Now we have central heating, supermarkets and no predators, but we have a built-in worry-capacity and nothing specific to focus it most of the time. This leads us to worrying about a myriad of relatively inconsequential things in survival terms, such as our weight, the mortgage or being late for the train.*

Thus we may be genetically predisposed toward anxiety, paranoia, and other manifestations of mania.

COMMUNICATION

The more manic people are the more they talk and express themselves, but - and this is a big but - they don't listen. They have to talk as fast as the ideas come to them. They describe their thoughts as being like a train in their mind going very fast, and out of control. Also, manics remember more, unless their thought processes are complicated by alcohol or other drugs. Cocaine mimics mania.

Sometimes communication by touch is more effective then language. It is the first communication we have, antedating birth, and far antedating mankind, and the most intimate we can have in adulthood, sex. One might say that all other forms of communication are **extensions of this medium, touch. By exposing the skin you get the largest organ (the skin) interacting with the environment and maximally open to various stimuli: heat/cold; pleasure/pain; light touch/deep touch; three-dimensional space (proprioception) two point discrimination; vibration sense**.

Perhaps the main immediately obvious difference between man and the great apes - man has only five percent of his fur - is relevant here: could the high degree of co-operation and communication, that distinguishes man from other animals, have stemmed from this exposure of naked skin to the environment? When there is good stimulation you emote OH, AH, When there is bad stimulation you emote OUCH.

A $\frac{1}{3}$ of sensory touch is in the mouth, tongue, pharynx.

A $\frac{1}{3}$ of motor touch is in the mouth, tongue and pharynx.

A $\frac{1}{3}$ of sensory touch is in the hand.

A $\frac{1}{3}$ of motor touch is in the hand.

This is the basis of language.

As cocaine mimics mania, so other drugs may have an effect here. People who are high are very tactile - Ecstasy is known as "the hug drug" - so hypomania often means greater physical contact (part of the disinhibition process that it leads to). The tiny body hairs - there are 5 million hair follicles on the body - register touch even before skin has touched skin, and the nature of the touch immediately conveys the emotion of the one touching. Thus we might expect that the hypomanic, whose thoughts constantly outrun his powers of speech, would be more tactile than another, "normal," human being.

CIGARETTES/ALCOHOL/COFFEE

Cigarettes punctuate thought, each puff being a full stop, comma or colon. We speak in bursts between sips of coffee and our nicotine hits. The conversation flows between beer and cigarettes. The brain is uninhibited and the stream of consciousness flows until we get drunk and unruly. We switch from wit to sayings to reminiscence to jokes. Bonding takes place with intellectual rigour, the nexus of minds probing the known, the unknown and the unknowable. Sex becomes more probable as people become more forward and women less inhibited, and with more testosterone men become more sexualised. But as more drink is consumed, irritability may come out and people get sensitive, envious or jealous and paranoid. Are these my friends? What did he mean by that? What am I doing here? Thus paranoia and disinhibition may lead to tragedy.

Sex assures one of company; but after alcoholic excess you wake with heightened sensitivity to sound and light and look for the hair of the dog that bit you. Hypomania increases in the morning, i.e. when the alcohol levels are low (Rebound Hypomania) Topping up keeps the alcohol levels up. This is when the hypomanic is most creative: the guitar licks, the vocals, the music, and the lyrics all flow. The brain is pouring out intellect, intuition, synthesis and emotion - the early morning horn.

Cigarettes, alcohol and coffee tend to make the mind manic and mania lowers inhibitions allowing people to voice radical and controversial ideas more easily than they might: democracy is a disease, socialism a sickness, and morality and Christianity mental illnesses. Thus hypomania reinforces itself and undercuts moderating influences. And if fewer cigarettes are being sold, Ireland now has the highest per-capita consumption of alcohol in Europe, and Starbucks has extended its coffee shops to Dublin.

"The coffee trade is worth 3 billion pounds a year in the UK. Its use started in the 1650s in coffee houses and by 1663 there were 80 coffee houses with no drink. In 1697 the Royal Exchange moved to the coffee house Jonathans with lists of stocks and shares behind the bar. It stayed there for 100 years. The modern day UK stock exchange turns over 300 trillion pounds a year."[72]

Functionally, alcohol is a disinhibitor more than a depressant. The first two pints are stimulants. In drink people often say what they mean without caring about what other people think: "In vino veritas". They spend more money and drink more. The gods of capitalism and drunkenness break out. People question the norms and are more exuberant, funnier, and wittier. They have a flow of ideas, inventions and intellectual thought. Thus the old Greek Dionysian festivals involved not just alcohol, but drama and mysticism - actual drunkenness was frowned on at such festivals.

However, Bacchus as well as Dionysus was a god of wine, and the two deities were not merely the same under different names. People may get into trouble with those in authority through drink. Bacchanalian drunkenness is a manifestation of greed, not a drive toward the mystic. People can let their anger out when drunk; they may become more aggressive and obstinate. Violence and crime are associated with working class drinking, but recently in Ireland it has come to involve wealthy middle-class kids as well, for instance the kicking to death of Brian Murphy in 2000. Murphy, like his assailants, was an educated, middle-class young man.

Thus in the Roman era Bacchanalian festivals were banned (186 BC) as a threat to morality and public order. A similar attempt was made with Prohibition in the USA but it was a miserable failure. It, however, constituted an impossible attempt to ban alcohol, rather than festivals.

As a disinhibitor, drink holds obvious appeal to the hypomanic, or anyone leaning toward hypomania. It may thus lead, directly or indirectly, toward hypomania, even if this is on the level where people may "run on drink," using its high calorific content to fuel their bodies in order to keep up with their alcoholically stimulated minds that are hypomanic when people drink to top up where coming off makes them manic. One unit i.e. glass of wine takes an hour to metabolise, 10 pints take 20 hours to metabolise. When you wake up you are buzzing from the night before, more sensitive and creative.

In *The Anatomy of Violence: The Biological Roots of Crime*, Adrian Raine

---

[72] UTV 31 March 2014.

argues is that broken brains are a reality we must recognise, whether their origins are genetic, accidental or social.[73] Twin studies indicate that half of our tendencies to antisocial behaviour come from our genes. Shockingly, Raine shows that the adopted children of criminals are not only far more likely to commit crime than other children, but that the more convictions the biological parents have, the more offending there is in their adopted offspring.

Raine argues, in part, for greater sympathy for those with a genetic predisposition to crime: is it fair to punish someone who, literally, may not be able to help himself? But when Raine started his career in the 1970s, it would have been completely unacceptable to suggest that anyone could have a biological tendency to commit crime. Academics who did so could be hounded out of their jobs. The sociological explanation, that people were purely the products of their environment, was the only permissible one in a world in which Marxism was in the academic ascendant - **Marxism, if it is to have any pretensions to credibility, must pretend that millions of years of evolution can be negated by a couple of generations of instruction in Marxist doctrine**. This approach has done nothing to stem worldwide violence and the physical reality of what goes on within the body can no longer be ignored.

The dangers from ideology were demonstrated when Trofim Lysenko postulated that acquired characteristics can be genetically acquired. This was a throwback to Lamarckism and had been discredited by Darwin's theories and the discoveries of Gregor Mendel. However, Lysenko "proved" that his ideas were congruent with Marxist doctrine, and fear of being seen to be anti-Revolutionary was such that this claim made his ideas sacrosanct. It is said that Stalin scorned Lysenkoism, but such was the power that the idea of the Revolution had attained that even he dared not criticise. Lysenkoism became the foundation of Soviet plant husbandry, and the consequence of that was the eventual all-but-total collapse of Soviet agriculture; the USSR's people came to be dependent on the charity of the EEC, whose beef and butter "mountains" and milk "lakes" went to feed the almost-literally starving. In the old Russian Empire Russia and the Ukraine had fed much of Europe.

---

[73] Reviewed by Jenni Russell, *The Sunday Times*, 2 June 2013.

MEMORY

We mainly remember the good times – "the good old days"; "school days are the best days of your life." To think of good times is good medicine for the soul; but when people are depressed they often find it hard to remember good times, and conversely, **when we are manic our memory works much better**. Also, we remember more when we are happy. We idolise the past in our memories and myths - some old Germans still look back wistfully on the Nazi era of their youth, even as they acknowledge the terrible side of it. It is no coincidence that "Yesterday" by the Beatles is the most recorded song, having been covered by some 5,000 artists.[74] NOVA radio 21st June 2016

Mnemonics of the past heightens the experience of recollection and can become part of our culture; relics are an important part of Catholic culture and were more so in the past, but in today's more secular times holiday souvenirs serve much the same purpose. The past can remind us of our innocence, or perhaps the innocence of others, as when parents save a lock from their child's first haircut.

Like everything else, memory has negative potential too. People may prefer to live in an idealised past than in the challenging present and thus fail to achieve their potential in life, or even run away from it. This very easily can lead to other problems, from loss of job to loss of family and friends, but it can also lay a person open to exploitation by unscrupulous others, who cash in on the person's vulnerability. This was perhaps at its worst in Britain after the Great War, when alleged clairvoyants cashed in on the grief of the bereaved, by putting them in "contact" with a dead relative or friend from happier times. Such charlatans often had a hypomanic or sociopathic streak that blunted the affect of exploiting people who by any standard had suffered enough.

Students sometimes take speed (amphetamine) for exams; it seems to improve memory. It is not known why this is so, but it may be due to increased blood flow in the brain, which might simulate hypomanic activity. Speed improves performance of the small tricky jobs, so memory and intellectual activity may work well together.

---

[74] Radio Nova, 21 June 2016.

People may take drugs because of a predilection to remember "the good things," which may be associated with such drugs. Cocaine, speed and perhaps ecstasy can give people a great rush of well-being, and the tendency to remember things in a similar environment associates drugs with "the good times" and may lead to increased dependency, physical or psychological, on a variety of drugs.

Smart drugs such as modafinil are being used more and more and have a positive and significant affect on cognition. It's been shown to improve the performance of healthy volunteers in several tasks-recalling series of numbers, decision making, problem and spatial among them. Modafinil is the safest smart drug. Long term affects are not known. David Adam Sunday Times 4th February 2018. One in four students, and one in five surgeons take Modafinil

Memory and association can mean that some people only learn if they read material out loud, a recollection of their "good old days" when they chanted aloud as they were reading.

Dementia may affect memory but can be improved by learning a second language, getting eight hours sleep or practising mind games. Useful occupational therapy can be to work with keepsakes, which stimulates memory.[75]

CHILDREN

Children are growing up faster too, affected by hypomania like everyone else. If childhood speeds up too much the children of today may be compromised in their ability to run the society of tomorrow, because childhood prepares us for adulthood by allowing us time to role-play and thus grow into our parents' responsibilities; to learn other life skills by other sorts of play; to learn constructive outlets for our creative endeavours through play alone; to learn social skills through play with others. Thus childhood teaches us how to move from the baby's utterly solipsistic world into the responsible, egalitarian world of a modern democracy. We don't lose our sense of wonder and of fantasy as we grow out of childhood, but we can discern the line

---

[75] "The Truth About Dementia", BBC 1, 24 May 2016.

between this world and the real one.

Children take time to grow into reality. When they are small the division between the objective and the subjective takes a very second place to making sense of their world. I used to think that there were small people in the T.V. who went to sleep every night, or so my father told me. He also told us that big rolls of paper on trucks were giants' toilet rolls. I was scared of earwigs thinking that they might go into my ears. I used to think that the Beatles were ants on the T.V., radio, records and tapes. My brother and his friends had a band and they used to use tennis rackets as guitars and a brush as a microphone. I thought the Beatles lived in a Yellow Submarine. I was very annoyed when I found out that Santa Claus did not exist. "People had lied to me". I had the same problem with God.

People reared without the necessary childhood experiences may have difficulty integrating into a fully socialised adult community - "putting away the things of childhood," in St Paul's expression. They may reject law and order if this comes between them and immediate, full gratification of their "baby's" needs, or if they have failed to learn or been educated in appropriate social responses. They may have problems discerning the boundaries between the real world and the fantasy world.

A strange situation is building up in China, which threatens to exacerbate the undermining of children's ability to grow up responsible adults. Every child allowed by China's strict birth control programme has two parents and four grandparents to spoil and dote on him. The child is treated like a prince, and this spoiled treatment may compromise his ability to perform mundane jobs as an adult. In 2016 it was reported that parents are camping outside the accommodations of their children when these leave for university.

To this dangerous solipsism is going to be added a severe shortage of women. Perhaps recognising the danger here, in November 2013 a new law was passed in China allowing two children per family, but much harm has already been created as an unintended consequence of the birth control programme, and the drama has yet to play out. Because sons are wanted far more than daughters, in this post-peasant society, there have been far more abortions of female foetuses, and the shortage of women is quite likely to lead to sexual competition and aggression, in an already angst-ridden society. Factor in traditional enmity with the Japanese and other neighbours, and a modern variation on the Rape of the Sabine Women could play out in our lifetime.

In the USA, also, many children are not prepared to grow up into mundane occupations. There remains a robust frontier mentality here, but since the late twentieth century there has been a marked turning away from blue-collar work. "Shop" classes have been dropped from many if not most high school curricula, so that those in the traditional trades can command high prices for their services. Simultaneously, technology is moving toward a throw-away economy to compensate: mechanics may be scarce but they are also increasingly specialised. No longer can a home-mechanic open the "hood" and do a routine service on his engine: when he opens the hood there's another cover over his engine and it takes a specialist with a dedicated computer programme to check the car's engine management system.

Thus modern Americans are educated to be helpless in the face of technology, something that produces custom for big business but also undermines the traditional American can-do mentality and creates a sense of alienation in white – notably - working class communities. This sense is exacerbated by the flight of traditional industry to the Far East and Mexico. Thus a "slacker's culture" has emerged, with the first generation that ever has expected to earn less than the one preceding.

The alienation manifests in two ways. There is, firstly, an affluent generation, the children of wealthy people who though they may not be able to find work themselves see themselves manicly as rock stars and film stars. Even of the more responsible young people, many are having an enormously extended adolescence. It is not uncommon for people to stay at home with their parents into their thirties and even longer. In some cases this may be because of an investment in expensive post-graduate education, but in other cases it is to subsidise expensive tastes in clothes, jewellery and other consumer goods.

This phenomenon is also seen in Japan, where young people buy brands, where the proportion of adult children living with their parents is becoming alarmingly high. No less alarming, a great percentage of these young people do not seem to have any sort of sex life.

The alternative manifestation of alienation in the USA is a darker sort. Not only are fewer plumbers, carpenters and mechanics emerging, the urban proletariat is more and more out of work, and the effects of this are backing up into rural America, where a violent vicious drug culture is well established. [76]

HYPOMANIC LOVE

In mania you have self-love and love of others. People feel great and are ecstatic, happy and confident and attracted to other people who are manic. People who are hypomanic often are very attractive: charming, funny, and intellectual; their self-love and love of others is contagious.

In manic society there is an outpouring of love but this love is quick and ephemeral. Sex with the same person gets boring and the more highly sexed will sleep around, mania facilitating encounters and short-circuiting courtship rituals.

It would follow that hypomanics have more children and have them with different partners and the huge increase in illegitimate births and one-parent families provide supportive evidence for this supposition. Often there are many children without a stable father figure and these children will tend to repeat the mistakes of their parents, imitating their role models and having more sexual partners and more adultery and divorce.

Romance is a manic archetype and is associated with spending money: Valentine's Day, "a diamond is forever". In *The Wonderbox* Roman Krznaric claims that love is "one of our most destructive cultural inheritances".[77] He informs us that romantic love was invented towards the end of the first millennium in Persia. It was brought to the west by the Crusaders, and also advanced through the Muslims kingdom of Al-Andalus in Spain. What became known as "courtly love" was celebrated by Andreas Capellanus and other nomadic troubadours who travelled mainly around France in the sixteenth century, and believed in love and unrestrained passion. They were regarded as heretical or semi-heretical in a straight-laced age, and it is tempting to speculate that they were successors to the

---

[76] See the memoir *Hiilbilly Elegy* by JD Vance; the novel *Winter's Bone* by Daniel Woodrell.
[77] See review in the *Irish Times*, by Padraig O'Morain, 22 October 2013.

Dionysians of the Classical age. In Bohemia in the 1400s there were nudist colonies, self love and free love and communal set ups - from which we still have the idea of a Bohemian life style - ultimately broken up by the authorities because it had become a threat to the established order.

That the "will to love" is everything is something one might expect to find more with Bohemians and hypomanics than with a random sample. The idea of courtly love was also advanced much later, through the influence of translations such as Sir Richard Burton's then scandalous *Arabian Nights*. More indigenous versions of the romantic ideal were dissipated through a rise in literacy and demotic literature like Jane Austen's *Pride and Prejudice*.

But popular fiction also portrays the darker and more paranoid aspects of the Id. In *Madame Bovary* Gustave Flaubert describes a wife's unhappy and eventually tragic affair; in *The Kill* Emile Zola writes about rape, murder and incest. Today romantic love is also portrayed in movies and on TV, while drama, fiction, poetry, music and lyrics continue to portray sex and romantic love, often with a grace, jealousy and passion impossible to find in normal human beings. Krznaric writes that romantic love "can usually only be found in our imaginations or on the cinema screen, where we are fed a reassuring diet of intoxicating romances with happy endings".

In the real world, and in literature, Morbid Jealousy is very common, dating back to the Bronze Age at least - Thou shall not covet thy neighbour's wife - and expressed by James Joyce in almost pornographic vividness and more clinically by Freud. The great psychoanalyst forbade his girlfriend from accepting helping male hands on the skating rink lest she be "tainted" by such touch, and the great Irish writer berated bewildered men for, he accused them, having slept with his wife. Mainly against an Italian count who was friendly with his wife Nora. Mormons and Muslims may have a few wives and the latter at least would seem to value sexual pleasure far above romantic love. Islam means peace. Among our nearest cousins the great apes the silverback gorilla, which controls the harem, kills the young that are not his own; this brings the female into heat and aids the new male in spreading his genes. Joyce's main character Leopold Bloom was cuckolded in a way Joyce was scared of.

The New Testament deals with love: "Love your God with all thy strength and all thy might"; "Love thy neighbour as thou loves thyself". Love is the greatest of the virtues. It would seem to have great power for good or ill. It can be seen as a delusion. What keeps people together, love or fear of loneliness or debt? Is it love that has domesticated man? Is it detrimental?

Five hundred years after Bohemia came a similar threat, in a similar guise. The 1960s were the decade of flower power: people believed in the sexual enlightenment that was possible with the development of the contraceptive pill, abortion and the greater availability of modern condoms.

The Sixties was the "golden age" of JFK's Camelot and the great age of hope, with Martin Luther King and marches against American participation in Vietnam and other perceived wrongdoing. LBJ promised a New Society and indeed did much to deliver it, with affirmative action still in place half a century on. The righteous indignation that marked the protesters is an almost clichéd characteristic of adolescence, and though many of the marchers were indeed adolescents, the phenomenon may bear out the onset of extended adolescence, alluded to above.

Marijuana, LSD, speed and heroin became popular in the Sixties "free love" and people experimented with their beliefs and expanded their consciousness, summarised in Timothy Leary's exhortation, "Turn on, tune in, drop out," said to him by Marshall McLuhan over lunch in New York city an expression of hypomanic self-gratification, and in "Leaving the Land of Cockaigne":

> Once syphilis and gonorrhoea had waved and gone away
> We thought the time had surely come for everyone to play
> With no more plagues on men and maids -
> But we had reckoned without AIDS.

The last line is as significant as the poem's title. As Iggy Pop said of the 70's the man with the biggest dick had the most sex. Culture is based on the fear of the man with the biggest dick or the best performance. In 1998 Viagra became available to complement the Pill, so in theory men were now empowered as women had been forty years before.

But the *best performance*, on the species level, is not gauged by the length of coupling. There is a dark side to survival - which is always of the fittest, no matter what faux-liberals may like to think - and there was more to the Sixties than Flower Power and Free Love. The reaction to LBJ and MLK included lynchings such as that of Medgar Evers and the shooting by state troopers of four protesting students at Ohio State University. There were movements both radical and reactionary and those that had elements of both: the Weather Underground; the Symbionese Liberation Army and Charles Manson's murderous Family. Along with Martin Luther King there was the angry Malcolm X and the Black Panthers. There was much against which protestors had to march - My Lai was only the most notorious of atrocities in Vietnam. The struggle of survival of the fittest goes on - across the world, within countries, within communities and across cultures.

There is more to survival than merely passing on our genes in coitus. Sexual activity does not necessarily mean that pregnancy will result, especially in this age of, not merely the Pill, IUD but abortion, effectively on demand, and availed of by approximately 5.000 Irish per year in U.K. In the long term survival of the fittest genes may be better ensured by those individuals who provide nurture and stability for their offspring, rather than by those who merely scatter their seed.

But even if this is true, it does not disprove the case that hypomania can be adaptive. Hypomania has a lot of positive traits that help in survival, notably energy and enthusiasm; it is when it is amplified into mania that chaos arises. There is a gradation from "normality" through hypomania to mania, and one suspects that it is the manic parents who are likely to see their lives and those of their children descend into the sort of chaos which terminates the genetic line.

Hypomanic traits are found in some ten percent of the population, mania only affects one percent and many manics remove themselves from the gene pool, either deliberately or accidentally. However, new medication is now helping people with MDI and they are not as chaotic as in the last century - far less than in the nineteenth century, when at least two people are documented as having died from manic exhaustion in a Kerry hospital. Might this very success in medication lead to a rise in the number of actual manics, as well as hypomanics, in the Brave New World of our children? When manic/hypomanic love is frustrated it turns to irritability and paranoia and sometimes manslaughter.

FLOWER POWER

The 'Sixties were seen as the new Renaissance in which everything was possible. Revolution was in the air; hippies were changing the world and thought they'd soon be running it. As in Bohemia in the fifteenth century, they had free love, nudity, dancing, and now there was drugs: coffees, speed, nicotine, alcohol, hash, LSD, cocaine, heroin - all were trying to get high. Total chaos seemed to be the aim, but in a quaintly anarchic sense, there was love of the world: "I'd like to teach the world to sing," as the New Seekers put it, albeit in the early 'Seventies (which some would claim to be "the real 'Sixties"): "I'd like to see the world for once / Go walking hand in hand." The sentiment of this song sold volumes of Coca-Cola all over the world, proving the universal love of peace magic. Why has it not being been repeated. Hippies were not driven by conformity, but rather a manic urge toward individuality - yet, of course, the hippie became a stereotype.

Hippies represented a manic dream, love of self and love of others. They dressed in comfortable brightly coloured clothes, a manic indicator. Politically they were socialists and anarchists, arguably manic indicators themselves. Music was a driving force among the hippies, as were drugs that helped them expand their horizons.

However, the hippies' pacifist belief that the world's problems would go away if people had a happy childhood in a happy family is a simplistic, manic belief: happy children were far less likely to leave happy families and throw in with the often sordid reality of hippie life. Also, when love of self meets love of others we may get paranoia, another manic trait. The student riots of the sixties came when people gave up on being pacifists and student aggression maniacally clashed with the authorities. Student leaders often become politicians and so were absorbed into the mainstream democratic mode.

Of course, it may also take a manic quality to become a successful politician, as politicians from JFK to Castro to Charlie Haughey would seem to indicate, and many of the neo-hippie leaders became politicians. Danny ("the Red") Cohen Bendit was one of the leaders of the Paris Spring of 1968; like Petra Kelly, he would become a significant force in Green and alternative politics in later decades. But others too made even higher waves. It has been argued that Jacques Derrida and other's of the "French School" developed their postmodernist ideas out of the failure of the Paris Spring; cynics have claimed that their rationale was, "We failed, but that doesn't matter, because there really is no objective reality so it wasn't really failure". If there is any truth in this idea, hippie-dom is alive and well in universities across the world. It takes no great stretch of the imagination to see the hypomania that's in postmodernism.

San Francisco was not the first centre of fashionable anarchy and socialism. The Fabians were hypomanic in many ways, with the sort of dangerous ideas associated more with the political right than the left. Virginia Woolf infamously decreed that those with mental illness should be euthanized; GB Shaw was of the opinion that "The majority of men living in Europe today have no right to be living". George Orwell wrote on Letchworth outside London: "The town attracted every fruit juice drinker, nudist, sandal wearer, sex maniac, Quaker, nature cure quack, pacifist and feminist in England". A temperance pub was there from 1907-1925. Today there is a centre for healthy living that offers yoga, tai chi and promotes vegetarian food, all arguably manic beliefs or traits. The people claim to love and respect each other and tend to be politically correct.[78]

Shaw lived near Letchworth and was attracted by its pacifism. Out of its eight pacifists during the First World War there was a Baptist, a Quaker, a Methodist, a Presbyterian and an Episcopalian, all hypomanic, and apparently attracted toward each other.

Pacifism is arguably a hypomanic trait. Belief that one's own peaceful intentions will be adequate defence against aggression is patently absurd, as GK Chesterton captured in a couplet more than a century ago: "Pale Ebenezer thought it wrong to fight, / But Roaring Bill, who killed him, thought it right". More recently the left has advanced the same sort of policy in CND, as if the West rendering itself defenceless would prevent the Soviets from taking over.

There is often deep inconsistency in hypomanics. The same pacifists who think it wrong to fight may think it admirable to euthanize "imperfect"

---

[78] Hugh O'Shaughnessy, the *Irish Times*, 28 January 2014.

specimens of humanity. In this the pacifist Fabians, some of them anyway, were at one with Eugen Fischer, Josef Mengele and Adolf Hitler.

PORNOGRAPHY

Sexism and racism, very different traits, are also examples of manic paranoiac beliefs, in these cases dysphoric mania. They may feed into yet another form.

Pornography increases testosterone levels but it may stimulate the sex drive in women as well as in men. Though it is mainly a male pastime, it is becoming more commonplace for couples to watch porn. Porn is sexual and is part of the manic archetype of sexual disinhibition.

Some studies suggest that people who look at porn have a better memory. On the face of it this seems doubtful, when we look at where soft port tends to be found, and indeed other studies provide more persuasive evidence to the contrary.[79] Trash papers have Page Three girls and smutty, suggestive headlines; they also have small words and small sentences, whereas broadsheets have bridge and chess and quizzes and crosswords, all requiring greater mental agility and better memory, and no soft porn. In such middle class papers sexual titillation and entertainment are looked down on and politics and intellectual discussion are given high regard.

But in the future even the establishment (middle class) papers may have such soft porn, as society becomes more sexualised. It is not so many years ago since sex was regarded as dirty, not to be discussed in "respectable" company and referred to, if at all in broadsheet newspapers, euphemistically. *Playboy* was introduced to the Republic of Ireland in 1995 having been banned for 36 yrs, but soon Holy Catholic Ireland was selling more risqué and laddish magazines. *Last Tango in Paris* was banned in Ireland in 1972, but forty-odd years later *Fifty Shades of Grey* played to packed houses, and the novel of the film, and its many imitators, became best-sellers.

As Irish Catholics used to be, so Muslims are now - or so it might appear. Muslims are not allowed to depict the human body and women have to cover

---

[79] For example: "Pornographic picture processing interferes with working memory performance", by C Laier, FP Schulte and M Brand; US National Library of Medicine.

themselves up, but this does not mean that they do not have pornography and are not as salacious as any *kaffir*: A Google survey of internet porn traffic shows that the highest consumption is Muslim countries, Pakistan being followed by Egypt and Iran. Muslim suicide bombers are told that they will have 74 virgins in heaven when they detonate their bomb. Islam allows men up to four wives and as many concubines as they wish. All this suggests fixation on sexual pleasure. Victorian men often obtained pornography in Egypt and other Muslim countries, where the "white slave trade", as it was primly called, flourished - as indeed it does today.

Pornography is not new. It was depicted in rooms in Pompey which Picasso visited and on which he based *Mademoiselle de Avigion*, his first cubist painting, and before the Roman Empire it was popular in Ancient Greece. Painters like Egon Scheil (who died at 28 of the influenza outbreak in 1918) and Gustav Klimt his friend were felt to be pornographic in their time; Scheil had his pictures burnt. Salvadore Dali based a lot of his work on masturbation. Surrealism made up by Apollinaire meaning illumination.

In the media of today, MTV is getting more and more sexual. The songs are coming second to the sexuality of the video that is expressed by the performance of scantily-dressed women in seductive and suggestive poses: Madonna, Rihanna, Britney Spears, Kyle Minogue, Jennifer Lopez, Pink, Lady GaGa and Andre Lavine. The Spice girls attracted young girls and showed off their knickers. Younger and younger children are being sexualized earlier and earlier, exposed through TV, film, advertising, music, video and concerts where performers grab their crotches in their dance routines; "twerking" being the latest craze.

High levels of testosterone, dopamine and cortisol are found with highly sexed people, people who are winners (stockbrokers and sportsmen) 2016-10-10 RTE 1 Henry Shefflin, and people who like violent movies. In *The Wolf of Wall Street* daily masturbation, in addition to sexual intercourse with women, is expected of high performers in the stock market. Criminals of every stripe seem to be more highly sexualised than the norm and perhaps to have a higher fertility rate. There is a higher rate of conception among rape victims than normal conceptions,[80] and while this may be due to the aggressive nature of the emotional catastrophe.

An old study in Denmark showed that recidivist rapists did not repeat rape crimes if they were physically castrated. Now we use drug / chemical castration such as Androcur to control sexually perverted criminals, but this is contentious in today's liberal and faux-liberal climate. A school of thought holds that only by reasoning with such offenders can they be rehabilitated.

SEX

Some people believe that if you use pornography to get a sexual thrill you demean your imagination. Some people do not believe in masturbation; they feel it takes away their sexual and creative experience. But pornography is a huge industry, and as we have seen, a very old phenomenon that crosses cultures and may well be most successful in repressed ones. Bob Guccione was the owner of *Penthouse* that in 1971 sold more copies than *Esquire*, *Time*, *Life*, *Newsweek*, *The New Yorker*, *The US News* and *World Report* combined. Its main market was the Puritanical USA.

Playboy sold even more copies than *Penthouse*.

Marilyn Monroe was its first centre fold back in the 50's. Allegedly she had several abortions and slept her way to the top, and she certainly led a promiscuous lifestyle, to which pornography aspires and by which it is inspired in hypomanic ways. *Playboy* also has a lot of jokes that are manic and a history of getting intellectuals to write stories and commentary. When the market turned to video and then the internet the market for men's magazines crashed, and *Playboy* now looks tame, but pornography is more rampant and hypomanic than ever, and the "dark net" allows for the sort of perversions that the "top shelf" could never have held.

Sex in the latter years of Roman civilisation was rampant. Though obviously an essential activity, not merely for the individual's health but for survival of the species, too much emphasis on sex, to the point where it becomes pleasure without responsibility, can be detrimental to society. Sex may be a

---

[80] See, for example, Danielle Dellorto, "Experts: Rape does not lower odds of pregnancy", *CNN Health*, 22 August 2012.

natural appetite but pursuit of it may also constitute abnormality - satyriasis and nymphomania are recognised aberrations, but on a level lower than this sexual activity may indicate a manic archetype. People become more sexualised and disinhibited when they are hypomanic. Such disinhibition and heightened sexual activity can happen with mania-proper, or by taking ecstasy, alcohol, Viagra, cocaine and amphetamines.

Whether pornography leads to abuse of women in prostitution is hard to say but it can lead to women being seen as objects and men in some countries can be found guilty of procuring sexual favours. This very fact, though, may suggest that society is still obsessed with sex, and those who see themselves as its moral guardians, today the PC, are as determined to mind the business and regulate the passions of others as were their puritan ancestors.

Heightened sexuality does not necessarily imply hypomania. Traditionally, the working classes have been least inhibited about sex; they have page 3 in newspapers (before that was stopped by a prurient faux-liberal PC). In Victorian times Freud catered for middle-class women suffering from sexual repression while Jung's more working-class patients tended to have no such hang-ups. Back then, anyway, the middle classes, to risk stereotyping, saw sex as something dirty that needed to be done clean; their preoccupation with this dirtiness, and with cleanliness being next to Godliness, meant that for them sex tend toward being a disorder. The upper classes, by contrast, were innovative and unhibited, almost to the points of being bored by sex. But the class least prone to hypomania is the sexually disinhibited working class.

De Clerambault's syndrome describes a condition of delusional love by the sufferer for a person of "higher rank" - in society, business, or the professions - a love that is not reciprocated. No matter what the evidence, the sufferer believes that the love object loves him or her. The syndrome's love of love can cause pain and ruin marriages. Princess Diana was the most famous sufferer, even though, on the face of things, her status was higher than that of the doctor with whom she was in love.

De Clerambault's syndrome's delusional quality reflects a manic state, and it is unusual in that the delusional love tends to exist without other aspects of mania being manifest, though the delusion may sometimes become more generalised. Some sufferers, for instance, may believe that they have written famous pop songs, and stalk pop stars. Stalkers with de Clerambault's syndrome can be highly dangerous: Jodie Foster's stalker shot President Reagan to gain her attention. They are all the more dangerous because they can be difficult to monitor.

John Lennon said "it was all cock"; Jack Nicholson interjects his conversations with "pussy". These and other everyday examples are evidence of what Freud claimed: that all our drives and needs are directed by sex in a subliminal way. He felt that sex was all. He caused controversy by saying that children had sexual fantasies that directed their actions, the Oedipus and Electra complexes. This suggests that Freud may have been suffering from Morbid Jealousy, like Joyce, two of the greatest intellects of the 20th century.

The casual way in which sex is treated today is a recent phenomenon. Bare female breasts were until long after World War II to be seen only in black-market pornographic magazines - or in *National Geographic* and other scientific journals, which had a sort of polite dispensation to show naked breasts of "savage" and "uncivilised" women, as they might the udders of cows, sure that no white man could possibly be titillated by such images. Today the feminist *Cosmopolitan* and other magazines, and even family newspapers, can deal with female multiple orgasms, sexual positions and even sex toys. The mythical G spot was once a widely discussed phenomenon.

Yet the same old prudery is still there - and even some of the same innocence. A friend had a patient who was pregnant and she did not know how it happened. "We did something up against a wall one night", she eventually recalled. There's an almost schizophrenic attitude toward feminine behaviour in today's "liberal" and "liberated" world. Complaints of sexual harassment are frequently invoked, while feminists insist that women have the right to dress as they like and go where they like so dressed, taking no responsibility for the consequences. They say they dress to please themselves, but one well-regarded study found a strong correlation between the amount of skin on display and pheromone count and expressed readiness for sex in a disco study in Vienna,[81] so "pleasing themselves" includes attracting men by sexual display. Another study reported that women who dressed "primarily for

---

[81] Grammer, Renninger and Fischer, in *Journal of Sex Research* 41 (2004).

comfort and practicality were more self-controlled, dependable and socially well-adjusted". [82] There is something of having one's cake and eating it in insisting on the right to put oneself on sexual display and to avoid responsibility for any of the consequences of such potentially risky behaviour.

In Ireland the widespread incidence of sexual abuse by priests has permanently damaged and disempowered the Church. Since the thirteenth century Roman Catholic priests cannot marry, mainly because their children might have rights over RCC land, but also because sex itself was seen as bad. Celibacy was seen as a higher state than marriage - itself an antidote to "burning", as St Paul saw it - but also as a way of controlling priests and nuns. But sex is as natural as breathing, and enforced celibacy all but ensured perversion. Other countries i.e. Sweden, Denmark and Finland have more liberal laws and attitudes, and these, significantly, are Protestant; the Reformation set out to replace Roman diktat with personal responsibility for salvation.

Roman Catholic priests and nuns tend to have manic traits, which may have impelled them to choose lifestyles of voluntary deprivation, or else developed because they were pressured into adopting such lifestyles (though intelligent maniacs would have been attracted to religious service in other religions). Because these people tend to have no children their genes are lost from the gene pool, and this suggests that since the twelfth century the manic gene has been bred out of the Catholic gene pool to some extent. Because of an association between mania and intelligence it is possible that Catholics in theory have a lower I.Q. But any such speculation must be tempered by the facts that the Catholic gene pool is regularly enriched by conversions, and that a great many Catholic clergy actually do have children. Fr Michael Cleary and Bishop Eamon Casey are notorious Irish examples from recent years, but the prevalence of the names McEntaggart and McEnaspaig - son of the priest and of the bishop, respectively - proves that they are hardly isolated examples.

While sexual repression has led to heartbreak and persecution, it is important to bear in mind that universally enduring attitudes almost had to have

---

[82] Sarasota Journal 38 (1981).

adaptive value. Prejudice and intolerance provided societal negative reinforcement for behaviour that endangered the individual and the tribe, and if they seem cruel to sensitive modern urbane minds, they must not be dismissed as "mindless" - they were no such thing. The welfare state is a very recent development, and before it provided material security a child born out of wedlock was at a very grave disadvantage, as was its mother. The taboo, social as well as religious, against premarital sex, remorselessly enforced, helped safeguard against such disadvantage. It also helped to hold families together: in early Jewish, and in strict Moslem societies today, adulterers were stoned to death.

Similarly, homosexuals were at grave disadvantage as their lifestyles deprived them of children to support them in their old age. Religious taboos were applied, as to heterosexual behaviour, and often even more savagely enforced by people who feared their own homosexual inclinations, or feared the homosexual as "the other".

But evidence also exists that homosexuality was adaptive, if not at the individual, at the group level. Bonobos use sex, homo- and hetero-, as social binders and to placate adversaries, and anthropologists speculate that hunter-gatherers may have done the same. Groups of men on hunting trips, highly-charged with testosterone, may have used homosexual activity as a release, or to establish dominance over rival bands encountered in the field. The latter behaviour would have conserved the gene pool of both groups.

Homosexuality is adopted by otherwise-heterosexual men in prison and in other sexually-deprived situations, such as in the armed forces, where, in the Second World War, some homosexuals were protected by their chums from exposure and persecution, and became unofficial unit mascots. Quentin Crisp reports widespread homosexual activity with American GIs in wartime London. RAF hero Lt Ian Gleed, DSO, DFC, who was killed in action in 1943, was revealed to have been homosexual by one of his former lovers, Christopher Gotch, who dismisses claims that homosexuality undermines morale as "a load of rubbish"; indeed, the Spartans believed that homosexual liaisons reinforced morale.[83]

---

[83] *BBC History Magazine*, February 2012.

In charged situations when men are facing death in combat sexual behaviour becomes notably more promiscuous. Men who were known to be homosexual were surreptitiously approached for sex by heterosexuals when battle was imminent; in both World Wars there was a marked increase in out-of-wedlock pregnancies and venereal diseases, with countless accounts of strangers copulating almost in public view (in the bushes of London public parks at least).

That homosexuals may have had social value in pre-agricultural times is supported by the fact that some American Indian peoples, though not all, regarded them with respect, and endowed them with spiritual power. They were called "two-spirit people", believed to incorporate the spirits of both a man and a woman and as such doubly valuable to a tribe, notably for their hard work and their gifts in caring and artistic endeavours.[84]

There may be a tenuous continuity from there to homosexuality in the Catholic priesthood, though the reasons for the presumed spirituality of priests were founded on the assumption of voluntary celibacy as a lifetime sacrifice to God, and early Church belief that virginity was spiritually good. St Paul famously - or infamously - claimed that "if they cannot control themselves, it is better to marry than to burn with passion",[85] but this is to damn marriage with faint praise. Priesthood celibacy was made mandatory from the Middle Ages by a Church unwilling to see its resources go to supporting the dependents of its ministers, but into modern times, as Irish surnames show, the prohibition was often honoured in the breach.

From 15 to up to 50 percent of priests are estimated to be homosexual, though many are likely to be celibately so. It is easy to see how, especially in less open times, a young man, terrified by his own sexual inclinations, would see the priesthood as a respectable alternative to not marrying, and also make a virtue of the necessity to stay celibate. While the Church officially rejects homosexuality in its ministers, there are claims that it uses guilt as a means

---

[84] Walter L Williams, of the University of South California, writes extensively on this subject.
[85] I Corinthians, 7-9.

of making its homosexual priests better ministers and more loyal to the pope.[86]

The greater acceptance of homosexuality today reflects a wider acceptance of Enlightenment values in a more tolerant society; but toleration may not always be species-adaptive - or even for the good of the individual. The taboo on homosexuality or extramarital sex may no longer make social or adaptive sense, but it clearly did so in the past, and to breach the taboo was not then for society's overall good. Bestiality is rightly taboo, in that it opens the way for cross-species mutation of various diseases - AIDS is rumoured to have so evolved - but bestiality shows are said to be popular in Belgium and perhaps elsewhere, and given the current disjoint between rights and responsibilities, how long before there is a clamour for access to this excess? For years paedophiles have clamoured for the "right" to have sex with children - something that was treated with palpable sympathy by Senator David Norris in an interview with Helen Lucy Burke in 2002: "there is something to be said [for] classic paedophilia" (though he also said that he personally would "not have the slightest interest" in such liaisons).[87]

THE UNITED NATIONS

The UN is a manic ideal: a group of countries, monitoring the world, exercising control. From small to big they have their share of influence, that of some small countries being disproportionate. The UN has its own "army" - peace-keeping forces made up from many countries - deployed notably in Africa, the Balkans, and the Middle East.

Representatives' from 180 countries sitting in one room, discussing the problems of the world, sounds pretty manic. Does the existence of such a group indicate recognition that the world is dangerously manic, and must be monitored, at worst, and protected from its own excesses, at best?

When the last Czar tried to establish the International Court of Justice at The Hague, the gesture was taken as a sign of weakness, and the Court had little

---

[86] More information in Fr Donald Cozzens, *The Changing Face of the Priesthood*, and David Berger, *Der heilige Schein: Ab schwuler Theologe in der katholischen Kirche*.
[87] *Macgill*, January 2002, p. 34; *the journal.ie*, 21 October 2011.

say in the events of the real world of the early twentieth century. But from the principle of arbitration arose the League of Nations and the UN, with peacekeeping forces around the world, and war criminals in the dock.

It is tempting to wonder if the world would ever have lost its Victorian sense of order - a manic-obsessive characteristic - and become the hypomanic place it is, if Serbia's request that the very last point of Austria-Hungary's ultimatum in July 1914 had been referred to The Hague. Thus the Great War, which brought down four empires and an ancient world order, might not have broken out if an arguably manic institution had become involved and people had not been paranoid about it.

AMNESTY INTERNATIONAL

Similarities can be seen between the UN and Amnesty International, a peaceful pressure group that concerns itself with political development in the world. It monitors political prisoners, institutionalised injustice, and oppressive regimes such as East Timor, Iraq, China etc and juntas such as formerly existed in Argentina and Greece.

Like the UN, there is a certain hypomanic quality to Amnesty International: the name *Amnesty* is manic in its own way, as is a world-wide popular peace movement of ordinary people who believe they can affect or even effect global developments, who believe in goodness and forgiveness, but are touched perhaps by paranoia too. Many popular artists, especially bands such as U2, back Amnesty International; they put Amnesty International's address on their album literature and have Amnesty International stands at their gigs.

Recently, I Ireland at any rate, Amnesty International has moved away from its original raison d'être to champion other left-wing causes, such as campaigning against the Eighth Amendment to the Irish constitution and for Ireland to bring in more refugees, arguably hypomanic causes in themselves.

GREENPEACE

Like Amnesty International, Greenpeace is supported by a lot of artists, e.g. U2; it is a popular, not primarily political, movement, another worldwide pacifist organisation, concerned with pollution, conservation of nature and countries' stances on "green" issues, whether it is nuclear bomb testing by France in the Pacific or nuclear electricity generation in Windscale /Sellafield, or "Save the Whales" and wildlife protection. **Its bible is *Gaia* by James Lovelock, a book that sees the planet as a self-regulating organism that controls its own temperature and atmosphere and everything that is affected by these variables - i.e. all life on earth.**

One can discern a microcosm of Global Gaia in the mind as self-regulating when in a state of health. As the planet is in trouble so are many individuals. One USA study indicates that four in every 200 people will deal with psychosis at some stage in their lives; one in 100 with Bipolar 1 or 2 or schizophrenia; one in ten with depression. More will be afflicted with problems of addiction, OCD and other neuroses.[88] In the long term the population always seems to approach the mean between normality and neuroticism, for instance in the Roman Catholic Church where unmarried priests result in the mania being lost to the gene pool.

Green parties have done well in recent elections, notably in Germany and Ireland - though after the financial crash their participation in a disastrous government cost them much support. Among their members are "deep ecologists" who claim that a world consciousness is building and people uniting in protecting nature. This something that no mainstream politician could have done 50 yrs ago, and the acceptability of such ideas may indicate the filling of a post-Christian vacuum in people's minds - the hypomanic appeal of religion remains.

The Greens are in decline since the recession, partly because traditional political parties have now adapted or even usurped strategies concerning Green issues. G7 meetings now discuss Green issues such as global warming. This could not have happened even 20 years ago, but now evidence for climate change is too compelling to ignore.

---

[88] *Aware: Your supporting light through depression*, http://spunout.ie/health/

In New Delhi in November 2016 people were wearing gas masks in a city polluted by manic industrial capitalism. The atmosphere contains 800 dangerous fine particles per cubic metre; the safe level is 60. Children and the elderly are the worst affected and city hospitals are struggling to cope with the endless stream of patients suffering from respiratory ailments. Schools were shut, construction activity stopped, a major power plant was closed and people told to stay at home. Licences of some 200,000 diesel vehicles older than 15 years have been revoked by the authorities.[89]

It would be wise, however, not to see in this evidence for imminent apocalypse - perception of which is hypomanic - for in winter 1952 the same sort of crisis led to hundreds of deaths in London. Then smog containing thousands of tons of sulphur and particulates from coal was trapped under a temperature inversion, and such events were commonplace. The crisis, however, prompted the Clean Air Act and other measures, so that today London air is clean and healthy, and salmon swim up the Thames after an absence of almost 200 years. Thirty years after London's crisis, Ireland suffered something similar, though on a much smaller scale, and again a law was passed mandating the burning of smokeless fuels.

The same could be done in India - in theory. But such anti-pollution measures cost money, and in the post-2008 crash the entire world's economy is increasingly reliant on the printing of paper money and extension of cheap credit. This in itself is hypomanic, and whether it subverts the healthy trust in which economies have flourished for 600 years remains to be seen.

DREAMS

We have on average four dreams a night, but are lucky if we can remember one; memory is aided if we are woken or disturbed while actually dreaming. When dreaming, we get rapid eye movement (REM), penile tumescence (erection in the case of men) and muscular tonus (paralysis) in men and women.

Freud saw dreams as wish fulfilment, the "royal road to the unconscious," and our wishes are our manic ideals. But nobody, from the Prophet Joseph,

---

[89] Rahul Bedi, *The Irish Times*, 9 November 2016.

King David to R.D. Laing, knows what dreams do, or whether they are good to remember and analyse.

One may speculate, though, on whether the extravagant nature of many dreams suggests a hypomanic potential, or quality, in the most normal of us. When people are asked what they would dream of doing or becoming them often says very manic things such as being a musician, writer or dancer, for example - the favourite dream of the English is supposed to be having tea with the Queen. These are very manic ideals, which are almost never realised.

Daydreaming is going figuratively out of our heads, temporarily, and fantasising about life. People daydream about winning the lottery - a one-in-seven-million chance! Such flights of fancy may suggest hypomania in imagining the things they could do with all that money. They imagine what they could spend the money on, and the National Lottery capitalises on such manic daydreaming, with ads for private Edenic islands and hypothetical questions like "What would you do with X million euro?" Expanding one's imagination is fine to a point, but daydreaming to the extent that speculating on the lottery takes higher priority than putting food in their bellies and their children's bellies can clearly be hugely negative, hypomanicly so. I had a patient mother who played the lotto and brought her children up on biscuits and cigarettes.

MUSIC

Music is commonly referred to as the "universal language." Singing heightens the levels of immuno-globulin protein and is associated with a better immune system, emotional arousal, mood, relaxation, and sense of humour. Just listening to music may lead to a tremendous release of endorphins and oxytocin and this release is associated with bonding people together. The parishioners sang more hymns in the vernacular after the start of the Reformation following Bach and Handel and an example was when James Brown was asked to do a concert on the night Martin Luther King was shot in order to keep the blacks off the street. This might reflect an awareness that they would bond in "soul" rather than in outrage.

Music appeals to the manic archetype of love of self and of others: the request to Brown perhaps reflects a dim recognition of this even by the authorities who we might not associate with great musical appreciation. This manic archetype may be seen in virtually any spontaneous display of traditional music, from a crossroads dance to a lone fiddle in rural Ireland of yesteryear, to jungle drumming or an Aborigine blowing on a dijeridoo, and with youngsters smooching at a disco. Music provides the casual listener with self-esteem and confidence-enhancing subliminal powers, which may rise to the point of frenzied dancing or even, in shamanistic ceremonies, falling into a trance. Manic spirituality, such as is seen perhaps at its extreme in black Baptist churches in the Deep South, Pentecostal and Evangelicalisms can manifest in shouting and quite violent movement as the congregation sings hymns. A sense of euphoria and community is evident in such congregations, and may even be felt by onlookers. Perhaps the apostle perceived the value of music when he wrote: "With gratitude in your hearts sing psalms and hymns and inspired songs to God".

We can discern appeal to different social groups in different genres of music. Classical music is associated with the middle classes as is opera.

Jazz is intellectual but was associated with drug abuse, mainly heroin, a century ago, and was perceived as a threat to the social order between the wars. Blues grew out of melancholy ditties of the cottonfields, and reflected the sadness of slave life in the ante-bellum South. Blues and jazz both fed into the post-WWII genre, rock'n'roll, the term a euphemism for sexual activity in blues talk - the rocking and grinding movements of copulation. The coining of the name in the staid late 'Forties may have been euphemistic, but also suggests a gleeful readiness to shock the establishment, and, like jazz earlier, rock'n'roll was perceived as a threat to the social order. Continuing the shock-horror tactics that rock 'n'roll always revelled in, some modern heavy metal bands can be quite Satanic, dysphoric and associated with tattoos and skin piercing; this is not good for impressionable teenagers, and can even lead to Satanic practises, self-harm (cutting of the arms), and suicidal ideation.

More recently rock'n'roll morphed into punk, a part-repudiation of it and of much else by an alienated generation in the depressed Britain of the 1970s. In their names and titles the punks set out to shock: Johnny Rotten and the Sex Pistols; the Stranglers. Their music was often deliberately grotesque, as well as anarchistic: the Sex Pistols' "God Save the Queen" and "Anarchy in the

UK", but they struck a chord with the disillusioned youth of the Callaghan and Thatcher eras.

The punk era soured after the death of Sid Vicious, and the later death of Kurt Cobain (1994) all but marked its end. It was overlapped and succeeded by the cloying disco craze. Many of the punks mellowed - Sting; Elvis Costello - but music found another way of appealing to disillusioned youth in the 1990s: rap. This was associated with gangs, especially black ghetto gangs, and they emulate prison garb with sagging trousers without belts, and lace-less shoes. Rap's lyrics are violent, while the beat is monotonous and menacing.

Music, and in particular rap, is becoming steadily more manic, as demonstrated by:

- More beats - up from approximately 120 to 150 per minute over the past ten years. This is related in part to the use of ecstasy in clubs and raves, giving people the energy to dance all night, making them feel happy, and leading them typically to describe their first trip as "the best thing that's ever happened to me." The disco beat is marked by a monotonous fast rhythm, with a strong bass. Earlier, aficionados of aggressive rock 'n roll with a similar monotonous beat were known as "head-bangers," perhaps a subconscious recognition of the mania at work.

- More graphically portrayed sexuality in the lyric and emotion, the accompanying dance movements and dress of many of the musicians in pop music that sexualise young people.

- A greater sense of spirituality.

But a more benevolent side is also evident. Music cannot change the world but it can inspire people to have a go: Woodie Guthrie sang about the problems of the dispossessed migrants in the Depression. He had Huntington's Chorea, a genetic syndrome that leads to depression and suicide and may have coloured his view of the world - though this was grim enough in the 1930s - and his music raised awareness of the Okies and Arkies and Mexican migrant workers, who took the brunt of the hard times. More recently Bruce Springsteen revisited the music of this time, perhaps with particular poignancy in "My Oklahoma Home", written by veteran American

Communist Cis Cunningham, about an Okie homesteader who falls victim to soil erosion and grasping banks.

Yet the hypomanic side of things cannot be discounted even here. U2 are involved with Greenpeace and Amnesty International and the problems of international debt; Bob Geldof set out to "feed the world" with Band Aid in 1985; George Harrison and friends had a benefit concert for the emergent Bangla Desh in 1971. While laudable, such ambitious undertakings suggest a manic or egotistical aspect that may blind the visionary to darker aspects of the undertaking. "We got a million off the Saudis!" shouted Geldof excitedly, losing sight of the facts that a million is small change to the Saud royal family.

Besides, while emotional engagement with any issue can generate enthusiasm and hard work - especially if the person so engaged is hypomanic - any long-term solution is more likely to become from intellectual engagement, and demographics and global resources demand *reduction* in population. In 1985, at the time of the famine, Ethiopia had a population of 40 million; thirty years later the population is over 94 million, and resources have been depleted in the meantime. While none could condone the drastic Malthusian measure of famine, ultimately controls will be imposed, some way. Band Aid was ironically no more than a Band-Aid on a haemorrhage.

Another uncomfortable fact about Band Aid is that a huge amount of the money raised for famine relief went to one of the rebel groups whose activities had contributed to the country's food shortage: up to $95 million may have been paid to the Marxist Tigrayan People's Liberation Front.[90]

We saw something similar in September 2015 when the corpse of a Syrian refugee child, Aylan Kurdi, was shown washed up on a beach in Greece. There was understandable emotional reaction, and two days later Angela Merkel unilaterally invited into Europe all Syrian refugees. The result was havoc at various borders, suspension of the Schengen and Dublin Agreements, and convenient cover for Islamist terrorists to infiltrate Europe. The ultimate result of all this may be collapse of the EU, because emotional reaction was allowed to supersede critical thinking. Any student of coastal

---

[90] Martin Plaut, "Ethiopia Famine Aid 'spent on weapons'"; BBC World Service, 3 March 2010.

geomorphology and wave action could have seen that the child's corpse was probably posed in a way to elicit emotional engagement, and ensure worldwide coverage of the photograph and propagation of the photographer's fame. (Wave dynamics would have rolled the corpse and almost inevitably extended the limbs, and the interplay of swash and backwash on the beach would have left the corpse at an angle other than the one in which it was photographed.)

The emotional reaction to human misery is natural and instinctive, and none would condemn the sense of outrage that decent people feel at sight of the starving, the desperate or the drowned. But while emotion can provide a very powerful point of engagement with a problem, it can get in the way of solving that problem. Problems are solved with intellectual rather than emotional application; emotional engagement can rather blind one to the best solution - insofar as there may be any solution.

The hypomania of any ideologue, however, favours emotional rather than intellectual engagement, because it's the emotional charge that mostly drives hypomania, and this factor tends to be exacerbated, nowadays, by the prevalence of fashionably-leftist thinking. This in turn is exploited by revolutionary elements who on the one hand exploit any situation in order to encourage disaffection, and on the other promise a Workers' Utopia after the revolution. The lyrics of John Lennon's "Imagine" indicates an idyllic view that few would argue is not hypomanic, and is certainly a post-Christian, post-Western Civilisation, Marxist world.

The danger from revolution is heightened by the infantilising of society in the past generation or so. People speak of "generation snowflake", young people who have been spoiled and never wanted for anything, and whose expectations are both unrealistic and immediate. Increasingly this generation is finding it harder to find work, and the level of independent living, in the USA, has gone down by some 5 percentage points in the past decade; the level in Japan is even higher. Many of these young people fail to develop emotionally, and this stunting can be aggravated by failure to have their expectations met; this can lead to resentment and, possibly, a paranoiac suspicion that "someone" is denying them their "rights". Thus a negative feedback loop is reinforced, and the naive belief that rights can exist independently of responsibilities makes the problem yet worse, and can leave a young person vulnerable to subversive propaganda.

A very different aspect of hypomania can be observed at any disco, which, with its musical beats and lights flashing in different colours, is exciting and sexy, along with wine, drugs, laughter, humour and suggestive talk. And then there are the girls, moving in unison to the manic high in tight or skimpy clothes. They're like birds preening their feathers, showing off the colours in the sexual dance of attraction before mating. In the rave culture people take Ecstasy and their heart rate goes up; they dance all night and feel brilliant: "The best time I've ever had," is a typical report after the first ecstasy tablet.

Dance is part of the physical manic archetype. Like music, it is creative and sexual. Both can be intellectual (ballet) and sexy (jazz). However, music has developed into a narcissistic culture, which of course appeals to generation snowflake: "I'm the greatest guy on earth" is the line of a song by the band Wheezer, a line that expresses both hypomania and the views of generation snowflake. People sing of *me* and *I* and less of *we* and *us* or *you*.

It would be very unfair to suggest that generation snowflake is responsible for this narcissism. That generation hadn't been conceived when the Boomtown Rats were singing "Looking After Number One" and Tina Turner's "Simply the Best" was adopted by hypomanic Loyalist killer Johnny "Mad Dog" Adair as his personal anthem. With "Private dancer" Turner got more sexual in her lyrics and many other singers did the same. Songs about following your dream are as old as song-writing, and "normal" people can think they're the best (grandiose delusions), but they soon grow up and lose their illusions. The way in which *some* of the "slacker generation" get frustrated and aggressive when they are reality checked and life does not work they have complacently imagined suggests that the *generation snowflake* epithet may have some validity.

ENTERTAINMENT

Shows are manic, the more manic the better: the music, the colour, the lights, beats per minute (this has increased from 120 BPM to180 BPM), while guns and all but overt sex have become part of the performance - and videos - Madonna being perhaps the best exponent but hardly the only one; Britney

Spears, Lady Gaga, Rhianna, and Beyonce have all followed her lead, and even creaky old Tina Turner got in on the act.

Ireland's *Late Late Show* was so successful in part because it was hypomanic. Gay Byrne was charismatic, obsessive and willing to question people about things that were not normally talked about at the time i.e. religion, sex, contraception, divorce and the infamous "Bishop and the Nightie" episode. Reviewing these early episodes one marvels that they could have aroused such controversy and outrage, but Ireland was a different place then and the Late Late helped change it. The show is poor today, arguably pathetic, but it still has humour, music, gossip, intellectual stimulation and, occasionally, (relatively) shocking guests.

The entertainer is a very important person and can sway public opinion, as we saw with the many Hollywood stars who campaigned, and continue to campaign, against Donald Trump. The entertainer's importance goes back to at least King David who used to be a musician in the court of King Saul, and in medieval times the court jester could be a powerful figure at court; possibly his importance went back to when the fool became king for a day and was sacrificed to the earth gods to help ensure good harvests, endowing him with a sacred role, and certainly part of his role remained to remind the king of his own mortality.

The entertainer gets a high from being on stage, where he expresses the manic archetype. Robbie Williams is a good example of the complexity of hypomania. He is good looking, comedic and very charismatic and he writes good lyrics. However, he often gets mildly depressed after the hit of the show and had to cut back on the drugs and alcohol he was abusing.

Here we see part of the price the successful hypomanic entertainer pays. Many entertainers have been bipolar, swinging wildly from creative high to wretched low. Examples include Spike Milligan and John Cleese and Robin Williams, described by music journalist and DJ Dave Fanning as the funniest person he had ever met. But Williams - and others - were not universally liked, their brand of comedy striking some people as just not funny, while their mannerisms and behaviour grate with others.

Entertainers often have problems with their ego. It takes a strong ego to become an entertainer anyway, and many, like Bono, are highly intelligent;

Bono is also grounded enough to return to his family for tea after performing in a packed stadium at Croke Park. But toadies tell them all the time that they are great, so that eventually they may believe the hype. Lead singers often get "Lead Vocalitis"; they look down on the rest of the crowd and often on other band members.

The successful entertainer does not let either ego or drugs control him, but in part because they are addicted to the hit of performing some may take drugs to keep the hit up; or they may turn to drugs to fuel the hypomanic energy that drives them - or to anesthetise feelings of failure, unworthiness, self-doubt or the underlying pain of depression. Perhaps underlying depression is in part what drives some to find and exaggerate the amusing aspects of existence: Tony Hancock's brand of humour was essentially very dark, however funny, and one of his punch lines was "You're all raving mad!"

Evidence for increased hypomania may be seen in the limited comeback in vinyl records. Vinyl registers sound waves that are lost on CDs, and while we might not consciously hear them they are registered by the brain. Vinyl therefore may be more stimulating of areas that are relaxing on a subconscious level.

ELVIS

Elvis is still known, as he was in life, as "the King". He was handsome, sexualised, and charismatic and he became a manic leader as King of rock 'n' roll, but perhaps of other things too: the modern, hedonistic, sexualised, hypomanic age, perhaps?

Elvis was the greatest living exponent of the rock 'n' roll popular movement, into which we might say the original rock 'n' roll music had metamorphosed. He was a white man singing black songs, shocking in the era of Jim Crow, and the sexuality of his voice and his stage theatrics made the girls scream, their responses simulating orgasm. One expected such animalism from what was then called negroes - and niggers - but not from respectable white girls. So much did Elvis put sex into rock n' roll that in his early days TV stations would only show his dancing from the belt up.

Elvis is a major icon of the twentieth century. He lived fast, died young and had a good-looking corpse - or would have had he not gorged on deep fried bananas and peanut butter. Ignoring the danger overeating meant to his health was not the only sign of his hypomanic activity. His twin brother died at birth, and he used to talk to his ghost. He sang manic paranoid songs such as "Suspicious minds" and "Baby, Let's play house", which included the line "I'd rather you dead little girl than be with another man". Though Elvis co-wrote very few songs he could sing and act, making several movies and following, at times, a hectic schedule, perhaps the sort of hypomanic activity necessary for modern entertainers to maintain. His schedule might have been even more demanding had his manager, Colonel Parker, not felt vulnerable to arrest in his native Netherlands - where he was a "person of interest" in a murder - so could not facilitate Elvis to tour Europe.

The Religious Right said that Elvis was evil and that rock 'n' roll was the "Devil's music." It is interesting to note how the Christian devil is most closely modelled on the Greek god Pan, from which the word panic, denoting hypomanic frenzy, is derived, and how Elvis - and after him, other rock n' rollers - inspired such hypomanic frenzy at their concerts.

ROMAN ORGIES

Pan was not the only inspiration of hypomania in the Ancient World. There were a lot of bars at the end of Roman civilisation, as well as brothels, whose mosaic sign was an erect penis, as may be seen in Pompeii to this day, preserved by volcanic ash. Orgies were commonplace, fed by food, alcohol and other drugs, the need for more and "better" sex, more and varied partners, hypersexuality being typical of hypomania, and carried over from the last days of Ancient Greece. There was wife swapping and incest, as in the case of Caligula and his family, and the breaching of many taboos, while circus games were organised to keep the plebeians at bay, and Caesar played to the crowd.

Modern-day sport developed in part for the same reason. The Marquis of Queensbury may have refined the rules, so that boxing is less bloody, and deaths in the ring uncommon, but a continuity with the Ancient World is evident, and men like Joe Frazier, their battered faces stoic in their corners between rounds, might have modelled for the Hellenist sculptor of *The Pugilist at Rest*. A great many people go to boxing matches, and to car- and motorcycle races, hoping to see carnage. Youtube is filled with clips that cater to this bloodthirsty craving.

Hypomanic decadence is evident in other ways in our own times. Gluttony and lust have always been powerful human appetites, and indulged in since the fall of Rome, even conspicuously, but today sex has become all but a spectator sport. Marriage breakdowns follow from infidelity and "swinging" lifestyles and online sex, and the "paralysis of choice" that internet dating offers leads men, in particular, to make their choices of supposedly-life partners on the basis of looks alone. The now-ubiquitous on-line porn, and even non-X-rated films, present unrealistically idealised sex and sexual performance as normal, and Viagra and other drugs offer the means to live up to artificial expectations. Ultimately, of course, everyone comes up against reality, but in the interim pursuit of the unreal causes huge heartache and disappointment.

Violence is as characteristic of hypomanic modernity as performance-sex. It often stems from intoxication, which is far more commonplace than formerly, given the low cost of alcohol and tolerance of public drunkenness. Intoxication infamously lowers inhibitions and distorts one's perception of reality, so fights become much more likely, and increasingly these are likely to involve knives or other weapons, as the hypomanic tempo picks up and young men perceive the need to be prepared for any eventuality - an arms-race in microcosm. Even without weapons fights can be fatal, one-punch fights often resulting in a man, already half-unconscious from drink, dropping to the ground with no means of protecting his head - the consequent blows suffered are becoming more commonplace, and may also follow simply from falling over, without violence.

Along with heavy drinking goes junk food binging, with obesity a major problem in the USA and quickly becoming one here. In the 1960's and 70's fat was blamed for obesity but it would seem now that sugar caused more trouble than fat. Six teaspoons of sugar used to be the average daily intake but in Ireland we now consume 25 teaspoons a day - there are eight in each can of Coke.[91]

Meanwhile, the excluded "barbarians" - Islamic fundamentalists, in this case - bide their time, hungry, fit and envious, beyond the Rhine - or rather, the Mediterranean, this time. Drugs and terrorism can be found hand in hand. Two different forms of hypomania seem set to clash and perhaps throw the whole world, not just Europe this time, into a new Dark Age.

ICONS

The more complicated society gets the more basic it becomes, in that it facilitates the availability of more and zanier icons to more and more people. Thus the Internet has made available the terrorist Bin Laden as an icon of freedom and heroism to millions of Muslims across the world.

When we repeatedly see people on TV or read about them in the papers, or listen to them on the radio and see them on the cover of magazines or posters in the street, we unconsciously tend to make icons of them and remember their names. We believe that their fame somehow makes them important, that they know better than us - may even be above the law - even if they are only vacuous reality TV stars. The cult of the leader was deliberately fostered in totalitarian states - Hitler, Mussolini, Stalin, Lenin, Mao - but in liberal democracies we have had the likes of John Lennon, Kurt Cobain, James Dean and JF Kennedy. We revere the dead, especially those who die young; we look up to them and aspire to their God-like status above us. Thus we tend to sanction corruption, or even robbery (Ronnie Biggs) and murder (Oscar Pistorious), if done by them or what they represent: there was relatively little condemnation of Ronald Reagan's illegal war on the Sandinista regime in Nicaragua, and Colonel Oliver North actually was a hero, despite his role in the drugs-for-arms scandal of that time.

This is a dangerous position in peace but even more so in times of war, when we tend to lose control of our critical senses and become atavistic. We regress to the id state of the spoilt child or starving adult, eating when hungry, not waiting for mealtimes. One can perhaps see this behaviour in the

---

[91] The *Irish Times*, January 2017.

election of Donald Trump, an icon of reality TV, and a dry-drunk for 30 years; he gave up drink after his brother died at 45 due to alcohol abuse. Trump's 2016 victory came down to fewer than 80,000 votes across three swing states. Trump's narcissism is all but legendary, and his rudeness reminds us of teenage louts'; but we might better look to the starving adult if we are to find an answer to why people chose him to represent them. Trump's constituency comprised in good part those whose jobs and livelihoods had gone, and he promised these back, along with restoration of American greatness. Here we see another hypomanic aspiration, along with xenophobia and paranoia: foreigners are taking over our jobs, seducing our women and trying to destroy our culture.

Trump's defeated rival provides another example of hypomania, if in different manifestation. Hillary Clinton has been an icon for decades, the good-looking glamorous consort of the most powerful man in the world through the 1990s, and an iconic feminist who broke through the "glass ceiling" when appointed Secretary of State by Barak Obama. In this role, however, she performed poorly, notably by advocating American interference in Libya. Fortunately Obama rejected her advice to establish a no-fly zone over Syria; such a move would have been a challenge to Russia and the consequence would have been either a major international incident or exposure of the USA as a paper tiger.

Such reckless behaviour suggests a sort of sophomoric hypomania, where fools rush in, full of adolescent bravado and overconfidence. Being lauded as a feminist and liberal champion must have heightened the rush, and given Clinton an arrogant sense of invincibility that led her to denounce people whose votes she needed if she were to win the election her hypomania deluded her into believing was hers by right.

Part of the reason Trump won was the complacent arrogance that stems from having "experts" on our team. We fall for the false-authority fallacy and forget that our opponents also have "experts" and that the reason why our "experts" say we're right is because we pay them to do so. If they said otherwise we'd hire others who would reinforce our hypomanic delusions. It was "experts" who were in charge of eugenics departments in universities all over the world a century ago, and those same experts endorsed Nazi pseudo-science, but for Michael Gove to say that "The people have had enough of experts" is enough to have him denounced as reckless and irresponsible. This he may well be, but presuming that experts are always right is hardly less so.

We would be wise to withhold critical judgement of our icons and look to our narcissism and our paranoia, rather than denounce those who disagree with us as stupid, fascist, racist and whatever other nasty names we call them in our hypomanic rage.

CENSORSHIP

The censor tries to control manic material such as sexually disinhibited material or gratuitous violence. The church, and later the state, used to have a lot of say in censorship - *The Life of Brian* by the Monty Python team was banned in Ireland for ten years, something that now seems bizarre if not quite a matter for concern, but in previous years great works of art such as *Ulysses* and *Lady Chatterley's Lover* were also banned under a puritan ethos. Philip Larkin said that sex started between the banning of *Lady's Chatterley's Lover* and the emergence of the Beatles.

Censorship is increasingly redundant; not merely changed attitudes, but new technology, the Internet, makes it almost impossible to enforce. However, people may need to be shielded from very violent films, as there is evidence they lead to a more violent culture, while in a separate yet connected concern, the internet may lead to mania and chaos.

In his book, *On Killing*, Lieutenant-Colonel David Grossman makes a persuasive case that the portrayal of violence in films, and even more so the desensitisation of people to murder by means of video games, is directly related to the frightening upsurge in violence over recent decades. The very games our children play for entertainment were designed to increase the "hit rate" of professional soldiers, after it emerged in the wake of the Korean War that a deep-seated taboo against murder meant that three in four soldiers shot over the enemy's head. Subsequent studies of all wars fought since the American Civil War support this statistic. The very video games our children play from kindergarten now "is one of the key ingredients in a methodology that has raised the [shoot-to-kill] firing rate from 15 to 20 percent in World War II to 90 to 95 97 percent in [the] Vietnam [War]".[92]

There used to be something obscene in violence - or at least in people's indulging in the portrayal of it. Newspapers used to spare their readers the more graphic details; now, in the struggle for sales, almost anything goes. Working class tabloids use small words and short sentences and cover crime, celebrity and pornography whereas broadsheets and tabloids like the *Independent* and *Irish Independent* have no pornography but cover politics, law, biography foreign policy, financial policy and business in more sophisticated English.

Here is another aspect of hypomania: our fascination with violence and the increasingly eroded bulwarks of decency and responsibility that used to prevent us from imaginatively engaging with it. We have become voyeuristic. Pornography has exploded on the Internet, to the extent that perhaps 35 percent of web searches are for porn sites, and paedophilia is an ever-present threat to our children. The fact that porn is now available on mobile phones means that parental supervision of the home computer may be easily evaded, and paedophiles may easily access children.

Voyeurism of another sort has also spread. At one time respect for public figures was such that, say, the sexual affairs of Roosevelt or Kennedy were never reported - even Roosevelt's polio was never, but once, revealed on screen. Now the paparazzi feel they have some sort of right to invade the most intimate privacy of public figures. And sadly, the public gets prurient thrills out of reading or seeing what would have deeply embarrassed their parents and grandparents.

Thus, in view of all the dangers, especially from the glorification of violence and the blunting of sensitivity that goes with that, there would seem to be a need for some censorship. But apart from any idealistic objection, there is now the practical impossibility of imposing any such control. Again, the self-indulgence, impatience with any form of restraint, demand for immediate gratification to the exclusion of any consideration for the future, betrays a hypomanic society.

---

[92] Lt-Col David Grossman, op cit, pp. 313-14.

FASHION

Fashion is a multimillion dollar industry, essentially concerned with glamour: furs and frills and ostrich feathers; colour, lights, sex and music on the catwalk. Such a fixation suggests either hypomania or an appeal to this. The rich play games of vanity, a lifestyle of Volvo cars and 2.3 children being endorsed by the perfect, smiling - or sulkily assured - models on display. Such vanity extends from accessories to the human body with face-lifts, nose corrections, and breast-augmentations. Even the language of fashion is manic. Fashion magazines try to make you high (by highlighting sexual attraction and sexuality) and make you want to buy something. People think of family and friends and how they would look before them. Sports, trends: do I fit in? I wear Yves St. Laurent! We try to look young and healthy and successful.

Music people want to be different and at the moment music is probably the most hypomanic of the arts. Musicians are creative and do not want to look like other people. They often wear a lot of coloured clothes and accessories and since the early 1970s "glam rock" stars like Marc Bolan and David Bowie use brightly coloured make-up. But paradoxically, in "not looking like others," they look more and more like their peers for the same drive is at work with them as with everyone else: the urge to look successful, glamorous (however glamour is measured in their worlds), "fashionable."

Clothes are an expression of our mood and of our thought pattern. When people are manic they wear brightly coloured clothes. They also wear a lot of makeup, red lipstick being perhaps most strikingly hypomanic. When people are attracted to each other their heart rate increases but more obviously, however subtly, so do their pupils. In the last century women used belladonna to dilate their pupils and thus make themselves more attractive. The beauty spot, favoured by Marilyn Monroe and Cindy Crawford, constitutes an artificial third pupil and further focuses attention on the face.

The French are very particular about their clothes, parading on the Champs Élysées and in restaurants and bars, and Parisian fashion has for centuries set the world standard. This may reflect a certain hypomania in the national character, expressed also in flair and panache and exaggeration of gesture and expression. It also is based on the Bourbon tradition, which created a whole industry in Paris to cater for the court at Versailles, but perhaps it took a certain national hypomania to establish and maintain Versailles. Fixation on fashion has generalised: slogans like "Because you're worth it" and "The best a man can get" suggest hypomania and when Diana Ross does a concert she changes her clothes about ten times during a two-hour concert.

Clothes and dressing comes from the creative right brain and have further biology connection: if you want to stand out you should wear clothes that are the same colour as your eyes. Red, black and white in combination make the most striking colours; these were the colours of Prussia and later of the Second Reich, and Hitler incorporated them into the swastika flag of the Third Reich.

Whether it is clothes make up or hairdressing, people enjoy shopping for clothes and when they feel low they get their hair done, or have some other appearance enhancement lift their mood; the term *facelift* is both literally and emotionally apt. But "retail therapy" may also indicate hypomania, as Imelda Marcos's shoes collection illustrates.

For some reason the icon of the cowboy is almost universal in Western culture. Films like *The Good the Bad and the Ugly* and *For a Few Dollars More* may be based on classical myths, but so is Joyce's *Ulysses*, and that is a very different interpetration. Cowboys sell Coke, Marlboro and Levis, but the myth that supports them is likely not Greek or Roman but a much more primitive one found in stories all over the world. Joseph Campbell would describe the cowboy as the mythic Hero, the bad man as the mythic Antagonist, and the ineffectual sheriff as the Trickster, all Jungian archetypes, and it is the universality of these that allows them both to resonate in the subconscious and to be turned toward hypomanic excess. In the Old West real cowboys were poor men and there's great irony in their image being used to sell expensive consumer goods.

Today, however, fashion is more and more tied in with popular music and vice versa. Songs with clothes are often successful: "Blue Suede Shoes", "Famous Blue Raincoat", "Lady in Red" (cheek to cheek).

Lady Gaga is the epitome of the hypomanic artist at the moment, epitomising self love, love of others and grandiose belief in herself and her sexuality and the love of her audience. Models look like pubescent boys and now the new trend is for boys who look like girls being employed as models.

There is a class factor in fashion. Only rich people can afford expensive brands like Rolex, Dior, Chloe, Gucci, Chanel, Cartier, Fendi, Coach and Burberry, and these brands help them stand out in the crowd. But the poor too have their distinctive garb. It would seem that a very working class fashion is the track suit and runners, though brands like Nike, Ellis, Adidas and Puma are expensive.

The wealthy are fashion-bonded by exclusive cars, hotels, makeup, perfume, luggage, and even shoes, scarves and jewellery. Annual international fashion shows in New York, London, Paris and Milan bring top models and photographers and magazines together to show the spring summer autumn and winter collections. Hauteur Couture clothes are very expensive and distinguish the super-rich from the merely wealthy.

They seem to come from French and Italian words with vowels at the end of words as seen in Opera i.e. clothes and perfume. Value of companies in Billions in 2014 are Louis Vuitton, bags jumped 14 percent to 26 bn, Hermes (scarf's kept by till) jumped 14 percent to 22bn,Gucci gained 27 percent up to16 bn, clothing Prada, watchmakers Rolex , jewellery producer Cartier, and fashion labels Chanel and Burberry next four of top eight. Giorgio Armani, Chloe, Dior, Hugho Boss, Jimmy Choo, Guess, Tommy Hilfiger, Mulberry, Miu,Miu, Chanel, make up, L'Oreal Esteé Lauder and bags by Louis Vuitton. Numbers also work such as Chanel No. 5.Vowels also sell jewellery such as De Beers and now Lady Gaga's black perfume that sold 6 million bottles in a week in October 2012.

Apple is yet again the biggest company in 2023 with a value of $2 trillion up 1%. Above valuations written by Andrew Roberts for Millward Brown Optimor estimated in its 2014 BrandZstudy, in Irish Independent 22 May 2014. Other names with vowels in the commercial world are Dunnes, Tescos, Aldi, Lidl, Ikea, Skoda, Audi, BMW, Merc and Honda. Manic names and manic culture.

Different countries in Europe say Yes using vowels Oui. Si Ja. Da. Vai Ano. Jah. Kylla.Ta. Igen. Taip. Jo. Iva. Tak. Sim. Da. Vai. Ja.

HYPOMANIC PRETENTIOUSNESS

One can see in popular culture the same sort of pretentiousness that often manifests in fashion. "Liberalism" is the only political affiliation for "fashionable" people to espouse, and this has been the way for many decades. The left has always been snobbish and exclusive, dismissive of not merely "the right" - anyone who doesn't share their "enlightened" views - but even their own constituency.

Hillary Clinton's disparagement of much of the American electorate as "a basket of deplorables" continues a long tradition. In "Working Class Hero" John Lennon dismisses the working class as "still fucking peasants as far as I can see" and invites them: "If you want to be a hero, just follow me" - a multi-millionaire who long ago left his working class background behind him. Lennon and other self-styled liberals rubbed shoulders with Michael and Malcolm X, and the proud Stalinist Ché Guevara became a "liberal" icon. Before Lennon the Fabians looked down on the people they patronised and championed Stalin's USSR.

Leftists' pretentiousness and arrogance permitted them to dismiss what the Nazis would term *untermenschen*. Virginia Woolf openly championed euthanizing mental patients despite her own mental problems, but in this she was far from alone in the Fabian Society: "in the first great enthusiasm for eugenics liberals were prominently to the fore, simply because what appealed to them was the rationality of science".[93] Margaret Sanger gave thanks for "the great outstanding service of Eugenics" in remedying "the vicious circle of mental and physical defect, delinquency and beggary [that] is encouraged, by the unseeing and unthinking sentimentality of our age, to populate asylum, hospital and prison".[94]

Liberals' belief in the "rationality of science" is, on the face of it, evidence for good judgement, but, like anything else, belief can be taken to hypomanic levels. Until recently most scientists held to the dictum that anything that cannot be disproven cannot be in the realm of science, and so largely eschewed engagement in theological matters. Einstein famously claimed that

---

[93] Michael Freeden, cited in, Gareth Griffith, *Socialism and Superior Brains: The Political Thought of George Bernard Shaw* p. 286.
[94] Margaret Sanger, *The Pivot of Civilisation*, pp. 174-75.

"God does not play dice" but he was speaking paradoxically, in the context of science. Recently both Richard Dawkins and Stephen Hawking have gone out of their way to denounce religion, and proclaim that there is no God.[95] This is something that simply cannot ever be proved or disproved, but the arrogance of men of science in a scientific age can lead them to conflate their opinions with facts.

This intellectual arrogance may constitute hypomania in that it exposes grandiosity of thinking - or, perhaps, the sort of paranoia that may stem from not knowing all the answers one feels one should in a scientifically-oriented world. Such paranoiac arrogance is replete with danger, and we saw the same in the Fabians.

George Bernard Shaw started off as a constitutional socialist but became an admirer of the Bolsheviks after the Russian Revolution, and while in theory he was a champion of full equality, in practise this was Orwellian: all are equal, but some are more equal than others. Shaw anticipated the Nazis when he argued, as far back as 1910, that those "who are no use in this world, who are more trouble than they are worth", should be eliminated in "lethal chambers". Elsewhere he wrote: "The majority of men at present in Europe have no business to be alive; and no serious progress will be made until we address ourselves earnestly and scientifically to the task of producing trustworthy human material for society".[96]

The arrogance of the intellectual is unmistakeable here. Earlier, at the very apogee of the British Empire, Shaw had given thanks for "the scientific massacre which has just happily rid the Soudan of its chivalry and heroism", and he goes on to recommend "a combination of America and the Western Powers to suppress civilised war by international force of arms, and to dispassionately extirpate barbarous races, whose heroism, chivalry, patriotism and religion forbid them to live and let live".[97]

Marxism made great strides in the West between the wars and during and following the Vietnam War 50,000 US soldiers died, 50,000 committed suicide (50,000 RAF died in the battle of Britain) and consequent

---

[95] See, notably, Richard Dawkins, *The God Delusion*.
[96] Cited in, Griffith, op cit, p. 57.
[97] George Bernard Shaw, in a letter to the editor of the *Daily Chronicle*, 13 October 1898.

disillusionment, but the Paris Spring was a failure. In the wake of this, though, postmodernism arose, driven by the ideas of Derrida and Foucault and other Paris-based intellectuals, as well as the politics of Spring veterans like Danny Cohn Bendit in the European Parliament. The idea that there is no objective reality but merely "competing narratives" and different "social constructs" is a subtle way of advancing the myth that all are equal - in a quasi-objective rather than legal sense. PoMo can make for clever conversation but, as has been remarked, stepping out of the window of the conversation room, should that room be on the tenth floor, settles any argument as to whether gravity is a social construct.

While it has produced some excellent literature like John Fowles' *The French Lieutenant's Woman*, postmodernism is pretentious nonsense at its heart, and scholars speculate, half-seriously, that the Paris Spring warriors, having lost the war, set out to prove that losing it was just one narrative competing with others, so they may well have actually won it. Arthur Scargill, perhaps employing the same logic, insists that "his" miners won the infamous strike of 1984: the historical outcome is merely one narrative competing with Arthur's.

Alan Sokal, a physicist at New York University, exposed postmodernism for what it is in a paper he sent in 1996 to the postmodernist *Social Text*. His concern was to test whether the supposedly professional journal would publish "an article liberally salted with nonsense if (a) it sounded good and (b) it flattered the editors' ideological preconceptions". The article was indeed published in the *Science Wars* issue of *Social Text* as "Transgressing the Boundaries: Towards a Transformative Hermeneutics of Quantum Gravity", and on the day the issue appeared Sokal sent another article to *Lingua Franca*, describing the hoax he'd carried out and describing his essay as "a pastiche of left-wing cant, fawning references, grandiose quotations and outright nonsense ... structured around the silliest quotations ... about maths and physics" he could find.[98]

Instead of hiding, the postmodernists came out in force to denounce Sokal. One described him as "ignorant" and "poorly read", and another claimed that

---

[98] Alan Sokal, "A Physicist Experiments with Cultural Studies" in *Lingua Franca*. Cited by Richard Dawkins in "Postmodernism Disrobed" in *Nature*, 9 July 1998, vol. 394, pp. 141-143.]

his article actually proved the postmodernist thesis. Postmodernists became much warier, but they continue to pump out fashionable nonsense, e.g. Luce Irigary's notion that hydraulics are only poorly understood because fluid dynamics, as opposed to "hard" engineering, are "female" and therefore feared and avoided by traditionally male engineers. This is as nonsensical and factually wrong (hydraulics are as well understood as any other aspect of "hard" engineering) as Irigary's contention that $E=mc^2$ is a "sexed equation" and non-universal.[99]

It is not considered intellectual heresy in some American universities today to argue that "non-traditional" societies, and minorities who belong to or emerged from them, should have "equally valid" ways of understanding the world than the scientific one. Some minorities, and their "liberal" supporters, argue, for instance, that American Indian creation myths be given equal status with archaeological discoveries, and that Afrocentrism be taught in history departments.

Is this evidence of hypomania in academe? It would seem to take a certain madness to believe that science and technology could be "sexed" as Irigary says, and more likely that her feminism has made her hostile to a profession, engineering, that traditionally has been very male-dominated. But that too is changing, and the lunacy is even more evident in her claim that any scientific formula could be "sexed", as she claims Einstein's is, especially as postmodernists insist that sex/gender are "social constructs" and natural laws precede society and humanity and are utterly objective.

There is another possibility, however. Sokal is not the only one to remark on the "left-wing cant" that characterises postmodernism, and there can be no doubt that academe is increasingly dominated by Marxist thought. Faux-liberalism is fostered by such thinking, perhaps toward revolution, and it is easy to see how pandering to "equally valid" ways of understanding the world would appeal to Islamic fundamentalists, taught to believe that anything not in the Koran is of the devil, and for many years openly at war with the West and its Enlightenment value system.

Nevertheless we may consider the phenomenon of postmodernism in isolation from Islamism - itself clearly hypomanic if not fully manic. PoMo champions

---

[99] Dawkins, "Postmodernism Disrobed".

may be considered hypomanic if they, for instance, argue that male sexual tumescence can be mathematically quantified as Jacques Lacan pretends:

$$\frac{S \text{ (signifier)}}{s \text{ (signified)}} = s \text{ (the statement), with } S = (-1), \text{ produces: } s = \sqrt{-1}.$$

This, and Irigary's claim that Newton's *Principia* is a "rape manual", or that E=mc² is a "sexed equation" because "it *privileges* the speed of light over other speeds that are vitally necessary to us",[100] would seem to bear as little on reality as a child's claim that a monster broke into the house and ate the cookies.

Alfred Adler, among others, made the point that mental health may be evaluated by the congruence of objective and subjective reality. If this is so - and commonsense as well as clinical practice suggests that it is - then postmodernists, in propounding that there is no objective reality, merely "social constructs", must be tending toward alienation from reality. Even if one accepts that PoMo more strictly claims that theoretical explanations for empirical statements are social constructs there seems something hypomanic in their advancing such solipsistic notions, *and in those ideas being entertained by academe and others* outside academe, suggests something hypomanic in society.

Such a development may bode very ill for the future of Western civilisation. One critic, Rob Weatherill, claims that the angst and anomie that has become so pervasive in recent decades can be traced to "liberal" anti-authoritarianism that emerged out of the protest movements of the 1960s and the publication, in 1972, of *Anti-Oedipus* by Gilles Deluze and Felix Guatarri. The result of hostility toward tradition, authority, morality and restraint - portrayed as fascistic - was that "the basic matrix of marriage and family" was rejected in favour of "free-wheeling individualistic modes of pleasure".[101]

Such pursuit creates all sorts of spiritual and social problems, but these are camouflaged under lofty aspirations and affirmations; the very deployment of *rights*, *choice* and *empowerment*, and other such terms, creates high ground

---

[100] Dawkins, op cit.
[101] Rob Wetherill, *The Anti-Oedipus Complex: Lacan, Critical Theory and Postmodernism* (Abingdon: Routledge, 2017).

from which to pontificate. "The 'right to choose' [is] the signifier of modern liberal democratic consumers", says Weatherill, but *choice* implies that something *is not* chosen, and the hedonism encouraged by nihilism and existentialism means that certain things *will not* be - that responsible choices will more likely be evaded. He instances abortion here, pointing out that the foetus, "literally unseen, has no rights" to worry about. In such a brave new "liberal" world, there are certain options that almost *must not* be chosen.

The ironic outcome is that traditional values are replaced by an ethos of "enjoyment unto death" and its associated irresponsibility, which can only be satisfied by embracing consumerism as an end in itself, and such consumerism ultimately benefits only the capitalist purveyors of it, consumers controlled more subtly than under fascism, but controlled nonetheless: modern "liberalism" allows no dissent: "The fascist trick was/is to hit those unenlightened few who question these forceful and emotive narratives of prideful righteousness and entitlement and shame them publically." Thus dissent is stifled, less brutally than in concentration camps, but perhaps no less successfully.

MONEY

What is always "fashionable" is what Orson Wells said were the three important things in life: Power, Sex and Money. Khufu a Pharaoh had hieroglyphics of sex, money and gossip on her temples. In April 2010 the President of China, Hu Jintao, gave a speech warning Marxist officials of the temptation of beautiful women, money and power after they were caught staying in expensive hotels in Las Vegas and visiting sex shows in the decadent, capitalist West.

Spending is a manic archetype. People get a thrill from spending money and if they do not feel well they will go out and buy something and get the hit. Woman will get their hair done. Making people hypomanic makes them spend; this is the basis of advertising. By stimulating people with the manic archetypes you make people hypomanic and they will buy and sell things, the basis of capitalism. But often people buy things they like when they're manic and after a few days they do not want what they've purchased.

Rakesh Khurana of Harvard Business School "has found that USA companies looking for a new leader seek charisma above all else".[102] But while charisma may lead to short-lived improvement it is not all that is required to run a successful business. Rather, it is one of the manic archetypes.

Arguably, mania and hypomania drove the Celtic Tiger and led to the almost inevitable recession that followed. In recession money is hard to get, but it may provoke some of the wealthy toward philanthropy - manic money makers are often do-gooders as well. Andrew Carnegie left much of his fortune to endowing libraries so that poor people could better educate and entertain themselves; Alfred Nobel, perhaps guiltily, endowed the eponymous Prizes.

This sort of charity appears to have a positive effect on society, which is, one expects, the intention. Questions have been asked, however, about the sincerity of some modern philanthropists. After all, cynics say, if they didn't give their money to charity they'd have to give it to the government in taxes, so philanthropy may be subtly undemocratic. Given the controversial history of the Clintons, one is hardly surprised by questions raised about the Clinton Foundation. The philanthropy of George Soros could, arguably, be used to promote a world without borders where cheap labour must favour creating wealth for those who already own businesses and industries, further enriching these elite.

When people are manic they try to expand their business; but when the economy goes into recession banks call in the money and people are made bankrupt. Stock exchanges are manic of their nature, with both buying and selling at fast speeds often using computers. The dealers make enormous profits, all on commission.

---

[102] Emma Young, "People with charisma are seen as good leaders but can be spendthrift", *New Scientist*, 23 June 2012.

This financialisation of the economy is fraught with danger. Not only does it substitute the trade of an artificial entity, money, for actual goods and services, it fosters a situation in which the great bulk of the artificial entity becomes a virtual asset, existing not even in vaults but on the internet, ethereal. Worse, its trade facilitates and fosters hypomania - finance isn't real in the tangible sense, yet it offers the same opportunities and dangers as real, concrete assets - and, most dangerous of all, it builds instability into the system. The 1929 stock market crash came at the end of a long period of financialisation, the crash of 2010 the same.

Another danger in financialisation is the enormous disparity in wealth the creation of artificial money fosters. After WWII the average American chief executive earned about six times what his janitor did; by 1980 he was paid 42 times the average factory worker's wage; by 2012 he was paid 325 times that. To make this disparity in wealth worse, avoidance schemes mean that taxes of the rich declined from 51 percent in 1955 to 17 percent in 2017.

By contrast to the stock market, the original form of transaction, barter, is more conservative and conducted at a far more leisurely pace, often over days rather than seconds. Until 1914 much of the world's currencies were gold-backed. Unlike shares, gold has an intrinsic value and this stabilised foreign exchange, but these very limitations led to its abandonment in the manic spending necessitated by the Great War. There was a brief return to the gold standard after the war but the collapse after 1929 led to its permanent abandonment.

People like gold, the feel and weight of it, and its glisten. It is magical and manic, and the clichéd image of the miser revelling in his gold probably strikes a chord with everyone - we can understand. Though its ductility and resistance to electrical erosion do have commercial application, beyond its measure of wealth, gold's beauty is its real attraction, and beauty and wealth are combined in the world's best jewellery. Despite its manic associations, gold probably does not have the same perhaps-genetic evocation that red, black and white colours do, and while it does feature in advertising, it tends to be used subtly, and in high-quality businesses, as one might expect.

FREEDOM, FREE MARKET, ART AND MONEY

Like money, for all its apparent negativity, hypomania may in fact be adaptive, not, as it has always been perceived, a maladaptive tendency toward debilitating, perhaps dangerous mania. Adaptability, at the end, is about ensuring our genetic survival, and hypomania, with its frenetic activity and avid sociability, must, on the face of it, ensure more human contact and opportunities to propagate.

Ultimately all our productivity - emotionally, physically and psychologically - is about getting our genes passed on, if Richard Dawkins' theories are correct. Stimulation gets us out there into the various social milieus in which this can happen, and the more stimulation we can engender in ourselves the better our opportunities to pass on our genes.

But is this entirely so? As freedom without responsibility may become a destructive force in society, at a certain level stimulation becomes too much; it overwhelms the individual and can't be accommodated by society, as we know it. At this point the graded threshold from hypomania to mania has clearly been crossed, however, and we are not built for a manic society: the body/cultural system overloads and collapses in chaos.

Rarely has society reached through manic, uncontrolled over-stimulation the depths of decadence and chaos that heralded and marked the fall of Rome; but there do seem to be signs of mania today in the proliferation of political (right wing, left wing, nationalism, internationalism) and religious belief systems on one hand, and on the other the abuse of alcohol and other drugs, higher levels of violence in society, a pace of life that is ever-increasing in speed. Huge fatalities are the result, in gang murders, traffic accidents (sometimes suicide, in single-car accidents), fights (one punch head bang), or dying from overindulgence, either through long-term illness or choking to death on one's vomit.

Is modern society heading for chaos? Or is the chaos merely the latest adversary that the fittest must fight to survive - the latest whetstone that hones the blade of humanity's energy and wits?

The link between hypomania and capitalism - through advertising - has already been outlined, and this link may be even stronger as capital is financialised. But will unfettered capitalism be able to withstand the reactions from the Islamic world, and establish a hypomanic New World order? Maybe capitalism, for all its manic aspects, is the cure even for hypomania's ills, as it is competitive, thereby fostering survival of the fittest, and wealth-generating, thereby better ensuring care of the less well-fitted who nevertheless have resources. Do you want a mediocre cheap doctor or a good expensive one, an ill-armed government or one with the best technology to beat fanatics of a different hypomanic mindset?

Many people who do not like capitalism and consumerism gravitate, not toward self-indulgence in wealth and drugs but toward such things as art and love as being the solution to our social ills. Yet in art too mania is manifest in some portrayals of the gods of Greece and Rome, such as Pan with a grotesquely large penis, and in the erotic portrayal of the many deities of Hinduism. This may reflect the manic notion of God.

Art is about the exteriorization of emotion (SWM); but it may also be therapeutic. There was a movement in this direction in the Sixties, when some saw art as a curative agent in mental illness - Dr John Cooney, a consultant psychiatrist, left his art collection to St Patrick's psychiatric hospital for this reason.[103]

Most practitioners would dismiss such use of art as futile - or at least of low value when set against capitalist-based conventional medication. Similarly, most would look askance on alternative methods such as positive thinking as a cure for cancer. And most of their patients would share these doctors' sentiments. There are few if any double-blind or otherwise convincing studies that prove such alternative systems of treatment work, and Dr James Randi has debunked homeopathy on a BBC *Horizon* programme. The best medication would still seem to be the best that money can buy, and when we look to the United States, we see how depressing the outcome of this approach is likely to be for those who cannot afford the best. By this

---

[103] Interestingly, Jonathan Swift, author of arguably-hypomanic - however ironic - tracts such as "A Modest Proposal", also left his money to St Patricks.

measure, nevertheless, if hypomania generates individual wealth, it is indeed an adaptive development in the evolutionary scheme.

This is not to dismiss the therapeutic - in the broadest sense - value of art. It is emotion that largely dictates thought. People tend to be more creative when they are high, and those with Manic Depression Illness and to a lesser extent hypomania are in a unique position as they experience highs (mania) and lows (depression). A clear correlation between MDI/hypomania and creativity has repeatedly been measured - one study indicates that seventy percent of the American Writers' Club are manic-depressive, as opposed to a norm of one percent. It is during their hypomanic phases, which come about when the manic archetypes are stimulated, that artists are most productive, and in the most fertile environment for them to pass on their genes - as long as they don't wreck this environment by maladaptive behaviour. Again within this constraint, they are at their most successful when they are in the hypomanic phase. If one considers that since Shelley's time the poet has been called "the unwritten legislator of the world," one can see how hypomanics may tend to create culture that reflects the hypomanic mental set; and if we look to how society has speeded up - in everything from the Internet, traffic to popular music - we may see evidence for this hypothesis.

Art, however, is at least as political as it is therapeutic. Political cartoons have been deployed for centuries, and in the USSR art was an important component in state propaganda. The CIA backed the abstract expressionists such as Jackson Pollack and his like. Young British Artists arguably revitalised a moribund art and took it out of the membership club and common room; now it is in pubs, cafes, gossip columns and glossy mag covers. YBA gave art back to the inexpert, but while on the face of things this is a good thing, for both the artist and the public, the "inexpert" include the uncultured and the philistine.

It is not difficult to see the Marxist agenda of equality at work here: all are equal; anybody can be an expert. At the same time the YBA led to new catalogue notes being more abstruse, more circumlocutory, precious, "jargonified" and pretentious - all are equal, but some are more equal than others, in understanding what "experts" mean.[104]

---

[104] See Elizabeth Fullerton, *The Sunday Times*, 8 May 2016, Culture Section.

It is essential to note that art may be as much a subject for consumerism as drugs, exotic travel, fast cars, or anything else. Hypomanic consumerism, like many things we like, may not be good for us. Neither may other forms of hypomania. Intellectual analysis piled on analysis may help lead us to as objective a perception of truth as we can attain, but taking this to its ultimate extension may lead to hypomania of a particular sort: the hermit isolated in his cave, or in our times, the ivory tower of academe. Politically we have seen the world change from a sort of hypomanic conflict between East and West with the fall of the Soviet Empire, but is the replacement any better?

Conflict between hypomanic socialism and hypomanic capitalism resulted in the victory of capitalism with the fall of the Berlin Wall in 1989 and the collapse of the Soviet Union itself in 1991 - man struggled with his conscience and won, the cynic might say. Most people would say that the world is better off without the Marxist utopia, but is the replacement for the Cold War really any better? Is it not just as hypomanic as was the prosecution of that war? And if hypomania can be held responsible for both the Cold War and the West's perhaps Pyrrhic victory, how does this affect the tentative thesis that it is an adaptive force?

Some people would say that American culture, which is probably the most hypomanic in the West, also dominates the West, from McDonald's to *Robocop* to *Friends*. Money is God in the USA. Spending money is a manic archetype; hence capitalism thrives in hypomanic societies and reflects success. You can buy yourself into the White House; at any rate, it is impossible for other than a very wealthy individual to fight a presidential, or any sort of political campaign, and even Abe Lincoln - allegedly a poor man, seen as Jesus, after his assassination, who saw himself as fighting for democracy of the world - was quite wealthy by contemporary standards. Ironically, the fact that money is the national God may protect America from extreme fundamentalist Christianity, another manic archetype. Bankers in China are told not to be flash with their profits.

WHERE TO TRUMP?

Will Capitalism survive, and will America continue to keep the peace? Bill Emmott, editor of *The Economist*, claims:

> At more than $600 billion a year, America defence spending plans for the first decade of the twenty-first century are ten times larger than those of any other country and exceed the spending plans of the next fourteen largest defence spenders combined. In the early twentieth century the sole aim was to control communism [but this] could blind policy makers. Our feelings about capitalism have always been and probably always will be mixed. Capitalism works. It appeals to our competitive instinct. Man, however, have other instincts. We are social animals, seeing both pleasure and benefit in co-operation. Capitalists combine competition with co-operative ventures. But we also have what Adam Smith described (approvingly) in the eighteenth century as "moral sentiment": emotions, feelings about fairness, compassion. Such sentiments can be, often are, affronted by capitalism.

In the USA, those defenders of pure market capitalism indeed argue for the abolition of Welfare, and they were able to force the Democrat Bill Clinton to drastically cut back on this social security measure during his second term. These people might agree that the hypomanic trait leads to more humanism and a more caring society, but they would argue that if people were left with more tax dollars in their pockets they would be able to offer more private charity and thus take up the slack created by the loss of Welfare payments. People's preoccupation with money can lead to private charities such as for illness, hospitals and housing at home and abroad. Rich people are often very generous. The problem with money is not money per se but, as was observed 2,000 years ago, the love of it. Furthermore, opponents of state Welfare argue, the personal involvement in such charity would be accompanied by encouragement to the recipient to better himself and become an economic asset rather than a liability.

The most amateur student of human nature must question the likelihood of this development - as idealistic as the Marxist slogan, "To each according to his needs, from each according to his abilities" and every bit as unrealistic - and it is all too easy, reading between the lines of such arguments, to discern the Protestant work ethic, taken almost to an article of faith. Might this be further evidence of hypomania, political/ideological in its overt form, as well as covertly consumerist?

However, capitalism - as a manic archetype - in tandem with paranoia that stems from it and then controls it, may lead to money being given away. Such apparently inconsistent charity is really logical: it is partly due to guilt, partly, maybe, to a semi-superstitious impulse to throw a sop to the masses who would take *all* the paranoiac's gains away from him if he didn't give them *something*. The King rules by giving presents away; if he clings to too much, he may lose it all, as King John and Louis XVI prove. King John protected himself by signing the Magna Carta at Runneymede on 15 June 1215 with the help of William Marshall, the greatest Knight of the time, who put his seal to the Magna Carta after John died. Marshall died a knight templar (My name sake)

The Magna Carta addressed the manic belief in people being equal and taxation being fair and was a vital early element of the unwritten British Constitution. *"To no one will we sell, to no one deny or delay the right of justice"*, as Clause 40 stated. After signing the Magna Carta King John rejected it and died soon afterward, but Marshall helped ensure that its ideas survived.

Such hypomanic ideas as the Carta expressed would have been seen as impossibly aspirational, unrealistically idealistic, or dangerously subversive of the "natural" order across mainland Europe, where a different sort of hypomania still reigned - the Divine Right of Kings. The idea that "No free man shall be arrested, imprisoned, dispossessed, outlawed, exiled ... except by the lawful judgement of his peers or by the law of the land" would have been seen as an affront to the right of both the King and God, to whom he answered. The idea of the Divine Right of Kings survived even in England up to 1688, and was only assailed in Europe a century later, when the *sans culottes* beheaded Louis XVI; it only died with the abdication of the Kaiser and the murder of Czar Nicholas II.

STOCKS AND SHARES

The professional moneyman, the stockbroker, lives in a manic world that can easily turn into chaos as more and more shares are sold and bought at very high speed. The more they sell and buy, the more money stockbrokers make. But as more and more share transactions occur, the brain and computer will be overloaded. The market is too manic. Modern day stockbrokers only last eight years at their peak, planning for their retirement but taking cocaine and drinking champagne on their way to manic stress-induced heart-attacks. Yet it may be instructive to observe how, out of what seems like screaming chaos on the floor, with millions of dollars changing hands every second, somehow an order emerges that allows the financial world to live on to fight again the next day.

All this hypomanic activity is not, however, a new phenomenon: rudimentary examples of options and futures contracts have been found on Mesopotamian clay tablets dating back to 1,750 BC. While modern lending practice goes back only to about 1500 AD, faith in the future, however cautious, is evident from this trade in the Ancient World.

Nevertheless the change in banking practices in about 1500 reflected enormously greater confidence in the future and in the common world view. Up until then the belief was that the world's wealth and resources were strictly limited, so that one could only get wealthier at someone else's expense. This meant that only small sums of money were ever lent, at high rates of interest and over short terms; it also meant that a moral shadow lay over the world of finance, and led to the attitude "neither a borrower nor a lender be".

The change in attitude and practice led to economic growth, and the perception that all people could benefit from this, that resources could be almost limitless. The change in attitude coincided with the discovery of America, and the fabulous wealth garnered there reinforced the new zeitgeist.

Thus we can see how consumer confidence leads to attitudes that affect the financial realities of the world. At the time of the soccer world cup in 1994, not long after a quite severe recession, people were following the Irish team all over the USA in a hypomanic orgy of consumerism that they could not afford. Despite this overspending, or because of it, the phenomenon of the

Celtic Tiger followed shortly. Though one cannot ever discount external factors, especially in an economy as open as the Irish one, in this instance, at any rate, we can see how hypomania may have been a force for economic good.

But there is a dark side to consumer confidence: confidence-tricking and overconfidence. Subprime property deals in the USA were broken up into "derivatives", loan packages in which the sub-prime mortgages were packaged along with others in what was presented as an overall-profitable deal and traded on across the world.

Low/cheap credit terms, including loans to subprime customers, led to property going up in price to unrealistic levels. In turn this led to rezoning of land for development, including patently unsuitable sites on flood-plains, and housing developments that did not have necessary infrastructures—the builders were in too great a hurry to move on to the next development to provide fully-functioning sewage and waste-water schemes; these could wait. In one instance in North Dublin a drainage system was installed but when tarmac was laid down it was decided that it would be quicker and more profitable to just cover everything and clear the drain-grills later; but this was overlooked in the rush to get on and heavy rain flooded the estate and damaged many houses.

The property bubble was effectively a Ponzi scheme and the problem was exacerbated by the incredible wealth created in the European heartland by the Euro, massive overconsumption in the PIIGS periphery, profit-build-up in French and German banks, and capital investment in the very deficit economies that could least afford to take a financial hit when this came, after the crash in 2008. Europe's own sub-prime packaging threatened to break the banking system, but this was rescued by shifting the bill onto the taxpayer.

There was more than breakdown in logic here. Moral, economic and engineering principles were all thrown to the wind. One Irish Cassandra had his concerns that what goes up must come down dismissed by the complacent assurance that "a new paradigm" was at work. The then-Taoiseach peevishly suggested that those who warned of the impending disaster ought to go and commit suicide.[105]

The end result was a frenzy of greed and people trying to catch their tails in the excitement of buying. The property boom was based not only on the belief in houses getting more expensive over a quick period of time but of the price increases continuing indefinitely. Newspapers and other media joined in the orgy of buying and selling, which provided extra copy and expensively-produced property supplements, which "somebody" paid for.

The wealth bubble corrupted everyone. Cynics noted, even at the time, how government was in bed with developers - symbolised in the infamous Fianna Fail tent at the Galway Races - and the judiciary was in bed with both. There is no shortage of evidence that white-collar crime was rampant during the years of the Celtic Tiger, but all that evidence has failed to send any of the crooked bankers to gaol. Some very questionable decisions were taken in the realms of government and judiciary. The financial regulator failed to regulate, the DPP failed to prosecute, and judges directed juries to acquit when it proved too much of an embarrassment not to at least go through the motions.

THE SHOPPING EXPERIENCE

Having made their money by whatever means, people have to spend it. Hypomanics spend more money than other people; conversely, spending elicits hypomanic behaviour. Shopping imitates the behaviour of the hunter-gatherer. Most people like shopping (a manic archetype and the basis of advertising and capitalism) and they even find window shopping enjoyable. Sensory stimulation from smell, colour, light and taste, and the noise of traffic and the marketplace, all appeal to people's hypomanic makeup. Dressing is a right-brain activity, as is appreciation of the music the shopper finds piped into malls and shops. It is not uncommon for women in particular to buy something when they are feeling down, thus stimulating their own hypomania.

---

[105] The remark was made by Taoiseach Bertie Ahern in 2007, when the banking crisis was looming and , as with every Ponzi scheme, collapse could only be avoided by inflating the bubble further.

Social class may be indicated by the brand of goods one shops for: Pia Bang, Yves St. Laurent, Armani, l'Oreal - the slogan of the last named is "Because you're worth it," an appeal to potentially grandiose delusion of the hypomanic. Gillette's advertising slogan, "The best a man can get," makes a similar appeal. There seems to be an appeal to selfishness in the marketing of many goods: in the summer of 2001 Pepsi's advertising theme was the ludicrousness of sharing a drink with anyone else, the message that selfish is smart. Less blatant, but still clearly setting the individual's personal concerns ahead of anything else, is the mobile phone company's "Your world, your way" slogan. Self-love and narcissism are traits of hypomania, just as reckless spending of money is.

CHRISTMAS

Christmas is a manic festival, a manic high to look forward to in the middle of winter. The very origin of the Christian festival, that a god is born as a human being, seems to the non-religious mindset clearly a manic notion, as is the antecedent pagan belief that the sun is born again. Around the same time people celebrate the New Year and ring it in, in another hypomanic event that may be, as in Scotland, more important than Christmas.

People are friendlier, money is spent, and more alcohol is drunk. Though Christmas is in the middle of summer in the southern hemisphere, it developed as a winter festival, perhaps originally a ritual entreaty to the sun god to return, perhaps one to assist his resurrection, and a celebration of that resurrection and return. The rock at the entrance to Newgrange has a carved left handed circle on one side and a right handed circle on the other side. This may indicate that there was roughly the same number of right- and left-handed people at the time, which would have both reflected and affected their culture. What's more likely is that the spirals symbolise the Celtic mystical belief of going into the mystery and bringing out what one finds into one's mortal life. The opposite direction of the spirals may symbolise what some occultists call the left- and right-hand paths - but it may also indicate the aesthetic appeal of symmetry.

Newgrange originally was a sun temple, designed to measure the sun's nadir and thereby, perhaps, aid in the timing of essential rituals. Thus Christmas came about to raise people's mood, in a time when people lived close to the land and the elements were crucial to their comfort and their very survival. It still is a happy time for the family and also for business.

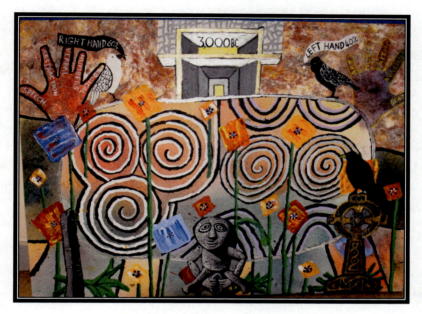

Newgrange by Stuart Marshall

Some people say that Christmas has become too commercial, but people have always had a festival in the depth of winter, and occurring as it does outside the productive season, this means, or certainly used to mean, a surfeit of time on people's hands. Today time has been replaced with a certain profligacy of assets - or, as we say nowadays, a commercial aspect. A lot of money is spent over the Christmas - music shops do a third of their business in the eight weeks running up to Christmas. But the very commerciality means sometimes enormous pressure, especially on families with small children who may be living from hand to mouth and put themselves in debt, sometimes to dangerous money-lenders, to meet the expectations of themselves, their children and their neighbours.

But Christmas is also a spiritual time, made so by the giving and taking of gifts and love. We may complain of the commercialism of Christmas, but it effectively forces us to think of other people when we buy them presents. The exchange of gifts means that people have higher self-esteem and they like other people more. People smile more at Christmas. This happiness is due in part to the very spending of money, the hypomanic state that this reflects.

There are other aspects of hypomania about Christmas. It is celebrated in song and hymn, reflecting the creativity of people at such time. There are songs of love and heartache, and of the spiritual dimension, concerns that occupy the manic mindset, but in recent decades Christmas songs have taken the message of Christmas to a crusading level. The best-known and one of the earliest in this genre is probably John Lennon's "Happy Christmas (War is Over)", but this has since been joined by others, of which the best may be Greg Lake's "I Believe in Father Christmas". These songs call attention to the fact that away from the smug self-satisfaction of the lucky ones in the Western World, children and others are being murdered in wars, sometimes fought in our name.

The other sub-genre is anti-Christmas songs. In the Pogues' "Fairytale of New York" one of the personae says "Happy Christmas your arse!" The hypomania manifested here is the depressive inverse of "White Christmas", when the slush melts in the streets and the *bon viveur* wakes up in the drunk tank with a hangover. But this sort of hypomania is very much a feature of the "festive season", with drunken family rows and terrified children calling help lines. In Ireland the Samaritans receive thousands of calls over the Christmas period, hundreds on Christmas Day; but significantly most come in the days following.[106]

The dark side of Christmas seems to be focused on its commercialism, and the inability of people to match public expectation in gift-giving. The season is marked by drunkenness, and the violence that can follow from this. This drinking and violence may be itself hypomanic activity, but it also is consequent to the rampant hypomania that commercialism brings: bright lights and extravagant advertising campaigns, that begin earlier and earlier each year as businesses seek to increase their market share.

The depressive effects of alcoholic overindulgence, and all this leads to, directly and indirectly, to oneself and to others, make this dark side of

---

[106] The Samaritans report that over the Christmas period in 2014 they received almost 200,000 calls.

Christmas understandable. People let their hair down at the office party and release their secret passions, so that one may end up in compromising or embarrassing positions even without being drunk oneself.

That the festive season can be terribly bleak and lonely is exemplified by the writer's experience of one Christmas many years ago: three packets of crisps and 18 hours of T.V. The late AA Gill tells a poignant story of visiting his parents briefly, collecting his expensive present and leaving under an excuse that he had to work, then selling the gift his parents had given him, spending the money on whiskey, and drinking it all alone in his flat.

A new sort of manic behaviour has come to associate itself with the festive season in recent years: a grim politically correct determination to secularise it to avoid "offending" any non-Christians. This development has the potential to tone down the hypomania, perhaps - "Happy Holiday" has an anaemic sound to it that falls far short of "Happy Christmas, Ho Ho Ho!" - but the humourless, crusading Calvinism is as hypomanic as anything else. The secular capitalism it endorses is what undermines what one may call the "real" spirit of Christmas, as so well portrayed by Dickens in *A Christmas Carol*, and by sports writer Thomas Hauser who was once called up by the late Mohammad Ali. Hauser was both amused and impressed by the universal humanity symbolised by a Moslem calling up a Jew to wish him a happy Christian festival.[107]

Coca-Cola dressed Santa in Red, black & white for an advertisement when he had been green and brown.

MEDICINE

Medicine fascinates people. They marvel at the body and its working, dread the prospect of its failing. They see technology advance and demand a cure-all for not only cancer and AIDS, but whatever may afflict them in the fearsome future.

Medicine goes back to the druids and the witchdoctors and the shamans when ingredients for drugs were passed on from father to son. There was often a

---

[107] Thomas Hauser, *A Hard World: An Inside Look at Another Year in Boxing*, p. 155.

psychotic element to the healing procedure with dancing, chanting, and talking in tongues, over-breathing and the taking of stimulants that make the shamans high. This is a long way from modern day practise, but a new way of working is the hippie-like alternative therapy where people wish for the cure-all without any proof of the drug's efficacy.

We cannot stop decay of the body. We can't live forever. We cannot stop death. Yet we wish for cures; we hope to be saved. The patient puts his life and wellbeing in the doctor's hands. The doctor gets the trust of the patient by the prognosis that confirms his knowledge of medicine. Thus the doctor is a sort of god, and also an icon. But changes are at work in a rapidly changing world.

Like hairdressing or massage, nurses, physiotherapists and medicine break the touch taboo, but there has been a change in recent years in view of the many scandals involving child abuse, a greater political correctness as regards treatment of women, and an increasing litigiousness among patients. Doctors will not interact physically with their patients in the way they used to; a "taboo of tenderness" has emerged.[108] They will not examine a patient without a nurse being present as a witness to their propriety. While this may be inevitable, and in some ways a good thing, it compromises the intimacy and confidentiality of the doctor-patient relationship, and conflates the problems brought about by the end of the "talk as cure" days. One could say that the need for such procedural safeguards, and the problems they bring with them, reflects the hypomanic world that makes them necessary, a world in which women are molested and children abused by those entrusted with their care.

The infallibility of the doctor-as-god has been further undermined by higher pressure on the doctor to see more patients than before. This pressure eliminates "talk as cure" and may lead, in many instances at least, to patients being denied the one thing that might well do them good, and must lead to a degree of alienation in at least some of them.

Today people's scepticism of conventional medicine is compounded by more choices in non-conventional medicine, such as reflexology, alternative medicine, herbs, tai chi, pilates, reiki and acupuncture. But perhaps the very

---

[108] See Dr Ian Suttie, *The Origins of Love and Hate.*

variety of these alternatives points toward an increasingly widespread hypomania: people seek, often maniacally, for a cure and are willing to try anything new. In their hypomania, scepticism is displaced by credulity. Alternative medicine has no controlling bodies and frequently very suspect methodology - no control groups, double-blind systems, etc - thus fantastic claims may be made without peer review or the possibility of refutation.

The far-reaching effects of this aspect of alternative medicine can be seen when we look to the extinction of the Romanov dynasty. This came about, ultimately, by the inability of conventional medicine to treat the Czarovitch's haemophilia, and the resultant dependence of the Czarina - and through her, the weak-willed Czar - on the machinations of faith healer and mystic, Rasputin. Rasputin represents a witch-doctor figure, an atavistic force in the courts and power-houses of modern Europe, both appealing to the hypomania of his followers and being himself clearly manic: his sexual energy and capacity for alcohol were far greater than any normal man's, and at the end, after swallowing more cyanide than would literally kill a horse, he was shot several times, bludgeoned apparently to death, but actually drowned in the Neva after being pushed through the ice. His infamous orgies maybe indicate the onset of modern hypomania as a somehow fashionable practise - more strictly, perhaps, resurgence of the sort of decadence that had marked the Roman Empire and the Bourbon and other courts. His death was quickly followed by the Russian Revolutions, and the orgies of killing that marked the subsequent civil war and Stalin's genocide and purges.

In one regard, though, mania can be a positive force in medicine. The search for a cure for cancer and AIDS, for example, is little short of manic (understandable, given the ravages of these diseases), and the now almost annual emergence of other illnesses - SARS and avian flu, for instance. Such research leads to many cures being put forward, sometimes spin-off cures for different diseases. Now we have Covid.

In another regard, mania in medicine is detrimental. In the past, medicine was often a family business, and there was a sense of carrying on a proud tradition; now it's for whoever gets the highest points. There is a lot of money in medicine and the profession is conservative, slow to change in certain ways for all the rapidity of its research and development. For example, the profession denied for years that Coca-Cola was responsible for hyperactivity - a form of hypomania - for all the anecdotal evidence.

This conservatism may have much to do with money. Many students enter the profession because of genuine altruism: they want to look after others (love of others is itself a manic archetype); but after exhausting years as overworked and underpaid interns they come out with an eye for money only - and many of them maniacally puffing cigarettes, which they took to smoking in order to withstand the pressure of their careers.

There is evidence that some doctors end up with lowered self-esteem (in one survey, forty percent said they would not do medicine if they had their choice to make again),[109] as a result of the high pressure of the training and the work itself, and perceived prostitution of a once-proud profession. It is difficult to see the doctors of our grandparent's generation, the stalwarts of society, suffering such lack of self-esteem.

Money plays another part too. Because medical problems are very important we pay more for the privilege of having them addressed, and are thus made willing prisoners in a closed shop. We get paranoid about our health and take out insurance - and the doctor takes out different insurance against malpractice, in an increasingly litigious society. The proud family tradition - which often respected a patient's ability to pay - is going, and for other reasons, much of the intimacy of the doctor-patient relationship along with it. Alienation of the patient may increase hypomanic activity in society at large, as sufferers seek alternative methods, many of which lack the professional standards of conventional medicine.

MARTIN LUTHER KING

Martin Luther King was manic; it took manic energy to persuade thousands to march on Montgomery and then on Washington where in 1963 he addressed a quarter of a million people at the Lincoln Memorial and told them "Free at last, free at last. Thank God Almighty, we are free at last!" King's hypomania is suggested by powerful speeches such as this, one of the finest pieces of oratory of the twentieth century. It is no coincidence that his

---

[109] *Irish Medical Organisation* magazine.

father was a preacher, some of the best speakers in American history having been influenced, directly or indirectly, by "pulpit oratory."

People who become preachers want to change the world, but King was a pacifist (he won the Nobel peace prize); had he been a revolutionary then the USA, ripe for revolution, might have degenerated into anarchy.

Such preachers as King love God and Love. They have a message to get across - in King's case, the need for black civil rights - and they are often good actors as well as orators, natural, charismatic and kind. Many rock 'n roll legends were close to preachers. His local Baptist priest fascinated Elvis and some say he learnt his stage performance from him. Neil Hannon of the Divine Comedy is very charismatic like his father who is a bishop. Notorious televangelist Jimmy Swaggart is a cousin of Jerry Lee Lewis - who surely must have been one of the most hypomanic entertainers ever. Swaggart, Lewis, Elvis are well known for their sexual exploits, but it is less well known, if hardly a secret, that King too had many sexual liaisons with women, besotted with his energy, his charisma, and his fame.

CIVIL RIGHTS

Man has fought for civil rights in the last two hundred years more than at any other time, a sign of popular mania. For example, the suffragette movement fought to the literal death - on hunger strike or, in Emily Davison's case, under the hooves of the king's horse in protest - and Martin Luther King was killed for his campaigning for civil rights for American blacks.

Women got the vote in 1920 in the U.S.A. But people have always fought for this or similar causes: Martin Luther fought for the right to a non-corrupt church; Socrates died for his democratic principles; the French Revolution was about the rights of the poor. When we can love each other, there will be no wars, no rape, no murder, no hatred and no jealousy; we can live as one with love - but of course this very idea is hypomanic in its simplicity, for love is always graduated downward from ourselves, and when a threat, real or perceived, threatens us or our loved ones, we react from the id.

One could, perhaps, trace the very notion of civil rights to fundamental Christian principles and especially to those that became widespread after the

Reformation had undercut papal autocracy. The New Testament admonition to "Render to Caesar the things that are Caesar's, and to God the things that are God's", was one of the principles that enabled a devout Protestant Europe - and America - to embrace secularism and separation of church and state. It was the devout Christian, William Wilberforce, who was instrumental in banning the Atlantic slave trade, and the sternly Protestant Victorians who later despatched gunships to Zanzibar to break up the largest slave market in the world. The remarkable, contradictory, elatedly Protestant General Gordon lost his own life because he refused to leave Khartoum without the entire garrison of the Sudan. Today, civil rights are taken almost to extremes in liberal Protestant Holland, where drugs are readily available and laws against their use are lax, prostitution is legal and bestiality is only recently outlawed.

But the id will not be denied. Civil rights, i.e. Equality, Liberty, Fraternity - democracy indeed, perhaps - is a manic ideal. It may be no accident that the same Wilberforce who broke the Atlantic slave trade also penned the gloriously manic hymn, "Amazing Grace," manic because it tells of one human being selected for salvation by God.

The whole plausibility of the civil rights struggle is suspect, however laudable its aims. Man is competitive by nature: it was by competition that he attained ascendancy in the natural world. He wants more power, sex and money: it is thus that he individually achieves success. (Orson Wells) - he wants flash red sports cars and blonde women by his side, not a used Ford and a harassed wife and demanding family, all making claims on him for the "rights" he owes them.

Yet it was the student protests in the United States that finally drove the country to withdraw from Vietnam. This was a reflection of the politicisation of students through the civil rights campaign, the seeking of freedom for all, showing how manic impulses may be channelled into positive channels.

For how long Enlightenment values will survive is a moot point. Rumours of the death of democracy have been, to borrow from Mark Twain, greatly exaggerated in the past, notably in the inter-war period and at the height of the Cold War when Khrushchev threatened to "bury" the West and its democracies. But today things are different. Demographics is destiny, it may be truly said, of nations and countries - and religions - and Western democracies are in demographic decline. Sheer pressure from outside is quite likely to eclipse them as surely as Europe did the indigenes of the Americas and Australia.

This possibility is particularly pressing today, with aging European populations being actively supplemented by immigration from the Middle East and Africa. On one level this makes sense: these people have a youthful population and the two demographics complement each other. On the other hand, they are arguably incompatible. Europe is an industrial and post-industrial society while most of the immigrants of recent years have few skills and are frequently illiterate, so are likely to be a further liability on an aging demographic rather than an asset.

More significantly, these immigrants are almost all Moslem, and ever since the extinction of Mu'talzilism almost a thousand years ago, Islam has been anti-rational and anti-progressive. Especially since the emergence of Wahabbism, fundamentalism has made headway in the Moslem world and this anti-progressive ethos presents a far greater obstacle to integration in secular Europe. The urbane and liberal Josef Joffe says: "The threat to Europe comes not in the form of uniforms, but in the tattered garb of refugees".[110]

Islam is the only world system in which politics and law are inextricably woven with religion, and this must present problems to Enlightenment politicians seeking to solve Europe's demographic problems. Sharia law is mandated by the Koran, by God Himself, Moslems argue, and secular legal - and political - systems are blasphemous because they seek to replace what God mandates with what man devises. It is any good Moslem's duty, the Koran makes clear, to wage jihad against such systems, not necessarily by violent means, but by *dawa* - "civilisation jihad". *Dawa* seeks to undermine the existing legal and political systems and replace them with sharia, or at any rate weaken them for an onslaught by violent jihad. Everything in sharia derives from the Koran, and everything not in the Koran is of the devil - at least since the decline of Mu'tazilism.

---

[110] Cited in Robert D Kaplan, *The Revenge of Geography*.

This is perhaps the most critical difference between Christianity and Islam. The Enlightenment grew out of the Reformation's idea of personal responsibility, and secularism is endorsed by the Biblical line "Render to Caesar the things that are Caesar's, and to God the things that are God's". The Koran says the precise opposite. How can this circle be squared to the overall benefit of Europe?

Yet must the Enlightenment fail? It is important to see that the above is a particularly gloomy prognostication that does not take account of human factors. Most Moslems are decent people, horrified by what is being done in their name, most – probably - unaware of the Koranic exhortations to force all infidels to "convert, submit or die", on which Islamic terrorists base their campaigns. Furthermore, as Moslems come to experience the advantages of the West some at least are likely to appreciate what they find. Since the decline of Mu'tazilism Islam has seen science as the work of the devil,[111] but the technology that Western science gives rise to is eagerly adopted by Moslems nonetheless. Cultural exchange is never only one-way, and in this there is hope that more and more Moslems will come to accept Western Enlightenment values, or at any rate accommodate them.

Perhaps more importantly, Moslem women are likely to more and more resent the way in which Islam treats them, very literally, as being worth less than men - only half, according to sharia law. The hand that rocks the cradle may yet rule even the Islamic world, as the West curtails the more savage elements of Islamic misogyny, and women take courage to express their views.

If democracy really is a manic ideal, no less than a world brought universally to *dar al-Islam* - the House of Submission - the world may be facing into yet another titanic struggle between rival manic ideologies, only one of which can win, so incompatible are they. If this is so, then in Yeats' words, "The best lack all conviction, while the worst / Are full of passionate intensity". The Enlightenment has led to so much tolerance that Islamic intolerance has immediate advantage; yet, as in the 1930s, after appeasement failed and war broke out, though totalitarianism had great initial advantages, its inherent

---

[111] Only two Moslems have won Nobel Prizes in the sciences - and both would be regarded as heretics by Sunni and Shia Islam both.

weaknesses, coupled to the meritocracy democracy fosters, led to its eventual defeat, just as the moral and intellectual bankruptcy of Communism led to its fall too.

DRUGS .

Both sides in World War II used drugs, Hitler was a drug-addict, Victorian Britain was awash with opium and cocaine and in post-war America millions of housewives relied on Benzedrine and Valium (mummy's little helper).

The proliferation of drugs is a sign of hypomania. Some 60,000 abusers die of Opiates every year in the USA the same amount of US soldiers that died in the Vietnam war. Speed makes you confident and in part works by increasing the blood pressure and heart rate. Some people believe that it releases dopamine in the brain. Ritalin is a derivative of speed and is used in Attention Deficit Disorder; it makes some people feel "normal," possibly not because it increases neural activity, but because it increases blood flow to certain parts of the brain.

Speed may also be a factor in speeding up the pace of cultural change and making it more manic and chaotic. Jack Kerouac took speed and this is reflected in the manic nature of *On the Road*, a book he wrote in a manic phase over a weekend on one roll of paper. The Beatles used to play in the red light district of Hamburg, doing two sets a day in the Reeperbahn Star Club, and taking speed to keep going. 250 gigs in 18 months.

In the Thirties speed was used for narcolepsy, slimming and asthma (Benzedrine). Seventy-two million tablets were taken during the Second World War. Hitler was a restless, frustrated, irascible man maybe due to speed injections from his personal doctor Dr. Theodore Morell almost every day with mainly "not just the opiate Eukodal but with testosterone, glucose, vitamins, animal hormones and cocaine" while the German soldiers took an early form of (methamphetamine) crystal meth called Pervitin. The German tank crews took speed going through the Ardennes.[112] RAF pilots were

---

[112] See *Blitzed: Drugs in Nazi Germany*, by Norman Ohler; reviewed by Dominic Sandbrook in the Culture section of *The Sunday Times*, 16 October 2016; also *Shooting Up: A History of Drugs and War*, by Lucasz Kamienski.

offered two Benzedrine tablets before a mission, while General Montgomery distributed some 100,000 amphetamine pills to his soldiers before the crucial battle of El Alamein.

In Vietnam American soldiers smoked marijuana, took hard drugs (mainly heroin) and used psychedelic substances. JFK got speed injections from his doctor, Max Jacobson (Dr. Feelgood), who was not a registered doctor and who also allegedly treated Jackie Kennedy, Marlene Dietrich, Nelson Rockefeller, and Tennesse Williams with injections of amphetamines, painkillers, vitamins and human placenta known as "fire-shots". Johnny Rotten and Sid Vicious, who started the punk music revolution, lived off the latter's speed dealing in1975 while they lived in a squat in Hampstead and ended with Sid killing his girlfriend Nancy in New York.

Drugs have been with humanity since we first drank fermented juice or chewed on cola leaves. Speed and cocaine make people manic: they move more, talk more, and think more quickly, are more sexualised, more confident, more humorous and more paranoid. But speed - in particular - can cause paranoia, irritability, anxiety, depression and insomnia. Cannabis can also lead to paranoia, a dangerous condition as a paranoid can kill without guilt, something that underpins the verdict of not guilty by reason of insanity in 40 out of 80 patients in the Central Mental Hospital. Mood-altering drugs may bring such a sufferer to very strange places. Cannabis in teenagers can bring on Schizophrenia more than normal.

Is the arguable increase in hypomania a function of increased availability of drugs? The high emotional state brought about by the endorphins and encephalin that may be exchanged across the placenta leads to a bonding of the mother and the child.

These are natural drugs that simulate opiates and are released at times of great emotion. Footage of the famous Nuremberg rallies would suggest a society living in a make-believe world of Teutonic myth and a madman's vision, but the high emotional state produced by participating in, or witnessing, such rallies may have bonded the German people together. Later bonding was through shared danger and hardship through the war, just as the shared experience of the hugely emotional Blitz may have bonded the British people.

Thus drugs, natural or artificial, make their contribution to societal hypomania, but also to social cohesion. The best example may be one of the oldest, alcohol, which by lowering inhibitions improves socialisation. Sometimes tragically, however, the same lowered inhibitions may also lead to strife and violence.

Thousands of years before the Nuremberg rallies, shamans took drugs such as psycillosybin, "magic" mushrooms, opium poppies and coca leaves, partly in order to have hallucinatory visions, and they influenced the culture of their society and were held in high esteem. Modern day Syd Barret. We may say that their aim was the best for their society; but was Hitler's any different? Did he not want the best, as he saw it, for the German people? Was his mythic guiding vision really qualitatively different from a tribal shaman's?

What Hitler gave his people was not a successful hunt, as the shaman did, but a convenient scapegoat for their defeat in 1918 and the almost supernatural ability to field the best army in world history, which almost beat the world.

Again, here, we may see a shamanistic parallel. The shaman's vision of a successful hunt often does lead to real hunting success, because by breaking hunting patterns in response to the shaman's vision - and we might expect that such rituals would be more often employed when hunting was bad - the hunters are more likely to be successful than by revisiting hunted-out grounds. Similarly, perhaps, Hitler's endorsement of popular resentment, and his presentation of both a culprit and a vision of themselves as a greater people than the Chosen People, gave the Germans the direction and ambition to make themselves, in a few years, one of the strongest countries in the world. Their very defeat, and destruction of their weapons on war in 1919, meant that they started without any of the inertia that restrained their enemies, ironically far more cowed by the prospect of another World War than were the losers of the First. The Germans' 88 mm field gun was the best in the war, as were their tanks and, at the outset anyway, the Messerschmitt Bf 109 fighter.

INTELLECT

Democracy, fraternity, liberty and equality make up the intellectual manic archetype: the essence of liberal minds comes from racing manic minds like a train. Intellect seeks truth, using left brain analytical skills to discover it.

But truth is elusive. And how does one measure it? There are three sorts of truth (or proof): mathematical, scientific, and what we may call "other" - such as that the Aryan race is superior to all others. The only form that is enduring across space and time is mathematical: two and two will always make four, wherever and whenever the calculation is performed.

Mathematical truth is pure and absolute. Scientific truth, though, is not, for it is always conditional on experiment continuing to confirm it, and the results of a scientific experiment may change depending on the variables. Thus classical or Newtonian physics ceases to be scientific "truth" at sub-atomic and astronomic levels; here one must employ Einsteinian or quantum scientific truth.

But left brain analytical skills, so essential to establishing "facts", must be integrated with right brain intuition if new "truths" are to be discovered. Einstein is said to have jotted E=mc2 on the back of an envelope long before he proved the formula. Singer discovered the working principles of a sewing machine in a dream, and the naphtha molecule was also explained in a dream as a snake with its tail in its mouth, thereby offering an explanation for the apparently extra atom.

Such visionary dreams need analytical skills to be applied to them if they are to manifest as useful realities. And this is maybe the best way to illustrate the "other" sort of truth, which makes discoveries by accommodating the sequential-analytical performance of the left brain with the holistic-parallelism performance of the right brain. When a scientist becomes too closely identified with his own field of expertise he is less likely to be able to step outside the box which it comprises, which can therefore become a prison for the intellect; furthermore, he tends to become professionally identified with the prevailing wisdom of his field. Thus people often make novel discoveries on the periphery, not at the centre, of any field. No mathematician is likely to discover new truths past the age of 26.

The problem with "other" truths - the third kind, after mathematical and scientific - arises when they cease to be tested by the intellect but rather are regarded as articles of faith, as enduring and eternal and immutable as mathematical truth. To insist that two and two make four is not only reasonable but essential, if the world is to work for its inhabitants; to insist that any article of "revealed truth" be as closely adhered to is a recipe for disaster, as the many holy wars have proved over the centuries. In hypomania, however, what often happens is that "revealed truths" regarding one's position, or how one is regarded by others (e.g. paranoia), cease to be tested by the objective scientific method, with sometimes tragic consequences.

Thus a healthy attitude to the intellect would seem to be that it should be respected for its worth but not worshipped for its own sake. It is an essential contributor to the acquisition of knowledge, and must be employed to test newly mooted ideas, but it should also be realised that it is not the only source of knowledge, and may even be an impediment to novel ideas. "Flipping the coin" in order to see what's on the other side should be an essential skill of the true intellectual, as it forces him to consider alternatives and prevents him from identifying too closely with his discovery—indeed, more likely prompting yet more discoveries. Such "flipping" is also a valuable means whereby the hypomanic may monitor himself. Overloading one side of the brain can cause it to flip to the other side.

STEALING

Stealing is probably a disinhibited behaviour - i.e. hypomanic - in that the thief refuses to acknowledge the right of the individual to his property. Some people steal because they need to in order to support themselves or their families; others do it for the thrill. These days thieves are often drug addicts, such as 5,000 heroin addicts in Ireland, hypomanics in themselves, who need £50 to £100 a day for their habit.

In the past people stole and plundered communities that came under their control through violence and war, mercenaries, like drug addicts, being hypomanics of a sort. Others were professional thieves: highwaymen and bandits and brigands, clearly hypomanic. If we look at possibly the most famous of these professional thieves, the James–Younger gang, we see men who had been traumatised by the Civil War. Jesse James was a psychopathological killer and a drug-addict, Cole Younger a larger-than-life personality and notorious ladies' man.

Today stealing is increasingly a high-tech business - as bank employees are told, no one comes in with a gun to rob them anymore, but rather does it on-line. Some security experts estimate that a great deal of the money needed to advance *dawa* (Moslem conquest by peaceful means, or "*sharia* by stealth) comes from on-line fraud. *Dawa* and *sharia* themselves, arguably, are hypomanic. Now we have hacking.

POLITICAL LIFE

Politics may exemplify the connection between the spending of money, which is the basis of capitalism, and the mania in modern life. Nowadays political success is determined in the first instance by money and the willingness to raise this by whatever methods. This calls into question the whole notion of democracy. Thus John Kennedy won the 1960 presidential election with 50.5 percent of the vote, but the margin was obtained from the ability his father, the richest Catholic in the USA, to deliver the Teamsters' Union, controlled by the Mafia, together with, according to some historians, the collaboration by Mayor Daly of Chicago, another powerful Irish-American. In the 2000 elections, when a similar question mark hung over George W. Bush's election in Florida, the outcome was challenged by his opponent; Richard Nixon, on the other hand, did not register a complaint in 1960, on the grounds that such an objection might undermine American democracy.

Does this change mean that democracy has suffered in the ensuing forty years, that self-centred hypomania has increased to the extent that it is now the inverse of what JFK urged at his inauguration? Ask not what you can do for your country, but what your country can do for you?

The Kennedy victory illustrated hypomania of another sort: the triumph of charisma, sexuality and intellect over stolid traditional Waspish values and appearance. Kennedy, a strikingly good-looking man - with a long string of sexual conquests - was dressed in a blue suit, had a healthy tan (caused by Addison's disease) and had his appearance highlighted with make-up; Nixon, on the other hand, refused make-up which he felt was only "for queers," had a dark five o'clock shadow, and his complexion was made appear paler by the grey suit he wore when they went head to head on a televised debate on TV which Kennedy clearly won by speaking as if to a friend.

A cynic might say that there are two types of politician: the caring, who is rare, and the ruthless, who enjoys power. Harold Wilson was photographed with a wedding ring and a pipe (a frugal, working-class way of using tobacco), though he smoked only cigars (associated with the establishment, wealth, the Tory Churchill), and with HP sauce on the table to make him look like the common man - a cynical, or at least calculating, pose in itself.

Because politicians control the finances of a country and can broker power, they are open to corruption, as the many ongoing and recent tribunals of inquiry in Ireland alone prove. Politicians may have delusions of grandeur if their power and high public profile lead them to think that they are better than other people. To want to have the power of a politician suggests manic leanings. Many politicians are publicans, teachers, lawyers, people who tend more toward hypomania than say farmers and housewives. They think they can change things, which they can't - or at least not immediately - but they behave as if they can. The IRA has committed itself to a United Socialist Ireland, a manic ideal, especially after socialism has taken a beating after the collapse of Communism, and one that has been pursued with ruthless barbarity ever since 1917.

The idea "to each according to his needs and from each according to his ability" is admirable in a misty-eyed way but it can never work because people are human and will take advantage of it. Lenin and Trotsky frankly acknowledged the need for state terror to make Communism work, and compromises with ideology meant that it never worked as well as any system that rewarded effort. The greatest reduction in world poverty in recent decades came when China abandoned Communism in all but name. Today a country that was marked by starvation, mass-death and cannibalism is one of the strongest economies in the world, and the USA's greatest creditor.

In the Communist Era Gabriel Garcia Marquez travelled to Eastern Europe three times and described how people there lived in terror and were "the saddest I had ever seen", even though he believed that socialism was the only way of getting rid of inequality of wealth. Even de Valera, one-time leader of Sinn Fein, acknowledged that the North would join the South only if unity were financially attractive. While he purported to encourage Irish people to stay at home he failed to provide the wherewithal for them to live there, and it's possible that he did not want migrants returning to Ireland as it might encourage dissent and dissatisfaction in the population, and introduce liberal ideas.

The connection between politics and big business - itself a manifestation of hypomania - might be seen in the CIA's involvement in the 1973 coup that brought down the democratically elected Allende government of Chile, the new democratic leader's leanings toward Communism being seen as too great a threat to capitalist interests in the USA. Recent scholarship suggests that the CIA ceased active involvement in Chile before the election, but it likely did assist domestic opposition to Allende after it, and there can be no doubt that the collapse of the Marxist government was in the USA's interests.

The connection - between politics and big business - may also be seen in the IRA campaign of 1994: they bombed the financial centre of London, costing the taxpayer hundreds of millions of pounds but more importantly threatening the existence of the financial centre. To kill a RUC officer was acceptable to the political establishment but to threaten the financial health of London's commercial activity was not acceptable to the business establishment.

If we look at individual politicians we can see signs of hypomania. Churchill, possibly the most famous politician of the twentieth century, believed, against all the odds, that a militarily weak and psychologically demoralised Britain could stand against the might of the Third Reich, and led it to do so. He was a charismatic man, convinced of the value and power of his own ideas, yet dogged by depression all his life, so prickly in his vanity that he once snapped at his grandson who had been about to take a photograph of him using a walking stick, and who destroyed a painting of himself commissioned by the House of Commons (because it refused to flatter him); he was also a functioning alcoholic.

Margaret Thatcher was the longest serving British Prime Minister of the twentieth century, the ruthlessness of her hold on power and the length of her term suggestive of hypomanic energy and a sense of destiny as strong as

Churchill's. She despatched a nuclear-powered submarine against a third-rate power in the Falklands War and sank the *Belgrano*, which was not an immediate threat and was besides outside Britain's own declared belligerency zone - all this to cover her administration's mistake in not anticipating the Argentinean junta's take-over.[113] In Northern Ireland, she refused to compromise with the IRA over prisoner status, leading to the disastrous Hunger Strike of 1981. If she wasn't motivated by hatred and ruthlessness she did have an almost Messianic conviction of the righteousness of her own position.

Eamon de Valera, though he had been leader of both Sinn Fein and the Irish Volunteers - later the IRA - executed IRA extremists when he had found his own way to constitutional politics. He once claimed that when he needed to know what the Irish people wanted he only had to look into his own heart, indicative of manic, almost messianic, fervour; he was also – apocryphally - credited by Einstein as one of the ten or so people in the world who really understood the theory of relativity.

Despite his religiosity and apparent asceticism, de Valera had his own relationship with wealth and big business. On his visit to the USA during the War of Independence he had raised vast sums of money for the Irish state, but he kept this and later used it to help set up *The Irish Press*. He raised the balance from shares sold to patriotic Irish people at home and abroad but these bought only A-shares, which paid no dividend and offered no executive control - they were officially called "Participation Certificates" and numbered more than 60,000. It was B-shares that offered both of these, and as "Controlling Director" de Valera controlled all 200 B-shares himself. The total value of the scam, in 1931, was about $250,000.

It is important to point out, however, that de Valera was not influenced primarily by personal greed for money but for power. One could even interpret his actions as being directed toward the well-being of Ireland. The money raised for the Daíl loan he may have felt in conscience he could not hand over to a government that had resigned itself to Free State status within the British Empire; that money had been contributed toward the foundation

---

[113] There was, as some of her advisers pointed out, the danger that the *Belgrano* could respond to orders from Buenos Aires and turn about, so if it was not an immediate threat it remained a potential one.

of an Irish *republic*, and *The Irish Press* was established to forward that aim.

If de Valera did not corrupt himself for money, one of his successors to leadership of his party did so with brazen and breathtaking audacity. The grandiosity of Charles Haughey is shown both by the manic way he lived beyond his means for years and by his success in doing so, till brought down by a drug-fuelled episode in another's hypomanic's life. His arrogance was highlighted by the contemptuous way he refused to answer journalists' questions on how he could afford to live the way he did on a TD's salary. He all but challenged them to expose his corruption, and a sad reflection on independent journalism was how Vincent Browne, one of Haughey's most persistent critics, cozied up to the old fox in the latter days of Haughey's life.

The cut and thrust of the political process is the mainstay of journalism. The journalist's clichéd dream is to call the editor and shout "Hold the front page!" Though many journalists are abstemious or even teetotal - Eamon Mallie, for instance - journalism is associated with heavy drinking, itself hypomanic, and hangovers have their own sort of hypomania, as neural activity tries to catch up on the depressive effect of the alcohol and the drinker tends to focus on seeking the truth.

There is far less toleration for heavy drinking in the profession nowadays; nevertheless many journalists tend toward hypomania of a different sort. Many favour socialism, perhaps driven into the profession by a wish to expose social problems and shortcomings, some perhaps overexposed to these by their work. Some may have a paranoid outlook - a paranoia that may be justified when one considers, say, the spate of killing of journalists in war zones and the hostility from an establishment anxious to conserve its power and privilege. Tapping of journalists' phones here and elsewhere prove that their concerns may be very real.

SPORT

Sports were important to the Greeks, Romans and Celts. Greece invented the Olympics, but they also placed more emphasis on learning than happens, especially perhaps with sportsmen, in the modern age. The Celts spaced their day into three parts: sports, games like chess, with drinking in the evenings. The modern Olympic motto is faster, higher and stronger, the pursuit of which is arguably manic in itself.

Competition to see who is best goes back to mating games, dancing, music, singing, humour and physical prowess in lights and drink of the night club. Men expressed their prowess and women picked the best, on the grounds that the best would be a good father, husband and breadwinner.

Expression of such prowess comes at a price. Far more men die violently, part of the reason nature sees more male babies born than females. Women break fewer amber lights than men, use seat belts more, smoke less, floss teeth more, take fewer risks and perform better at hedge funds.

Playing sports is a sublimation of man's basic instincts to win and to kill; it is controlled aggression. But some soccer players are now better known for their loutish behaviour than for their skill, and off-the-pitch hooliganism and sexual antics have long been associated with the game; in recent years the Leeds team in particular, perhaps, has acquired notoriety for fighting and causing trouble off the pitch. That sport is a form of displaced warfare is evident in the hate for the opposite team by some football fraternities. This hatred can almost be psychotic e.g. Rangers and Celtic where the Celtic manager got bombs in the post. An associated factor here is there is the narcissistic ego-driven love of one team and the hatred of the other by the paranoid id.

The violence extends further: in January 2002, Thomas Junta, the father of a child hockey-player from Massachusetts, was jailed for beating to death the referee of a game. Traditionally the GAA has been characterised by good humour and sporting behaviour, on the part of both players and fans, but even the GAA is experiencing violence on and off the pitch, the game becoming "more physical" and several referees savagely beaten after recent matches.

All this suggests a rise in hypomania. We seem to be getting to the stage where gladiators, back-street fighters as depicted in the film *Fight Club*, will fight to the death, a sign, prefigured by ancient Rome, which may anticipate the end of our manic civilisation. In Britain there are such fights organised outside the control of the various boxing boards.

There is a class element in sport, originally set by the nature and resources each called for. It is no accident that horse-racing was called the sport of kings; very few could afford a horse to work, and almost none could afford to risk the life or limb of one in sport. Falconry was stratified, according to the 1486 *Boke of St Albans*, with eagles for emperors, falcons for lesser royalty, hawks of one sort and another down the social scale with, at the bottom, "a kestrel for a knave", or servant. Soccer developed in the nineteenth century as a sport for the urban poor, in which virtually anyone could join in and all competed to kick a home-made ball of rags toward improvised goals. One can still pick out what were the most prosperous counties of late-nineteenth century Ireland by identifying those that have a hurling tradition: when the GAA was established to revive ancient Irish sports, football was as accessible to the rural Irish poor as soccer was to the urban English poor, with all competing for a single ball; but to play hurling one needed an individual hurling stick, which not everyone could afford. It's significant, in this regard, that Antrim is the only Ulster county to have a hurling tradition, though Antrim is also anomalous, because the necessary wealth here came from Belfast industry, not from farming.

Entertainment of the masses can be exploited in order to gain control of the masses, to some extent at least, as the Coliseum games were designed to do. Sport, especially snooker, boxing and soccer, are ways that permit the working class to become upper middle class. In part for this reason, where most sportsmen and - women were amateur, now an increasing number are going professional, and starting to play sports seriously at an earlier age, attracted by the fame and the money, or pushed and coached by ambitious parents. Tiger Woods exploded onto the fairway at nineteen to command winnings and merchandising worth millions of dollars, but the same hypomania that drove him on the greens also drove him to sleep around and his wife left him. Mike Tyson was groomed from the age of thirteen for the heavyweight championship. Twenty years ago people would not have dreamt that Rugby Union would become professional (the capitalist side being looked down on league).

The physicality of sport has increased, almost as in the decadent days of the Roman Empire. Gaelic games are certainly played at a faster pace than they were in the days when players had less time to train and were less well-nourished. Helmets are now usual in hurling, and one almost expects to see American Football padding on GAA players. Field games and cycling have also picked up pace, while boxing, "the nobles art of self-defence", with its Queensbury Rules, has been joined by cage fighting, in which nearly anything goes, and one can almost hear the baying of Coliseum crowds.

Further evidence of hypomania can be seen in how sports are becoming more technical as well as more violent. People are getting bigger, fitter, faster and stronger leading to more concussion in rugby and NFL. Ireland now has centres (Brian O'Driscoll) in rugby who are built like forwards in the past (Willy John Mc Bride), and helmets are commonplace in hurling.

As the stakes increase, so do the risks of one sort and another. Drugs are being used more and more in sports, enabling people to run faster and jump higher than before. We can do better than God or nature. Testosterone is the new winning hormone; it's a natural hormone too, of course, but seems to go with hypomania. People who win have a higher level of testosterone, and women who train intensively often stop having their periods. Thus a quintessential part of the female's life is done away with in the hypomanic quest to be the best. Careers are ruined, Michelle de Brún being best known in Ireland, her Olympic medals now a mockery of sport in the eyes of many.

Sports are going to the extreme of danger as in bunji jumping, bare knuckled fighting and the increased popularity of martial arts. The sportsman is portrayed as the new muscle-bound hero, the new Apollo. As people get more manic they enjoy the penalty shoot-out more than the actual football, fascinated by the tension.

We also see in the world of sport a sort of global hypomania - or rather, a particular sort of hypomania that manifests as globalism. Everywhere there is more migration and sports people are becoming part of a bigger European sports super league, with different nationalities playing in various countries. Racism may be undermined when people support a team that uses coloured players, and racism must be on the wane when coloured players such as Cole and York can play with prestige clubs like Manchester United. But such ideas need to be approached with caution.

Initially boxing broke the colour bar, and Jesse Owens became a hero in a still-racist age when he won gold's at Berlin in 1936; but it was Jackie Robinson who really made history when he signed for the Brooklyn Dodgers in 1947. Tennis player Arthur Ashe and Mohammed Ali were at the fore in the fight against racism in the Sixties and Seventies.

That said, however, Jack Johnson faced race hatred when he became heavyweight champion of the world in 1908, and his victory over James L Jeffries provoked race riots. He almost certainly threw the fight with Jess Willard in 1915, in the face of death threats. Johnson flaunted the immunity his position gave him, appearing conspicuously in the company of white women when this was enough to have him lynched in many American states. A couple of decades later Joe Louis had the tact and good sense to keep his affairs with white women secret. However popular the Brown Bomber was, he had to know his place in a white man's world, and arguably part of his popularity lay in his great rivalry with Max Schmeling, at a time when race theory was itself a core component of Nazi ideology, and Nazism was seen as hostile to American democratic values.

Mohammed Ali was probably the greatest sports star of the 20th century. He maniacally said, "I'm the greatest!" and certainly he was the black Apollo with a great physique, good looks, and a glib tongue. Ali did more than any sportsman to transcend the race barrier in sport; he was treated like a god by whites as well as blacks. Men loved his boxing and women loved him as an intelligent sensitive good-looking man. But while his racism was never personal, he was never able to transcend it fully.

More tragically for Ali himself, popular adulation fed back into his hypomania, ultimately to the detriment of his health. His hypomanic belief in himself led him to become the only man in history to have captured the world heavyweight title three times; it allowed him to take on, toe to toe, the "invincible," ferocious Sonny Liston, and later, more "hopelessly," the younger, stronger George Foreman. On this occasion Ali disregarded his own trainer's screamed advice and beat Foreman his way, taking brutal punishment from the younger, stronger man in order to wear him out.

This same hypomanic self-confidence, however, which empowered Ali to defy his trainer's "sensible" advice, and to absorb terrific punishment yet stay on his feet long enough to wear out a younger, stronger man, must have been a factor in driving Ali to keep fighting when he was far past his prime, which may have affected the onset of Parkinson's disease. Con Houlihan, the best sports writer in Ireland, told me that Cassius Clay was the greatest sportsman in the world.

Huge income, as well as huge ego, tends to fuel hypomania, and a hypomanic lifestyle, and a negative feedback loop often develops. Sports stars, the gods of the new age, as film stars were the gods of the Thirties and Forties, are paid a lot more money than in the past: David Beckham used to get £100,000 a week at Real Madrid, but sports stars also get more money for merchandising e.g. Beckham's boots and Roy Keanes' crisps.

This illustrates another connection between big money and advertising, which we claim drives the hypomania of modern times: sport is controlled by a few TV stations e.g. Sky Sports, and a 30-second advertisement slot during Super Bowl costs $1,000,000. Thus there is very expensive exposure to a very large potential market, so every microsecond of exposure must be made to count in terms of product placement and exposure. Hypomania is, effectively, a requirement to deliver this, and advertising and PR executives have to be the best in their field.

But the best do not come cheaply, and expenses in executive salary and in exposure have to be recovered somehow - in sales. In the last ten years people have been wearing expensive, cachet tracksuits and runners e.g. Umbro, Nike, Adidas. These firms have largely taken over the youth market of fashion, and are charging young people premium prices while the young people both reimburse the firms' costs and advertise the firms' goods. Couple unscrupulous merchandising with the adulation youth has for athletic superstars, and a hypomanic buying frenzy can result. Air Jordan sold one million trainers in their first year.

Another aspect of hypomania also of necessity emerges here: ego and associated paranoid insecurity. The cost of branded clothing and footwear is many multiples of its cost, and far above that of generic items, so a social cachet needs to be attached to the brand if it is to sell. Young people tend to feel insecure at some level, and peer pressure reinforces both the solidarity of group membership and emphasises "otherness". Thus an "other", already socially marginalised by relative poverty, is likely to feel marginalised further if he tries to gain membership to the "group" by wearing otherwise identical generic items. The brand, utterly incidental to the effectiveness of the clothing, then attains disproportionate weight in continuing to exclude the "other".

Always associated with sport has been betting, and like so much else in this field, the stakes have been getting higher - but also the opportunities to bet have been expanded by the internet. This makes it possible to bet from a mobile phone while riding the bus or on a toilet-break from work, so it becomes more difficult to get away from a hypomanic compulsion, and this moves the world toward hypomania. Enormous money is generated, making sporting events more easily affordable to run, creating a positive feedback loop which increases opportunities for the gambling industry. The rising tide lifts all boats in this marina: advertisements for casinos can now be heard on Irish radio, and social media supports such innovations as Betfect, which is associated with Ladbrokes. While one needs to be 18 to gamble legally, children as young as 16 can play gambling games in amusement arcades.

The end result is a fostering of hypomanic engagement with betting, and this is heightened by various "free bets" offered on various web-betting outlets. The temptations are immense, and endanger careers and lives. Traditionally boxers and jockeys were most open to corruption, but while team players may not be able to throw a game they still can, individually, becomes victims of the gambling industry. Oisin McConville, former Co Armagh football player, is one high-profile gambling addict.

ART

Art is the exteriorisation of the emotions so that they can be shared with other people and the exteriorisations can be assessed in as close to a rational or objective way as such things can be. Good art resonates with an inherent sense of beauty. But art is also the product of interplay between the left- and right-brain; between rhyme and reason; between exteriorising the uniquely subjective and making it accessible to others. Yet at the same time it is *neither* rhyme (left hand) *nor* reason (right hand) but exists uniquely, somewhere between the right and the left where one could say chaos lives (nonsense).

Art is also subjective representation of the human condition and the more it departs from this the less it becomes art and the more it becomes commercialism or propaganda. Yet the more intensely subjective its expression the less accessible to others it becomes, to the point of being solipsistic. A danger here is of art becoming isolationist, of artists convincing themselves that they are somehow superior beings. Such an attitude, however expressed, is bound to alienate "ordinary" people, some already perhaps suspicious of art as the work of wastrels or subversives. In fact, all can gain from deeper understanding of the human condition, which art offers.

Perversion of a rather opposite sort can also occur when art is mandated and conscripted toward some cause. For centuries this was the case, when art almost exclusively - in Europe anyway - represented Christian or kingly values. (Islam was different; it forbids the representation of God's creation in any way, so Islamic art is exclusively abstract.)

In the USSR ideology made regimented art a public spectacle and a political statement, reflecting the hypomania of the culture, which saw even the personal as subjected to the demands of the ideology, to the point of public enforcement. Marxism's theory that any system can work according to the principle, "to each according to his needs, and from each according to his abilities", is a manifestation of manic love, and in the essential corollary, that it can only be implemented by state terror - acknowledged and endorsed by Lenin and Trotsky, long before Stalin made it notorious - we see the paranoid manic archetype. So Soviet art was part of a hypomanic pattern that exalted the worker as the hero of the revolution.

Such regimented art compares unfavourably with the freedom of abstract expression of, say, Jackson Pollock, Mark Rothko and William de Kooning who made New York rather than Paris the centre of modernism. Yet the CIA directed this art toward their own ideological ends, through capitalistic sponsorship rather than state directive - again, in keeping with politics and arguably another way of prosecuting the Cold War by sponsoring capitalism and consumerism. The Rockefeller family championed Pollock. Andy Warhol, a commercial designer, was the manic artist who created pop art with Robert Rauschenberg, not through abstract expressionism but using the imagery of advertising, the supermarket and the city. It was Muriel Latow, an art dealer, who advised Warhol that he should "paint something people see every day like a Campbell's soup can", and Warhol did exactly that with *Campbell's Soup Cans*, a regimented painting of 32 of them, in an exhibition held in Los Angeles in 1962. Andy Warhol's picture of Marilyn Monroe sold in May 2022 for US$160million.

But even "pure" art may impose its own regimentation. Cubism, the art of the early twentieth century, was about shapes and patterns. Patterns are associated with right-brain activity, which is creative and non-linear; but cubism was not freedom but an artistic straightjacket, as it appealed specifically to male artistic urges and seemed to underline the impersonality of the world left behind by the Great War. Men are good at spacio-receptive geometry i.e. lines and angles. "Intelligent" art tends to be more truly intuitive - it is hardly an accident that not one of the many cubist artists and sculptors was a woman.

Creativity is a manic archetype. Lots of creative people are and were manic-depressive, like (poet Robert Lowell) or the modern Irish artist Michael Mulcahy, who is hypomanic, disinhibited, creative, funny and sexualised. Art and emotion are mainly right brain activities. Apparently dancing improves creativity as does thinking of shapes in your head - pyramids, cones and spheres - a device used by Yeats and others of the Golden Dawn.

Some people feel that drugs such as cocaine, speed and alcohol improve their creativity; both Francis Bacon and James Joyce used to create when they had hangovers. The creative hangover happens when you drink for a while (say a week) and you get up the next day when the alcohol wears off and you get the shakes (slight withdrawal symptoms) and sometimes epileptic fits (severe withdrawal DTs - very dangerous, a cure might be alcohol). The brain is overactive and very sensitive and therefore songs and stories become easier to write. Withdrawal DT's can cause increased blood pressure and death.

In the early stages bands often live the rock and roll lifestyle, with drink and drugs and having disturbed sleep. Then with some success they sleep in and the manic drive is dissipated and they don't have the creative hangover.

For creativity you need energy, confidence, mood and self-belief - all manic archetypes in themselves. You need the energy to create and the confidence to pursue your dream. Artists seem to have a high sex drive, e.g. rock 'n roll stars, Picasso, Rodin and Francis Bacon. They tend to create when they are high (Van Gogh) but this high can be dysphoric, where the person is irritable, aggressive, anxious, paranoid and suicidal, like a teenage spirit.

Sylvia Plath, in a letter to her brother Warren before her breakdown and suicide attempt in 1963, describes signs of manic depression (for which she was treated with ECT): "I have been very ecstatic, horribly depressed, shocked, elated, enlightened, and enervated....all of which goes to make up living very hard".[114] Plath poured her emotions into poetry; Van Gogh expressed his in colour and manic brush strokes with black crows screaming in the distance. Picasso was prolific, something perhaps suggestive of hypomania: in his lifetime he did 50,000 art pieces, three a day, including paintings, photographs and ceramics. The very name *Picasso* is a good one for an artist: there are three vowel sounds, and these, with their musical quality, appeal to the right brain.

After an epiphany in Dun Laoghaire, Beckett realised that art tended to be about positive culture and that few artists expressed the depressive position which he did. Beckett put himself in the mindset of the depressive and expressed the depressive's world view. He set out to eulogise the underdog and the "mad": e.g. people in barrels or buried in sand. Beckett always clung to his governing aesthetic that the artist is forever doomed to fail, to attempt to create and to fail again, yet to keep on trying and "fail better".

Creative people may be more productive - "fail better" - when they are bored and their rather well-known tendency to indulge excessively in alcohol and drugs may stem from the same drive to escape boredom. When they are depressed they are not creative, though the emotions they experience during depression may inform their creativity when they recover, or enter their manic phase, and there may be a parallel here with Hemingway's admonition to "write drunk, edit sober". Left hand, right hand.

But for other artists, activities that are "fun" or "exciting" foster creativity less than just allowing the mind to wander and engage imaginatively with the human condition. Joyce Carol Oates, one of the most prolific writers today, describes her life as unexciting and even uninteresting to the point of being "boring". Is her creativity a way of escaping this "boredom"? Or is she proof that "creativity" can be excuse for self-indulgence?

---

[114]Cited by Maeve O'Brien, in review of *The Letters of Sylvia Plath, Vol I*, edited by Karen V Kukil and Peter K Steinberg, in *The Irish Times*, "The Ticket" supplement, 4 Nov 2017.

INVENTIONS AND THEORIES

Like art, inventions and theories come from the synthetic, parallel, over-inclusive right brain - though implementing the ideas may call for logical left-brain application. Inventing means putting ideas in association with other differing ideas and in this regard intuition becomes important.

Intuition comes from many sources, but dreams are often cited as examples. Elias Howe, the inventor of the sewing machine, could not work out how to shuttle thread through fabric until he dreamt of being attacked by savages wielding spears that had holes in the blades; this inspired him to put the hole in the point of a needle, which made the invention possible. August Kekulé discovered the chemistry of the benzene molecule when he dreamt of a snake with its tail in its mouth.

Probably these are merely examples of the Eureka phenomenon, the process of incubation, the brain working on the problem at a subconscious level until a solution emerges into consciousness by whatever means. "Intuition", therefore, may be no more than a natural process, with nothing mysterious about it. Nevertheless, it does seem better developed in some than in others.

Ideas bounce into each other, by intuition or open discussion, and develop new areas of thought. Rationality and creativity are synthesised at a conscious or subconscious level. However, over-inclusivity, which forms apparently strained connections, is found in both schizophrenia and mania, often leading to confusion in diagnosis, and it also manifests itself in humour.

RD Laing and other "anti-psychiatrists" hold that madness is a logical response to an intolerable reality. The manic mind is intellectual and creative, and can find ways of "reconciling" intolerable reality with a tolerable *modus vivendi* by seeing "non-existent" connections and including what, to others, is not there. Yet while the manic mind looks forwards and has no fear it also looks back in paranoia, as it worries about people trying to control it.

Creative people have racing minds, are more sensitive to information, and have better memories that allow many conflicting thoughts and ideas to mix, possibly because of the manic energy animating them on a cyclical basis, but in some cases because of intrinsic gifts like a photographic memory. George Russell - "Æ" of the Irish literary revival - had such a memory, and also incredible energy that allowed him to mentor writers like Patrick Kavanagh (and, indeed, Robert Frost, indirectly, as "The Mountain" suggests). But Æ's left brain was hardly less influential, for he played a central role in setting up the Irish Co-op Movement, which transformed the Irish rural economy after the 1890s.

It seems impossible to avoid concluding that Æ very effectively synthesised left- and right-brain activities toward constructive ends, but he also "saw" fairies and painted them in vivid colours - he was a minor painter as well as a minor poet - and claimed that there were several sorts of fairies, not all of whom were aware of others. This would seem to be evidence of over-inclusivity, but Æ was a fully-functioning member of Irish society and in no way "mad".

The creative man often thinks of new inventions and new theories; he works away in the hut at the back of the garden, cutting up golf sticks and putting new material into the head, or making 1,000 failed light-bulbs before he gets one that works. But the successful inventor is one who is *realistic*; he will see what there is a need for, and he will apply scientific principles in getting the thing right - as Edison did - moderating the soaring flights of fancy of the right brain with the logic of the left brain.

The Renaissance was a great time for creativity in inventions as well as in art. Da Vinci had many ideas including the helicopter and the tank. Giotto in the 14th century; the architect, sculptor and theorist Filippo Brunelleschi in the 15th century; and Michelangelo in the 16th century, a superstar artist in painting, sculpture and architecture, were all truly great creative men.

The Renaissance blossomed from the collision of Western Christian society with Eastern society through trade by the Italian city-states. Trade with the Spice Islands and Cathay exposed people like Marco Polo to Mongolian, Confucian and Buddhist ideas, while transit through the Abbasid Empire exposed them to Moslem ideas. Until about the 12th century, the Abbasid Empire was the capital of world science and technology, and also the repository of Ancient Greek scholarship.

Such shaking-up of medieval thought and systems of belief were unquestionably manic by the standards of the time, and such hypomania was given impetus by the Great Voyages of Discovery - prompted by the Moslems' closure of the overland route - and in turn this challenged previously held ideas about the earth.

Galileo's theory about the heliocentric universe was only accepted officially by the Vatican in 1992. His *Dialogue* was banned from 1664 till 1966 when the Index of Prohibited Books was abolished following the Second Vatican Council. His persecution shows that control of thought by vested interests - the Christian Church's interest vested primarily in Revelation rather than Reason - is to the detriment of scientific discovery. A modern parallel is the (American) Foundation for Scientific Creationism, which states boldly that science may only be true if it is in conformity with the word of God, a logical nonsense by any critical measure.

PARTIES

Parties are manic mating rituals. People drink, talk, dance, joke, sing and try to impress the opposite sex with what their plans are in the hope of having sex, and perhaps less procreating, doing what they like in a hedonistic way. People express their taste in clothes and dance, often flamboyantly.

Students notoriously live for parties, settling down to more staid lifestyles after graduation. With the increase in wealth, however, and arguably an increase in hypomania throughout society, people party well beyond college years, every weekend. They go to night-clubs and stay up all night, increasingly using cocaine and other stimulants to do so. This all amounts to infantilising behaviour. People are staying single for longer, living at home and postponing marriage, in part a reflection of the real price of buying a house, but in part a reflection on the amount of time and money spent partying and in Japan on Branded goods.

Infantilising is not the only downside of such irresponsible behaviour. More and more alcohol is being drunk and use of it and other drugs leads to an increase in fights, traffic accidents, abortions, use of the morning after pill.

Such simplification of complexity is another manifestation of infantilising of society, and that it can lead to real injustice is proved by the witch-hunts of the 1990s. In 1988 some child-abuse survivors formed a support group in

New York and published *The Courage to Heal*, variously described as an abuse-survivor's bible and a propagator of False Memory Syndrome. One of the book's most dangerous claims is that anyone who believes she was abused, and whose life shows the symptoms of an abuse survivor, "probably" was abused. This remarkable sweeping statement led to one man, George Franklin, being found guilty of the murder of a child killed 20 years earlier, on the sole evidence of his psychologically erratic daughter - her erratic condition being "evidence" of the trauma she had suffered from witnessing the girl's murder.

Manic people, with their higher sex drive and confidence that the opposite sex is attracted to them, party more than normal people as they have more energy. But a partying lifestyle may create mania in what might otherwise be "normal" people. Many people today take drugs such as coffee, nicotine, alcohol, cocaine, speed, LSD and E that make them manic, and lead to increased confidence, sexual disinhibition and sometimes paranoia. Also, they will be influenced by their peers, in a party atmosphere for the worse, as the group dynamic here will more likely foster mob mentality.

People can be misled into making obviously wrong decisions in many situations. In the Asch experiment three people were shown lines on a screen and asked to select the longest. But only one of the people was the experimental subject; the other two were experimenters. The longest line was always obvious, but after a few rounds the two covert experimenters began deliberately picking the wrong line. At first the subjects were confused, but almost always they eventually would go along with the patently wrong opinions of the other two. If people will do this with strangers, they certainly will be influenced by the opinions of their partying friends. In this way "normal" people may be made hypomanic.

ROMAN ORGIES

Roman orgies were the parties of the Empire and showed the manic nature of the culture, with partner swapping, the need for more and better sex. Like the parties of today, these orgies would have been fed by food, alcohol and other drugs. In this hypomanic society Roman leaders became very decadent and carefree, thinking they were gods. Hyper-sexuality, as in the earlier Greek Empire, would have been rife.

Parallels with our own times are obvious. A sense of moral rootedness is being lost today; increasingly people live for the moment, with no sense of responsibility and much less concern for the future than their parents' generation had. One measure of this attitude is the amount of credit card debt. Another is the high levels of anomie and angst so prevalent today, especially among young men, who with no faith in the future can easily see no hope in it either.

May we see another parallel between the virile, sternly disciplined, highly principled (by their own measure) Fatwa warriors of today, and the tough, hard, hungry Huns, Ostrogoths, Visigoths and Vandals who brought down the decadent Roman Empire? Cheap technology and cheap international transport mean that the "barbarian hordes" of our own time may have already "crossed the Rhine." In the aftermath of Iraq, Syria and latterly Libya, we see refugees crossing the Mediterranean to Europe. Some are fleeing Isis and other intolerable conditions, but some, beyond a doubt, are Isis, and collapse of the so-called caliphate is sure to bring more.

Social controls of hypomanic tendencies, including, perhaps, hypomanic thought, may be necessary if society is not to descend into chaos, as Rome did. But how are we to police ideas, or even keep tendencies in check, without producing the sort of fascist state that is another form of hypomania? Maybe control of alcohol and smoking might be a way of controlling this artificially induced hypomania, but such control would also constitute legislating for morality, which is always bound to fail.

LOVE

Linked to parties and orgies is falling in love, a universal behaviour, and highly adaptive for a species as well as an individual level, but when it occurs serially and rapidly it suggests mania. We are surrounded by love in papers, magazines and music - part of the advertising blitz and instant gratification that characterises hypomanic society - but when we become obsessed by it, love becomes a manic delusion.

This may well be what the medieval troubadours brought to Europe: the erotic Courtly Love, which undercut the prevailing system of pragmatism in affairs of the heart. This pragmatism was alive and well in Ireland through much of the twentieth century, in certain rural areas, the matchmaker fulfilling a vital social service; dating agencies, and chat-rooms now provides something similar. Benjamin Disraeli often joked with his wife in their later years: "I only married you for your money" - which was true; but her reply, "Yes, but if you had to do it all over, you'd marry me for love," was equally true. Perhaps love is too serious a business to be left to the heart alone.

Friedrich Engels, the son of a wealthy industrialist, wrote of love in *Das Capital*. He said that the greatest thing that could happen to two people was falling in love with their ultimate partner and that religion, tradition and class structure (money) came in the way of people finding their ultimate love. It's still true, if maybe less so than in Engels' middle-class Victorian society, that people of different classes and religion do not marry.

Engels felt that getting rid of monetary and religious differences would facilitate true love, but soaring divorce rates undercut this notion, and as we watch people fight custody battles across the world it seems evident that "ultimate love" is not that between man and wife but between parent and child. Children need economic security and a strong tradition; they need money (capitalism) and tradition (religion) to give them the sense of certitude and security they crave in their essential weakness. Certainly if the species is to survive, then parental love is the one essential requirement, human babies, unlike those of most mammals, being entirely helpless at first, and having an uncommonly long neonate period. All this suggests that parental love is the absolutely biologically-essential sort, not based on socialism.

The idea that serially falling in love is maladaptive manic behaviour is therefore strengthened. Falling in love, on a species-adaptive level, is merely a stage on the road to "real" workable love, and terminating the process to start all over again not merely defers and endangers ever reaching that "ultimate" sort of love, but casts doubt over the paternity of such children as may result. Even when paternity is not in doubt, the absence of either parent, as a consequence of the end of the love affair, compromises the situation of such children as may have resulted. Such uncertainty as to paternity and financial and emotional support, tends to lead toward social chaos. Ensuring paternity by marriage may have originated as a cynical exercise by newly-settled Neolithic farming communities in the interests of passing on property, and homo sapiens may well be naturally promiscuous, but marriage did serve to impose some sort of social and economic order once we settled on propertied ground.

However, it also seems that the manic male, in his serial affairs, will pass on more genes than the sedentary, responsible type. In the short term this will be so; but in the longer term, babies needing a lot of care and attention to get them to the stage where they may pass on their genes, children of the serial-lover are likely to be at a disadvantage if, as is more likely than otherwise, their mothers are single. Even in today's socialist economies single parents have a difficult time; in the past this was even more the case.

This explains the brutally harsh intolerance of sexual promiscuity and "bastardy" - the brutal treatment of unwed mothers served as disincentive to endanger the well-being of a child, and to burden the community with rearing it in pre-social security times. For many years now society has been more tolerant, to the point of indulgence of promiscuity, critics being dismissed as religious arch-conservatives or even fascists; but social workers who actually work with problem families and children - as opposed to tenured academics writing up "research" - report a very strong correlation between lack of a father-figure, literacy problems, and delinquent behaviour.[115] Steve Biddulph 12 May 2018 Saturday Irish Times magazine. Compared with a girl, a boy is nine times more likely to end up in jail, three times more likely to use drugs, three times more likely to take his own life or die in a car crash. The science is getting clearer that for most boys, and most girls, there are glaring differences we have to address. Sampling umbilical cord blood at birth some have high or low testosterone and the high testosterone boys have more trouble with reading and speaking. Boys are three more likely to be problem readers than girls. And those are mostly high-testosterone boys. Most boys at five(and some girls too) aren't ready to stand still-in fact it harms their brains development if they do. And they are not ready for rote learning or being forced to read or write.

---

[115] The University of Melbourne's Institute of Applied Economics and Social Research reports that adolescent boys are much more likely than girls to become delinquent if they lack a father figure in their lives.

Tenured academics, often Marxist or neo-Marxist, have recently addressed this observation with the claim that "one meaningful adult can make a difference" in a child's life. This is obviously true, but it would seem to be the social equivalent of half a loaf being better than no bread, and it ignores the obvious fact that two meaningful adults must be even better than one, and that the chances of a child finding one meaningful adult are doubled in a traditional two-parent family. The "enlightened" academics, however, thus manage to subtly undermine the traditional family while inflating the non-traditional and advancing the Marxist ideal of uniformity (usually camouflaged as "equality").

JEALOUSY

On a continuum of pathology there is anxiety, jealousy and paranoia. Like paranoia, jealousy is a manic archetype. A link may be apparent between it and insecurity. Drink and drugs can bring it on and jealous people may be willing to kill their lover with no guilt. In France such a murder may be viewed as a "Crime of Passion." Jealous partners are sometimes dangerous. A patient who killed his wife and two children, said that he was glad his wife was dead while he was in prison so that she could not have relationships, the rationale being, "If I can't have you, no one else will".

In mythic and ancient times wars were fought over women, notably the Greco-Trojan war; more recently wars have been over territory. Jealousy is in everybody but only becomes pathological in a few cases where it might end in murder. It is seen as atavistic behaviour that might be maladaptive, certainly when killing one's spouse endangers one's own children and genetic heritage.

Christianity recognises the importance of jealousy: the commandments prohibit covetousness of wives and property in an attempt to avoid the problems it may cause. Such avoidance, the sense of certitude it may bestow, may actually increase individual freedom, by allowing one to be oneself on one's own terms (within society's dictates). By contrast, free love in the Sixties attempted to control jealousy by denying it - by allowing people to sleep around. Jealousy was seen as a weakness in that it undermined the ideology that there should be no societal controls on love. Like Iggy Pop said "the guy with the biggest cock got to sleep with the girls".

This disinhibition was often driven by either a leftist or a pacifist ideology, and was of limited success at best. The leftists look to undermine traditional society by advocating alternatives that allegedly have no jealousy, but man is not the only mammal that feels jealousy - and the Rousseau romantics were wrong.

For almost 60 years social science was dominated by the teachings of Margaret Mead, an American anthropologist who, at 27, published *Coming of Age in Samoa* (1928), which described a Noble Savage world. Mead argued that war was "an invention" of civilisation and that in the natural order peace prevailed. In Samoa there was no jealousy and sexual freedom was for all. Rousseau had been vindicated. But in the 1980s Mead's informants, by then old women, confessed that her obsession with sex meant that her sources, half embarrassed and half thrilled, "just fibbed and fibbed to her". In 1984 Derek Freeman challenged Mead's claims with police records that proved that the rate of violent death in Samoa in the Roaring Twenties was higher than it had been in the USA. Sexual jealousy was as commonplace there as elsewhere.

Meanwhile, in 1964, Napoleon Chagnon had investigated the Yanomami and found that violence and murder were not merely commonplace but genetically adaptive.[116] Some disbelieved him and denigrated his work, even accusing him of complicity in murder, just as they had denigrated Mead's critic Derek Freeman, who challenged her conclusions after living in Samoa and realising what the actuality was.

The enlightened lefties, after their savaging of Chagnon and Freeman failed to shut them up, called on postmodernism and claimed that all anthropologists' data collections are really "creative fictions", but the real problem was short time-spans of study and too-small samples. Rousseau's vision of utopia had been exposed as a mirage, but even into the twenty-first century Mead's champions kept up the fight.

Jealousy is what drives a male to defend territory and mate, and a female ape

---

[116] Ian Morris, *War—What Is It Good For?* p 56.

will often kill the offspring of other female apes so that her offspring will have a higher survival rate. Silverback gorillas also do this.

Away from the jungle and Pacific islands, "keeping up with the Joneses" may be a spur to improvement of one's material welfare, and therefore adaptive. Capitalism is somewhat driven by jealousy; snobbery is a factor in the us-them social, economic and political divide that can lead to either mutually advantageous, healthy competition or mutually destructive war. Class increasingly is distinguished by ownership of goods, whether a house, land, address, school, holidays and culture.

At the petty level there is a lot of jealousy in the workplace where people want bigger offices, better car perks and expense accounts and better promotion prospects. People try to outdo each other. Clothes are a main part in the mating game: they show whether you can afford designer labels and live the lifestyle that requires money. We are jealous of the stars and their comfort. We are jealous of happy marriages and wealth.

Despite its ubiquity and its arguably-adaptive consequences, jealousy is seen as a negative quality, especially by feminists who feel it is an excuse for men's controlling women. People can play on their partners' insecurity and manipulate their relationship. But jealousy can cement a relationship too; it can bring people together, and its positive survival advantage is the protection given to a partner by a male driven to fight to hold onto her, if largely so that he can be more certain that the children in the relationship are his.

Who is the father? is a main question in the paranoid state in the modern age. DNA testing can now show paternity and thereby marital infidelity, which an unfaithful wife in the past might have been able to conceal. This new technology, which will become more popular, may impose extra stress on relationships.

As with so much else, emotions may extend beyond the individual and become cultural constructs. Jealousy may have been a factor in the many nationalist movements of the nineteenth and early twentieth centuries, as well as in the imperial rivalry that marked the decades running up to the Great War. While one – nationalism - just might be regarded as adaptive, the other reminds one of the psychopath who destroys his partner and anyone else who gets in the way. Germany, a Johnny-come-lately European Great Power, jealously wanted to have its "place in the sun" like the others - an overseas empire - and become a World Power. But the need for a navy to maintain such an empire aroused the fears of Britain, adaptively jealous of its own navy, which was essential for an island nation. This jealousy led to devastating war, after which the Germans projected their jealousy onto the Jews who were blamed for having "stabbed in the back" the German armies that otherwise would have won the Great War.

The Jews, successful and rich as a result of their cultural tradition as bankers, diamond cutters, jewellers, furriers and moneylenders, provided the Germans an enemy on which to focus their hatred (id). The Germans made up a mythical cultural belief to counteract their humiliation after the Treaty of Versailles and redeem their self-esteem, even if this myth flew in the face of actual facts. Many of the pre-war German financiers and businessmen were Jewish, and one of them, Walter Rathenau, was even *Reichsminster* in charge of materials distribution, invaluable to the war effort. Jews had been awarded the Iron Cross and other military decorations; it was a baptised Jewish officer, Ernst Hess, who endorsed Hitler for one of his Iron Crosses and - surely irony of all ironies? - it was a Prussian chemist, Fritz Haber, who supervised the first German gas attack at Second Ypres in 1915, and later synthesised Zyklon-B, the gas used to exterminate six million of his fellow-Jews during the Holocaust.

DISINHIBITION

Over-inclusiveness is found in schizophrenia and mania where there is a lack of physical, social, emotional and intellectual boundaries. A sign of mania is disinhibited behaviour both sexually and intellectually. "Rapid cyclers" are very disinhibited; their mood-swings are rapid - over hours if not minutes. When disinhibited people experience more stimulating physical, mental and emotional states they look for something new to do or think. Disinhibition is the basis of creativity: new thoughts, new experiences and new emotions.[117]

---

[117] One of the essential points emphasised by teachers of the "composition process" is not to be concerned with grammatical or spelling correctness in the first stages, as such inhibitions will interfere with the essential creative process.

Disinhibition leads to new associations of intellect (humour), physical (sexual) and emotional (creative) experience; but the uninhibited right brain may undermine society - or at any rate social mores. Impulsiveness, creativity, emotionalism all tend to lead to a drop in moral standards; the jokes get cruder, the sex gets weirder. People are more physically and mentally-emotionally receptive to each other's advances. Disinhibited people have more sexual relationships; incest moves in as the boundaries fall. Diogenes showed his "freedom" by masturbating in public.

Such behaviour militates against the corollary of individual freedom: social responsibility. Freedom only works effectively within certain constraints which we "freely" agree to uphold. Public masturbation would be an affront to the sensibilities of others, a sign of individual madness, and if enough people imitated Diogenes their exhibition of personal freedom might lead to political exhibitionism for its own sake, and indicate a crumbling empire.

Masturbation in history was blamed on haemorrhoids, tuberculosis, paralysis, emaciation, listlessness, asthma, acne, warts, cramps and blindness.[118] Dr. Kellogg developed corn flakes because spicy food in his opinion made you masturbate and bland food did not. If people masturbated in public, at present, they would be charged with offences against public decency and removed from society. But if these same people did not have to go to work on Monday it would be a different world, a permanent weekend, a holiday every day as opposed to two weeks in the sun; and on such holidays, as has already been noted, inhibitions are lowered. To some extent society is more tolerant of misbehaviour by holidaymakers, but whether this toleration would extend beyond public drunkenness to public masturbation is doubtful.

Does this suggest that it is public or circumstantial pressure that keeps people in line? Without societal pressure would we all indulge in permanent holidays, and masturbate or fornicate in public? Semi-public drunken fornication did occur during VE Day celebrations in London, all but a blind eye being turned to it.[119]

---

[118] See Mels Van Driel, *With the Hand: A Cultural History of Masturbation.*
[119] See "People had sex outside Buckingham Palace on VE Day", *The Telegraph*, 17 March 2014.

The fact that society is now much more tolerant of social misdemeanours than it was in former years might indicate that the world is reducing societal pressures on its members. Social control by peers can be a feeble check; alcoholics and drug addicts take no heed of advice from friends, AA and when people get a lot of money they often squander it in a short time, whatever friends may advise them. Should there be more stringent controls, "for the people's own good"? Greater enlightenment, and economic and social change, mean that we cannot go back to such regimes. The injustice of the death penalty for sheep-stealing is too patently obvious for such a penalty to be used any longer to maintain privilege in a class-divided society, and the counter-productivity of harsh penal regimes offers empirical evidence to justify a more enlightened, rehabilitative approach.

Yet there does appear to be greater expression of hypomanic behaviour in modern society. Is this because modern society is more permissive? Or might not our more permissive regime be due to greater hypomania in society?

If the latter is the case, when did the change begin to occur? Disinhibition was found at the end of the Egyptian, Greek and Roman Empires and now it is being seen in what one might call the Post-Christian Empire. Social control was lost during the days of Caligula's reign; the rich partied all the time; but hypomania also drove the Renaissance, the Reformation, the Enlightenment and the French and American Revolutions. The turn of the twentieth century saw a hypomanic conflict between the Great Powers, including a punitively expensive naval race between Britain and Germany, but those years also saw Liberal reforms in the 1908 Children's Act and Old Age Pensions Act and the 1911 National Insurance Act. Around this time, too, Einstein developed his theory of relativity and Picasso painted the first Cubist painting *Les Demoiselles de Avignon*.

In the 1960s a political awareness developed that centred on Flower Power and the hippie belief that homosexuality should be made legal and the death penalty outlawed. By the end of the 1960s these aims had been largely achieved and today some of the former hippie idealists are now in positions of power in the European Parliament - Danny Cohn-Bendit, for instance. Outside of those, Bill Gates, formerly a slacker of Silicon Valley, is set to give most of his money to charity and a few million to his children. Richest man Elon Musk, worth US$210billion

Philanthropy is a manic trait; people on bi-polar highs may give away much of their wealth and possessions that they might have made through mania. The previous great philanthropical period was the Gilded Age, when people like Andrew Carnegie and Alfred Nobel endowed libraries and various other good causes. However, the beneficence of philanthropists needs to be set against the fact that their "generous" gifts would otherwise go to paying taxes, so is philanthropy really a manifestation of hypomanic generosity or shrewd calculation?

Humour is a special state of disinhibition that is shared by society as it can break down boundaries or reinforce them. Freud saw humour as a reflection of the unconscious mind but he never made the link between humour and sex in advertising and mania. When people are manic they can be very funny and it is recognised that a lot of comedians are manic-depressives and their humour is infectious - e.g. Tony Hancock, Freddie Starr, Ruby Wax and Lenny Bruce, Spike Milligan, Robin Williams.

It has been found that dancing can cause disinhibition and increase creativity; Dervishes use it to prepare themselves for "unnatural" feats such as walking on hot coals and broken glass, and – formerly - to whip warriors into killing frenzies. Some Pentecostalists and some Baptists use dancing and chanting in their church services to get closer to God, a religious experience described by Van Morrison in his songs e.g. Astral Weeks – "being born again." Snake handlers go through the same frenzy.

TV

Overall TV may be good for people in providing both information and entertainment but its utility declines if it displaces other, more real, more important aspects of their lives. Unless we pick the programs we really want to watch, TV may come to dictate our needs and wants; become the altar in the corner dedicated to the great god of hypomanic consumption. BBC has its own culture but does not have advertising.

TV is getting faster, more creative, gossipy, funny and intellectual - but also anti-intellectual and vacuous in much of its reality shows. There are more channels, digital, satellite, terrestrial, colour TV, wide screen TV, Cefax, computers, Google, video, stereos, video games, the Internet, Natflix and DVDs. People see more violence and sex which increases their testosterone levels, testosterone being known as the success hormone.

But even "information channels," like Discovery and History Channels, may subtly become sources of "information": information-as-product; another measure of what we have rather than are; another reflection of hypomanic possessiveness. Soaps, once wholesome, family entertainment, seem more and more concerned with crises and with sexual affairs, stimulating the manic archetypes and encouraging hypomania. The news is very paranoia-driven with rape, murder, death and job losses being the main ingredients, not unlike the story in soaps. Tik Tok is everywhere.

Humour has been successful at selling as sex is also used to sell. The ads are getting "better" than the programs: more clever, more amusing, more erotic. They are becoming the new art medium - if not the new entertainment, a reflection on the quality of many programmes. More money is spent on them and they (ads) are getting more creative. On average a three-minute ad costs €30,000 to produce, the same as an hour of TV.

TV shopping is easier, cheaper and people buy more on credit. People spending hours on the phone and using the Internet more, and thereby avoiding personal contact with real human vendors of products. What's happening in America will happen in Ireland and Britain.

TV helps people who are lonely but too often their favourite program takes over their life. As one of its writers said, *Coronation Street* - watched in the U.K. by 11 million people, with the highest rating on T.V. - is for "people who have no lives". Benjamin Shapiro claims: "I think entertainment matters more than politics: that's what convinces people what to think and how to feel".[120] "You'll find out that the box in your living room has been invading your mind, subtly shaping your opinions, pushing you to certain socio-political conclusion for years."

---

[120] Benjamin Shapiro, *Primetime Propaganda: The True Hollywood Story of How the Left Took Over your TV.*

This influence, according to Shapiro, shapes the world's political thinking. He says that Hollywood shapes "America's styles, tastes, politics and even family structure". Popular programs such as *Glee, Friends, The Simpsons, Sesame Street, Will and Grace, Sex and the City* and *the Mary Tyler Moore Show* were started to push their liberal agenda by producers who believe in liberal democracy and left wing politics. You are either for or against same sex marriage and if you are against you will not work in Hollywood. Leonard Goldberg, a politically-moderate producer, says that liberalism in television is "100 percent dominant and anyone who denies it is kidding or not telling the truth".

Shapiro asks Martha Kauffman, the creator of *Friends*, about criticism that the show promotes a liberal agenda. "How could it not?" she responds. "You have a bunch of liberals running the show...we're going to put out there what we believe. These characters mirror who we are."

BRAINSTORMING

Brainstorming, by encouraging people to break away from the dominant, rational left brain to the intuitive emotional right brain, broadens our thinking. New ideas come up, and these then are examined by the rational - left - brain, so that in the end logic and calm evaluation determine whether any brainstormed "solution" is in fact adopted.

There is a manic element in brainstorming, with ideas just thrown around. It is very creative, basic and intellectually stimulating. The margins of thought are opened. The idea of over-inclusiveness, normally an impediment to adaptive behaviour, comes constructively into play here, where we try to "think outside the box"; normally we are encouraged to restrict ourselves to "the box" in order to focus on specific targets.

Over-inclusiveness is seen in both mania and schizophrenia but I feel it is mainly a manic idea, because over-inclusiveness is the basis of the creativity which makes people willing to look at anything in a way that may be opposite the agreed truth of a modern culture. Over-inclusiveness allows one to put different unusual ideas side by side and out of this comes a new idea that has not occurred before. Simple coding such as skipping A-D-G-J-M illustrates, at a basic level, creating new "words" in a creative manner that helps us to solve problems.

Sometimes these ideas are very intuitive. Einstein is said to have written down $E=MC^2$ on the back of an envelope years before he could prove the theory. He used to meet his friends after work in a cafe in Vienna and it was here that new ideas were discussed. He used to get the tram home after seeing his friends and wondered what it would be like if he travelled at the speed of light and what time his watch would show in comparison to the town hall clock he was moving away from, as the light from this followed him—an over-inclusive way of thinking.

Such thinking is perhaps more natural than we imagine; it merely gets stunted as we discover how things "really" are. A friend's small son, asking the are-we-there-yet question and told "Soon", responded "Why is a grown-up's *soon* short and a little boy's *soon* very long?" Such a perspective on the subjective nature of time's passage is the sort of over-inclusive thinking that may lead to discoveries like Einstein's. Perhaps it's no coincidence that Einstein liked the spontaneity of children and hated dinner parties because he said people ate him, where convention rules. He loved to play music the violin, which would have stimulated his intuitive right brain, and he did this with his friends.

AGGRESSION AND VIOLENCE

Some people feel that aggression has increased among juveniles and young adults over recent years. Measuring whether this is really so objectively is difficult but there seems little doubt that it is the case. The relatively recent popularity of weight-lifting and body-building leads to elevated levels of testosterone, and often this is augmented and heightened by consumption of steroids. Fist-fights at weekend dances were usual in the 1970s and before, but they seldom resulted in death or serious injury. Fatal outcomes of fights between young men are commonplace now, where in times past they were much rarer and more likely to result from calculated malice than almost random striking out.

Reasons for the increase in such violence have been put down variously to food additives, increased alcohol consumption and drug abuse, and video games that simulate shooting dehumanised targets - probably the phenomenon has more than one cause. It is hardly outlandish, however, to at least postulate a parallel between the increase in violence and that in hypomania in modern society.

Colonel David Grossman makes a very convincing argument that the increase in violence is due to a deliberate blunting of human sensitivity, in particular to the increased availability of violent computer games that have a high "kill" rate, a method that was developed by the US military after the Korean War. According to Grossman, up until the Vietnam War perhaps a quarter of soldiers in actual combat actively tried to kill their enemies, the taboo against killing being so strong; but in Vietnam, this figure increased to over 95 percent. Grossman attributes most of this remarkable increase to the sort of simulated computer games soldiers were made play, and to the desensitising effect of watching violent films. He attributes the increase in violence in society to exactly the same games and violent films that now have trickled down into virtually every home.

Violence per se, however, need not be maladaptive: it stems from the overactive physical archetype. This can be channelled peacefully into games like football and boxing, but this may not be enough. People like violence and this is exemplified in the rise in popularity of cage-fighting and mixed martial arts, which replicate the desperate nature of street-fighting far more than "the noble art of self defence" ever did. Women too can now be found in the boxing ring - is this a manifestation of some perceived need to demonstrate "equality", or of an increase in actual violence?

It is important to remember that violence was always evident in society. Coliseum crowds called for fallen gladiators to be killed if their fight had not already done so. The legend of the Amazons suggests that women always had the capacity for violence, and one of Kipling's poems speaks of a soldier "wounded and left on Afghanistan's plains, And the women come out to cut up what remains".[121] By many accounts society has never been safer than

---

[121] Rudyard Kipling, "The Young British Soldier".

now,[122] and it may be significant that only today does bullfighting look like following cock-fighting and bull-baiting into the dustbin of opprobrium.

But there has also been an upsurge in random violence across the West. Gangs attack strangers for no good motive. Recently whole spates of murder in Ireland occur after the pubs have shut and every weekend there is a new victim, alcohol both providing disinhibition and the hypomanic energy that fuels the excess that may lead to tragic violence.

Violence may also be ordered and calculating. In modern day executions and amputation of limbs we see a form of social control in Muslim cultures and regimes. Arguably Islamic culture, with its perceived God-given mandate to convert the world, is intrinsically hypomanic, but state-sanctioned violence can be seen in some states of America, where the death penalty still exists - as it does, of course, elsewhere.

As a deterrent to violent crime the death penalty has been argued to be no more effective than incarceration, a less-violent expression of state control. There is a correlation between those states with a high incidence of fatal violence and those with the death penalty, so it would seem that the latter does not deter the former, but one must not confuse correlation with causation. Guns are widely available in the USA and this in itself may up the aggression stakes but the availability of guns does not seem to be the critical factor. Per capita, the USA comes perhaps seventh in the world; first is Switzerland, second Sweden, and neither of these countries is associated with violence (the reason for their high rate of gun ownership being that most adults belong to the national militias and must, by law, maintain an assault-rifle in their homes).

In the USA, there does seem to be a correlation between regions with high rates of gun ownership and violence - the South is almost a synonym for gun-happiness and for violence and murder - but the correlation is not complete. Vermont is unique in that it has no prohibition on carrying concealed weapons, but it has a lower crime rate than the adjacent Maritime Provinces, though Canada overall has a much lower incidence of violence than the USA. North Dakota has a very high rate of gun ownership but is one of the safest places in the world to live - or was until recently, when coal-mining began to

---

[122] For instance, Ian Morris, *War: What is it Good For?*

attract young men to the state and violence increased. Always and everywhere young men, driven by high testosterone levels, are the likeliest perpetrators and victims of violence.

Wider social and demographic factors, specifically hypomanic tendencies, may better explain different levels of violence. Sweden and Switzerland both have long traditions of peace and international non-aggression, as well as a strong Protestant work ethic. Sweden also has a powerful Lutheran tradition as does Germany where Chancellor Dr. Angela Merkel is the daughter of an East German Lutheran pastor and the President Joachim Gauch is a former Lutheran Pastor.

History is another factor. The American frontier was like almost all frontiers in that it was advanced against great dangers from nature and usually other human beings. These dangers all but needed to be met with violence, and this violence is of recent origin in America. The Indian Wars ended only in 1890, and even after that "wild" Indians like the Paiute Willie Boy and the Apache Kid created widespread fear and paranoia in their brief rampages.

The situation in Canada was different than in the USA because by and large the Crown treated Indians better and the rule of law preceded settlement. The USA broke every single treaty made with the Indians (one of the very first, signed by George Washington, was broken in 1966) and after the Civil War brutalised veterans, many of them outlawed Confederate guerrillas, moved West ahead of the law into the land of hostile Indians and often came in contact with the law later in the form of former Union veterans wearing tin stars, like the Earp brothers or Wild Bill Hickok.

Cheap weapons technology of the Industrial Revolution created a certain Western egalitarianism: God made man, an old saying had it, but Sam Colt made him equal. New technology and other changes made some weapons redundant and cheapened them further. Brass cartridges became widely available after 1870, so earlier cap-and-ball revolvers became relegated; smokeless replaced black powder in 1890, with similar results; and after the great herds of buffalo were effectively wiped out in the 1880s, expensive and very powerful and suddenly useless buffalo rifles were dumped on an already-glutted market.

The end result was a heavily-armed population of mostly young men, many brutalised and traumatised by war, in a land with no law and few women, but full of guns and enemies and paranoia. A violent culture was almost bound to emerge.

Most USA descendants are German not Irish. Yet there is another element in the American mix. The Germanic/Teutonic culture is manic, OCD, Protestant, Lutheran, hard working, saving money and building business. It is musical - Bach, Beethoven, Mozart - and based on ideas and philosophies such as Kant's and Nietzsche's. Lutheranism is the dominant religion in North Dakota, a predominantly rural state, and the main reason for the high incidence of guns here is hunting and vermin control. Vermont has a Yankee Puritan tradition and a long history of rural conservatism (in the "best" sense).

The South, on the other hand, and the West to a lesser extent, has a different ethos. No less Protestant, Protestantism here is of a more manic sort: conservative in the reactionary sense, impelled by evangelical fervour and informed by the Old Testament. Yet simultaneously these areas have high alcohol consumption and a tradition of xenophobia and intolerance, including, counter intuitively, for Yankee Puritanism. Also, the Bible belt spans most of these areas and society here expects eye-for-eye retribution, hence the death penalty persists in Southern states, unlike in Northern states - Minnesota, for instance, abolished it in 1911.

Perhaps the high incidence of both social and state-sanctioned violence reflects a social attitude that, to some extent at least, tolerates violence. The South and West of the USA were settled by violent war against the Native Americans, and these areas have a tradition of manly honour that needs to be defended by duels, if necessary. Thus society almost expects a young man to use violence, even as a first resort, if he imagines his honour to be impugned; high alcohol consumption lowers inhibitions and inflames tempers, and the South and West are and always have been known for high alcohol consumption.

The USA, unlike Canada, was settled by primarily violent means. Furthermore, again unlike Canada where settlement was accompanied by the Northwest Military Police, settlement in the USA was a far more laissez faire business, and usually preceded the law. To make matters worse, after the Civil War, hundreds of Southern guerrillas, denied amnesty, took off for the West, bringing with them the casual violence to which they had been hardened by their experiences. The brutalising effect of the Civil War, the greed for gold that was the impetus for much Western settlement, the many range wars between rancher and homesteader, the genocide Indian Wars all fed a hypomanic frenzy that is still to be discerned in these parts of America.

Man is a potential killer and is naturally violent. Violence is actually species-adaptive because it ensures that the strongest take the best resources while the losers are driven out to colonise more harsh environments and thereby improve their stock or go extinct. The commandments say you should not kill and this is a way of controlling the id; but the word translated as "kill" more closely means "murder" i.e. the killing of someone from one's own tribe; the Koran's prohibition is closer to the Old Testament's than the Christian's.

Violence is a basic instinct, normally subsumed into controlled aggression in sport, so the id can be controlled. Murder, rape, incest, cannibalism, infanticide and paedophilia were possibly widespread in early human times. Infanticide stopped dissemination of the genes, and something similar can be seen when a new alpha male takes over a pride of lions. Incest may also have had long-term beneficial consequences because in-breeding fosters critical genetic change, such as language development, which thus would be concentrated in a group, thereby acquiring a certain critical mass before being passed on to the greater population.

At the same time language may have developed, in part, as a way of stemming violence in early human society. Language allows for more subtle expressions of violence or friendship than non-verbal communication might have made possible. Touch is important in communication - light touch, deep touch, hot-cold, vibration sense, propio-reception, two point discrimination - but words allow for fine distinction that otherwise might not be possible. As well, the need for such fine distinction fosters development of vocabulary.

Considering man's potential for same, there is a low level of murder and violence in modern society. Through the violent 20th century about 1-2 percent of the world's population died violently, a tenth of the rate in pre-industrial and pre-modern societies.[123] Whether modern culture and civilisation have domesticated man permanently, however, remains not proven. As HG Wells once put it, scratch the most urbane of us hard enough and the hot red eyes of a caveman will stare out.

WINNING

Modern culture is all about winning. Manic people have a high confidence level and this is what often separates the winner from the loser. Confidence is seen as being very important and psychology is now being used in sport to bolster confidence. Self-belief is important in all walks of life. U2 were known to have such a high level of belief in themselves even when they were unknown that people in the business now evaluate new bands by their confidence in comparison with the young U2. It is not surprising that U2 came from a liberal co-ed school such as Mount Temple where the majority of pupils are educated Protestant and individuality is championed. A band of two Protestant boys (4 percent of the population in Southern Ireland) Adam Clayton, the Edge, Bono - whose Protestant mother died when he was 14 years old at her father's funeral due to a brain aneurism four days later - and a fourth a Catholic Larry Mullin. My uncle William Marshall was a teacher in an early part of this school called Mountjoy.

People will overcome obstacles because their belief in themselves and their persistence makes them immune to criticism and drives them on to their goal, the nonentity Austrian corporal who became the most powerful man in the world being perhaps the prime example. Furthermore, people like confident people; even the famously shrewd Lloyd George found himself charmed by Hitler, as late as 1936.

In particular, confident men attract women. "Winners" have a higher level of the male hormone testosterone (the success hormone), and this peaks massively in the winner even of a chess game immediately after the win. Conversely, testosterone levels plummet in the loser. This is purely animal reaction. Within a couple of days of being displaced, the erstwhile-dominant gelada baboon loses its distinctive and distinguishing colour.

---

[123] Ian Morris, op cit, passim.

We love to win whether it's monopoly, chess, cards, football, climbing Mount Everest, driving a rally, or even by proxy: the same pattern occurs in followers of the game, e.g. football supporters. We like the euphoria caused by endorphins and encephalins, the manic high; but this seems to be triggered by testosterone. We also love the entertainment and are willing to spend money to see our football team or local hero win for *us*. We like to see the best people fight it out, on the chessboard or in the boxing ring. Mohammed Ali was manic and charismatic in his personality and he was voted sports star of the twentieth century. "I'm the best."

Champions are high up in the pecking order of society, rewarded with wealth, status and love. But at the end it may end up, as Solomon, whose study was of madness and success, said, "All in the wind." The price is high: Hitler died at 56, Napoleon at 52, Alexander the Great at 33. Though Churchill died at 90, his childhood was wretched and he was dogged by depression all his life. He and Michael Collins shared bipolar disorder illness (though Collins died before it could fully manifest).[124] Tiger Woods was hot-housed by his father; he held his first club at six months and was playing golf at four years of age. But at what price to his childhood did this inculcated hypomania come? The Jackson Five were similarly hot-housed by their father and Michael Jackson is almost a synonym for manic delusion and disappointment at what the real human being became (post-mortem photographs revealing him to be balding were somehow shocking and sad). By any reasonable standard, trying to change one's skin colour and to look like Diana Ross is unreasonable behaviour at best. His obsessive examination of his own concert performances on video after the gig indicates both fixations on winning and perhaps manic-compulsiveness. Conversation with his lighting engineer.

GOSSIP AND CONSPIRACY

Gossip is manic; it deals with fame, sex, money, power; who's doing what to whom. It is digested and read by people with little conviction and what would seem to be empty lives, who live through *OK* and *Hello* magazine.

---

[124] Eoghan Harris, the *Sunday Independent*, 14 January 2018.

Yet to some degree everybody gossips; they want to know about emotion. Princess Diana was the doyen of the gossip columns with whom she flirted and who followed her everywhere. When she died there was an outpouring of emotion on an almost unprecedented scale. Even politicians who were republican and anti-monarchist such as Fianna Fail publicly grieved. Her story had all the ingredients of a fairytale: the beautiful misunderstood princess who transgressed in love and whose husband had a mistress; a victim of the all-powerful in-law family; a mythical modern day tragedy. Diana was an angel in people's minds; the pretty princes we all long to be.

The empathy and transference of emotion at this level has rarely been seen. **It was as if a fertility sacrifice had happened and; people's id had been satisfied**. People cried openly in a mass-hysterical type of way. The absolute coverage by Sky News made it a global happening on the level of Live Aid in 1985. People felt as if a person in their immediate family had died. Millions from across the social classes mourned as one. Elton John rewrote his song "Candle in the Wind" to commemorate the death of Princess Diana and it became the biggest selling record of all time with 37 million sales. (To compare, "Rock Around the Clock" came in second with fifteen million and third was "Yesterday" with 1.5 million.) Jackie and JFK and Marilyn Monroe were others who had similar beauty and charisma and ultimately tragedy.

The public and the gossip press like to make stars of people but their love may turn to hate. This may be because of simple disappointment, when the idol is revealed to have feet of clay (the "unbeatable" boxer is knocked out; the "invincible" team is defeated; the national heroine is revealed to have probably gained her Gold Medal through cheating); but in a manic world it may be due to something else. Escalating levels of manic love may lead to paranoia, where the emotional projection is reversed and the once-loved person is perceived as threatening. Thus the media turned public adulation for comedian Fatty Arbuckle into public hatred and contempt.

Gossip can feed public paranoia in another manner, when conspiracy theories emerge to account for the death of Diana or JFK. Though it is, on one level, a healthy indicator of democracy when questions are raised, and the official version of events is queried, it is anything but healthy for an individual to persist in rejecting rational explanations in favour of far-fetched suppositions. A rather empty life lends itself to fascination with, say crop circles and gossip mentality. It surely is significant that even when the men who started making these circles admitted their prank many people refused to believe the simple truth - even after the pranksters demonstrated how they had made the circles. Whether this indicates hypomania or mere stupidity is moot, but the whole conspiracy theory mentality surely gives cause for worry to those who look on humanity as rational: "Evidence? That was planted by the conspirators!" Or: "Of course there's no evidence! That's a measure of how successful the conspiracy is."

Another darker aspect is that conspiracy theorists are the opposite of winners - losers in the literal sense. Having lost the war in 1918, Erich Ludendorff blamed the "November criminals", notably Jews, for "back-stabbing" the victorious German armies, and the *dollstoßlegende* was born. The consequence for the Jews of Europe was unimaginable at the time, and a warning of the power of the lie. After the next war the Holocaust was denied by David Irving and other conspiracy theorists, whose anti-Semitism drove and still drives them to proclaim what the evidence plainly shows to be a lie.

Fake News, Trump – *"I won"*, so gossip is not harmless. It gives spurious validation to what may have fatal consequences. The "justification" that "there's no smoke without fire" can create the belief that even blameless people have "a case to answer". Few Germans believed Jews should be exterminated, but enough believed they had "a case to answer" to provide the Nazis with a mandate.

Nor is this danger an historic one. Today in this country some people genuinely believe that Catholic priests deserve to be somehow held to account for the cover-up of crimes by the Catholic Church, even if the priests were unborn at the time those crimes were committed. Justification of such a position is founded on guilt by association, logical fallacy being the essential building stones of conspiracy theory.

The danger is not restricted to Ireland, as the dismissal of Steven Galloway by the University of British Columbia in 2016 proves. Galloway was accused of sexual molestation and other offences and suspended in November 2015, but "the university went public in the national media before there was an inquiry", demanding the accused sign a confidentiality agreement. The

University "would not [even] disclose the nature of the allegations" and Galloway was left with everyone free to attack him publicly under "the impression that he was a violent serial rapist", since under the confidentiality agreement he couldn't say anything to defend himself.[125]

The truly grave aspect of this case was that a retired court judge brought in to conduct the investigation was able to sustain only one of the allegations made against him, yet Galloway's dismissal was upheld. His single "crime" was to have had a two-year affair with a married woman some years older than he - hardly taking advantage of some vulnerable young girl.

Yet what's arguably even more disturbing than the persecution of Galloway on the basis of accusation alone is the outrage of extreme feminists at the defence of due process by the veteran feminist Margaret Atwood.[126] *Witchhunt* is surely not too strong a term to use for such persecutions.

HUMOUR

Gallows-laughter might seem the most appropriate response to such disturbing developments - some people feel that incongruity is the essence of humour. Freud felt that laughter was a release for aggressive impulses whereas a lot of it is sexual. Verbal humour lights up the parts of the frontal cortex involved in resolving ambiguities, flexible thinking and seeing situations from a different point of view - being able to laugh at oneself has always been regarded as a sign of mental strength and this would therefore seem to have neurological support. With laughter the funnier the joke is found, the more activity is seen in the brain's "reward centres" which create pleasure feelings, and these feelings are contagious. "Laughter is social, being 30 times less frequent in solitary than social situations".[127] Being contagious, laughter helps us bond and communicate. It also eases our stress,

---

[125] Marsha Lederman, "Author Steven Galloway fired from UBC after investigation of 'serious allegations'", in *The Globe and Mail Online*.
[126] Margaret Atwood, "Am I a bad feminist?" in *The Globe and Mail Online*, 15 January 2018.
[127] Professor Robert Provine, *Laughter: A Scientific Investigation*; reviewed by David Derbyshire in *The Irish Independent*, 25 May 2002.

lowers our blood pressure and reduces our anxiety and makes us live longer and healthier lives. It may well truly be the best medicine.

There is a link between humour and hypomania. Manic people tend to be funny, deliberately or unwittingly. Humour is anarchic; it brings people together to have a laugh and is associated with drinking at the pub, parties and weddings. We greatly enjoy jokes and put comedians who are often manic-depressives high on our popularity lists. As its neurological coordinates suggest, humour is often about new associations of words and ideas; thus it is linked to over inclusiveness (different associations) that is the basis of creativity and in itself is creative.

When girls are asked what they like in boys they put humour high on the list. Humour is often about sex and unravelling of our preoccupation with it and it also reflects our unconscious desires and thoughts such as race. Humour is often about foreigners: Americans tell jokes about Poles and the British about the Irish. Jokers clowns and jesters were important people in the king's court as are comedians more recently, but nowadays the focus of public humour is in the media, especially TV and more recently in concerts where comedians can make millions such as Peter Kay who made £20 million touring in 2012. More recently it has been used in advertising, underlining the manic connection where humour sells. Humour is associated with irrationality and intuition.

SELF HELP BOOKS

Self-help books are usually written and lectured about by very charismatic hypomanic people, gurus of health, wealth, and intellect. The field has been explored from Aristotle's time, notably by Seneca (first century AD), and Robert Burton (1577-1640), who talks about self-help books in the *Anatomy of Melancholia* (1621). The self-help movement really began to expand in Victorian times, and over recent years books like *I'm OK, You're OK* (on Transactional Analysis), *The Road Less Travelled*, and a whole slew on "Creative Visualisation" comprise much of the best-seller lists. You can do it, you can succeed, is the message. In these authors promulgate an ancient manic message more in keeping with twentieth-century American mores.

What seems to be more evidence of mania is the type of people who read these books. On one level it is self-evident that people can improve their circumstances - it is intrinsic to our survival instinct to maximise our opportunities. But often people who are fixated on their perceived failures are exploited by self-help gurus.

A distinction exists between genuine popular science and New Age flake. Self-help books often use modern psychology to help the reader change, usually through transactional analysis, gestalt or cognitive therapy, demonstrably effective methods. New Age "self-help" books tend to focus on such things as "creative visualisation" of a more effective self and a happier future. Their authors often adapt magic and shamanistic rituals, which, if they work at all, do so by the shaman's imposition of will on another. There is evidence that such approaches not only do not work, but rather may exacerbate the problem, as the failure of the therapy drives the person trying to improve himself to see this as evidence of further personal failure, and the disappointment drives him deeper into despair.

Self-help books have been associated with manic Americans, all but comically addicted to psychoanalysis, as exemplified by Woody Allen in his numerous films; but increasingly Europeans are taking to them, Andrew Weil's books selling widely here as well.

CURSE WORDS

Curse words are musical and they come from the right brain.[128] They switch you from your left rational brain to your right intuitive, creative brain. The right brain is more manic and as we get more manic, we use more curse words, though they are frowned on despite this. They used to be rare in books, plays and films, and even the suggestion of them, as in "f—," or even "b—x" or "d—n" was frowned on, but now they are commonplace even in PG movies, indicative of greater tolerance of hypomania. *Coronation Street* and *Eastenders* do not have curse words despite their popularity and being set largely in bars, where one would expect such language. This is possibly because the watershed mark is 9pm. However, it has been remarked that even

---

[128] Professor Breathnach lecture, St Patrick's Hospital, 1987.

these soaps have become far more salacious in their subject matter in recent years; how long before curse words infiltrate?

"Don't take the Lord God's name in vain" - the Second Commandment. Curse words were perceived as highly dangerous in superstitious, spirit-centred societies, invoking the gods' presence and possibly undermining both morality and authority of the tribe - later of the state. Many still view them, atavistically, as bad and evil. Rap music uses curse words, reflective both of the musical quality of the words and rap's disrespect for society. Children like rude words because they upset their parents and because the children can sense the power of the words, if only because adults, powerful people, use them.

Popular opinion says that people who use curse words have a limited vocabulary and cannot find the right words to express themselves. But this may not be true of every instance. Curse words are very powerful, if less so and in a different way than primitive societies imagine. People use them when emotionally aroused. If you are having a problem you can often be helped by cursing as this will make you think in a different way flicking from a full left brain to a right brain and thereby get a solution - perhaps by helping to articulate the anger and tap the emotional power. Curse words, like jokes, are often about sexuality, and together they are a reflection of the unconscious drives.[129]

ARISTOCRACY

Mania tends to afflict the upper classes more than others. The aristocracy famously live lives filled with wit, humour and sexuality, in blissful unawareness of the problems of the day. A friend who married an aristocrat remarked once she knew him for ten years and the woman she was speaking to retorted that her family knew his for three hundred years.

Aristocracy is close to royalty. Aristocrats got their land and position through war and as gifts from the king or queen for their support. They have money so they do not have to work; yet they can be high achievers. They have their own language and dress code. They know their position in society

---

[129] See John C Parkin, *Fuck It: The Ultimate Spiritual Way*.

and they do not have to be pushy. They tend to have their own semi-exclusive pursuits: the Henley regatta, coming-out Balls, Ascot, Wimbledon, polo and fox- and stag-hunting.

The aristocracy is a very small collection of people who have a disproportionately large influence on culture and politics. They tend to be well educated in the best private schools and this gives them confidence above their intellectual abilities and get jobs for the boys such as Lloyds where you have to invest a lot of money to gain a position of authority.

One must understand that free education is only a relatively new concept. It was quickly seized on by Catholics in Northern Ireland as a means of escaping generations of oppression by an establishment of industrialists and craftsmen. Prior to 1947 higher education had been the preserve of the wealthy, and they used it to advance themselves, as might be expected.

But plutocracy is taking over from aristocracy; in Ireland the plutocrats and their antecedents, the Gombeen men, have been the only native aristocracy since the end of the clan system. In the USA obscene amounts of money are needed to run electoral campaigns so plutocracy is eroding true democracy and money makes more money, so "dynasties" like the Kennedys, the Bushes and the Clintons emerge. Like the aristocracy, the plutocracy seems to be able to grasp wealth and power by hypomanic force of personality and strength of both limb and character.

LEARNING

Learning is necessary to survive, and ubiquitous in nature. We learn how to survive in the jungle and in modern western civilisation. We like to learn about new things and we absorb the information, whether from books, films or the modern media. Children love learning and when they are about two years old they can learn 70 new words a week. But learning, along with being necessary, is manic. Mania can lead to an increased memory (hypermnesia) which, with over-inclusiveness, can lead to greater creativity, which, in turn, improves learning.

Recent socio-economic changes across the world mean that learning is a much more ongoing process than it was in the pastoral or even the relatively recent past, when a school certificate might be enough to provide a person with the wherewithal to obtain a "job for life." Now we expect to change jobs more than once in our working lives, and we expect the jobs themselves to change over time. Does hypomania confer an advantage in the workplace?

We are educated to suit employment availability. At the moment in Ireland there is a lack of school graduates in the science subjects. As a result, they are not capable of filling all jobs in the computer and technological industries. Furthermore, apparently ten percent of school leavers are functionally illiterate so their entire education is deficient. On the other hand, people are now in a situation where things are changing all the time and they need continuous education.

Essential to learning is communication. It is through touch that language has developed. When apes are grooming they touch each other a lot and express their feelings vocally, having recognisable sounds for such emotions as pleasure and pain. Apes cannot express vowel sounds, though, as their vocal cords are higher up the trachea.[130] What is said is not important; it's the emotion that is recognised. Consonants tend to communicate meaning whereas vowels express emotions. Chimpanzees make a "ha-ah" panting noise when tickled but they cannot make more than a single sound in one breath. It differs from the "ha-ha" sound of modern human laughter, which emits a series of short vowel-like sounds.[131]

Certain people like Tom York of Radio Head can sing about nonsense and it sounds great. He just has a good salesman's voice that can connect with our emotions, despite lyrics about plastic watering cans and fake Chinese rubber plants. Pop deals with pure emotions such as love and loneliness, whereas rock may have a political content or context. Pop relies a lot on vowel sounds - la-la, humming - whereas rock uses more consonants: "Sweet child in time"; "Time waits for no man."

The pop star is always in the news or gossip-columns; the rock star does few interviews. Van Morrison is notoriously reticent; Bob Dylan is a mystery, giving very few interviews: the only interview Dave Fanning could find for a

---

[130] But man pays a price for his vociferousness: because of the low placement of the vocal cords in the larynx, he is far more prone to choking than other animals.

[131] Provine, op cit.

recent RTE radio programme was from 1984. One day I was driving into town on Clare St. when I noticed a man on a bicycle coming the other way. He looked up. It was Bob Dylan. He was with a minder cycling behind. A few days later I heard that Dylan was in town but he'd managed to keep it from the press.

Such reticence reflects a certain mind-set. Some authorities believe that Dylan's famous withdrawal from public in the late 1960s was due not to a motorcycle accident, as was given out at the time, but to mental breakdown. Journalist Eamon Carr (a drummer with the highly rated Irish band Horslips that fused Celtic Rock, hypomanic in its own way) reports that Dylan definitely did have a breakdown, during which he "saw" and "talked to" Jesus and even had a Messianic delusion.[132] At very least, Carr claims that Dylan "needed a motorbike crash to save himself [; to] rescue his music and salvage his integrity" after the concept album made philosophers of "dullards" and pop music fell into the hands of the squares".[133]

John Lennon called his people together in Abbey Road studio to tell them that it had been revealed that he was Jesus. Sunday Edition Observer. Front page.

Though it may be far from being pop music, Italian opera is also emotional rather than cerebral or intellectual, and it evolved in a country whose language has a higher than average percentage of vowel sounds.

Language comes primarily from the mother; it is she who lays down the word and the ability to express emotions.[134] A two year old can recognise 250 sounds that make up all the sounds of all the languages in the world and is potentially born to speak them all. This ability decreases with age. A sound that a two-year-old makes depends on 40 facial muscle movements. To an extent, therefore, we can see how the nurture/nature mix becomes biased in favour of nature that follows Naomh Chomsky's theory of linguistics.

It is possible to learn; the impetus and ambition to do so can be inculcated. It is equally possible to discourage learning. Thus, some generations ago, "book learning" was regarded as a waste of time in many instances in

---

[132] Personal conversation, but reported also in the *Evening Herald*.
[133] Brian Boyd, "The Beatles, Bob Dylan and the Beach Boys: 12 months that changed music" in the *Irish Times*, 4 June 2016.
[134] *Secret Life of Babies*, director Barny Revill, 2014.

working-class households; now it is rather regarded as a necessary and expensive investment. Learning, therefore, has vital cultural determinants.

Old cultures are based on achromatic teaching where the teacher chooses the pupil because of his qualities and passes on "the secrets" by word of mouth. This leads to verbal elite among the people, an elite that directs and creates culture; Socrates, Plato and Aristotle are obvious early examples. Learning performance depends on cultural as well as genetic factors that affect IQ, therefore any faction that feels itself isolated culturally may have learning difficulties, real or imagined. In the 1970s H. J. Eysenck "proved" that Irish schoolchildren are less intelligent than their English counterparts, citing as evidence the earlier findings of another investigator, McNamara; but McNamara's study had rather indicated that a lower IQ score, a perceived lower intelligence, actually reflected how rural Irish students had been alienated by the details of a test designed to suit urban English kids.

Such cultural, certainly individual, determinants may not be uniquely human. Among baboons there is a class system. The alpha male, all but by definition the most hypomanic of the troop, works out problems and passes on knowledge; he will show the rest of the troop how to do things. If he is taught something artificially - as opposed to working out a natural problem - he will be able to teach others. The beta baboon will learn to get a banana out of a cage but he will not show the other baboons how to do it. Perhaps this says more about the ability to teach than to learn but it does show that learning affects more than the individual: it has vital cultural consequences. The challenge may be, in this increasingly hypomanic age, to identify and separate out those manic elements of the hypomanic condition that lead to improved learning performance, and incorporate them in a learning and teaching strategy.

GAMBLING

Gambling is a way of controlling a changing environment. It is manic in that people get excited, believe they can win the prize against sometimes immensely long odds and spend a lot of money they cannot afford feeding their children cigarettes and biscuits. They get a downward mood-swing if they lose, upward if they win: the HIT.

Gambling can be taken to extreme as shown in the film *The Deer Hunter* where they play Russian roulette for money, but for most people it is a relatively harmless vice. Yet it remains a system based on chance and, because of carefully worked out mathematical formulae, the punter rarely wins; it is an addiction to spend money and a treatment is Gamblers Anonymous which is necessary for 1 percent of the population.

But it is also a component of the liberal capitalist democracy. Professional gamblers are quite conservative and they are obsessive in the way they bet. They are more controlled then the average punter. The stock market is essentially a huge gamble, and, as at the poker table, bluff plays a role - which is fine and well until reality calls the traders' bluff and the entire stock-market collapses, bringing ruination to the gamblers and all whose lives they touch.

Both the occasional flutterer and the professional punter gets a manic hit from the race. Some people say that there would be no horse racing without betting. In Las Vegas casinos provide free food and drink and have oxygen pumped into them so that gamblers will be less likely to leave through hunger or tiredness, and there is 24-hour lighting so people lose track of time - always easy to do when one is utterly caught up in something - the aim always being to keep them gambling.

In the old days people bought indulgences; now they use other methods to try to control an uncertain environment, one of which is the sudden acquisition of fabulous wealth, which will cushion them against life's knocks. Once a year on Grand National day people who would never gamble otherwise have a flutter. The chance of being a millionaire drives the National Lottery, a seven million to one gamble. People not only get the manic hit from winning, they like the dream of winning a lot of money and they fantasise about winning, being free to do what they like, indulging the manic archetypes.

The National Lottery's advertising campaigns express various extravagant and even flippant consequences of a successful win: buying a tropical island or following a favourite band to concerts across the world. Such inconsequential ambitions, and living by chance at seven million to one, suggests irresponsibility and may even signal incipient breakdown of culture and society.

Northern Presbyterians will not gamble on a Sunday - which is when southern Catholic priests go to the races - and many Christians see gambling, like alcohol and other drugs, as the devil's realm. It is interesting that gambling and drink are outlawed in Islamic countries, where a similar manic brand of religion as is found in Northern Ireland often prevails.

TAROT CARDS

People feel insecure, especially about money and relationships, and they don't like uncertainties. We like to think we know what is going to happen. We have sayings and stories (Æsop, the Bible) that we live our life by.

The mind is made manic by the unknown and the unknowable, and not only gamblers seek to control their circumstances: some who say they are psychic claim they can control the circumstances and lives of others as well as their own. Tarot, a very old method, deals with love, money and the future in general. How the random fall of cards can be used to predict the future defies logic; maybe the cards work as a prompt, together with betrayed emotion and body language.

But people who attend fortune-tellers believe in actual psychic ability of certain individuals who can foresee the future and tell about manic things. The nearest to a logical accounting for such a phenomenon might be that time is actually not the plastic, unidirectional thing it seems, but something rigid and already laid out in eternity, and that some people can fleetingly gain access to a perspective on the future and the past. Perhaps, if this theory is correct, we all have - or once had - this ability but such sometimes terrible knowledge became intolerable to sentient beings, so evolution removed it.

This is fanciful, however, and it is more likely that neatness is the sign of an orderly mind, and neat stories can be woven around the draw of Tarot cards. We have an apparently-intrinsic need for closed narrative with satisfying endings,[135] and like people to say things are all right, even when we have our doubts. The problem is that, like Chamberlain and his bringing of "peace in

---

[135] Anyone can test this by telling a small child the story of, say, Little Red Riding Hood and trying to pretend it ends with the wolf taking leave of the little girl in the wood. "But what happened then?"

our time," self-delusive certitude is as likely to do harm as good. One who sets out to better and enrich himself by his own efforts - by "blood, sweat, tears and blood," as Chamberlain's domestic nemesis memorably put it - is far more likely to do so than one who relies on a fortune-teller's prediction that wealth will come to him.

There are other hypomanic aspects to this sort of behaviour. The ability of the fortune-teller to cold-read from unconscious responses of another whether the "fortune" being read is being endorsed or otherwise is beyond the ken of most people; and the conviction of the sincere ones who truly believe in their ability, and the self-confidence of the charlatans to carry off their bluff also suggests hypomania.

MANIC DEPRESSIVE ILLNESS

This seems to affect men and women equally but any analysis needs to take account of national and cultural differences in diagnosis. That caveat understood, it seems the lifetime risk in Western countries is 0.6 percent to 1.1 percent for mania, as opposed to perhaps 10 percent for hypomania. The average age of onset is mid-twenties so teens and adolescents are seldom manic. Manics are probably sexualised earlier than their normal peers and this, together with their characteristic disinhibition, means they are more likely to have children earlier, and to have through their lives more partners and children than the normal person. In this manner they partially overcoming the limitations of their illness a little in the way a cuckoo propagates by having other birds rear its young. The baby cuckoo pushes the other eggs and babies out of the nest.

Mike Oldfield, a prolific and genius composer, has had seven children by different women. While in his case he looks after them all, were he not so successful he would be less capable of doing so. Oldfield has had mental health problems, and while these may be linked to LSD use in youth, he seems hypomanic in several ways, not merely in his artistic output but in a fondness for fast motorcycles and light aircraft, and a certain footlooseness.

Mania is more common in the upper social classes i.e. classes 1 and 2. The eccentricity of hypomania in the upper classes is more acceptable than in the working classes. The Virgin Prunes, a working class band, included Gavin Friday and Guggi as front men, and they were often beaten up for wearing woman's dresses and other unconventional clothes not acceptable to the controllers of rock. Such colourful eccentricity may have been a way of coping with internal dissonance - Gavin had sayings such as "If you've got hassle in your head get rid of the hassle not your head" - but it seems to have threatened the working classes. The idea of a working class hero is a myth, as John Lennon made quite clear in his often-misunderstood song.

GENETICS

There is a definite correlation between mania and genetic influence. The manic gene is so strong that it overcomes almost any sense of nurture. In bipolar probands (family) there is an increased risk of both bipolar and unipolar disorders in first degree relative (combined risk of 18-20 per cent). There would be a spectrum of the disorder (mania) and of hypomania in the extended family.

The dominance of nature over nurture is evident in twin studies. The concordance ration for bipolar disorders in monozygotic twins as opposed to dizygotic twins is 79:19; that for unipolar disorders is 54:24. The likelihood of inheritance of bipolar disorder from a biological parent is 28 percent, as opposed to 12 percent from an adoptive parent.

That genes rather than environmental factors are predominant may be explained by the apparent link between low levels of serotonin, essential to neurotransmission, in mania and depression. But more work needs to be done in this area. The positive neurotransmitters like serotonin and dopamine make up 5% of neurotransmitters in the brain whereas negative neurotransmitters such as acetylcholine make up 95% of neurotransmitters in the brain.

SOLUTION?

Freud claimed that all problems originate in the subconscious, in the often-conflicting demands of id, ego and superego. A remedy for such problems might be found, however ironic it may seem, in a compound of manic-depression (hypomania), obsessive-compulsive disorder (OCD), and a psychopathic nature. The manic-depressive has the drive to accomplish; the obsessive-compulsive the urge to finish a task; the psychopath the lack of guilt of one who doesn't care and makes firm decisions. The combination can contribute to the success of any venture as it fosters a certain confidence, however reckless. This "synthetic" condition could be set up through a series of tests and initiations (with, obviously, various checks and balances), initially on people whose control of their lives had slipped - because they were "victims" of any of the above conditions - so as to use their condition, their own nature, to restore control to their own lives.

It might be foreseen, however, that even "normal" people might benefit from synthesis of some of the elements that could give them the drive to embark on a worthwhile venture, and the confidence to complete this.

FUKUYAMA

In *Consequences of the Biotechnology Revolution*, Francis Fukuyama argues that in the "post-historical" world people will be enhanced by biotechnology to improve their genetic inheritance and to remedy, pharmacologically, their mood, the aim being universal enhancement of individual self-esteem. Individual self-esteem may be the single motivating thrust of the human story and, as one reviewer puts it, "if Prozac has it in its power to alter history, what could be made of the influence of alcohol, cannabis, money, religion and sexual attraction in the boosting, or dampening, of human motivation?"

The criticism that "[Fukuyama's] insistence on reducing a highly complex process of emotions, relationships and meaning to the status of a procurable buzz" is a valid one. "By linking self-esteem with a specific neurotransmitter, serotonin, Fukuyama makes common cause with psychobiological reductionists who treat every emotion and human capacity - love, violence, aggression, intelligence - as if they are molecular entities that can be explained, manipulated, appropriated and fixed, in biotechnological terms."

Eighty percent of serotonin is found in the gastro-intestinal tract is made in the brain from tryptophan by tryptophane hydroxlyase. Into TH-5. Serotonin is a sleep and mood stabilizer. Antidepressants such as selective serotonin, reuptake inhibitors inhibit the reabsorbing of serotonin and so can increase the high from cocaine and MDMA. Thyophyline in tea is a mild a mood stimulator that may be used in self-medication. A manic patient admitted to St Brendan's psychiatric hospital had been drinking 20 tea bags in a tea pot. The late Dr. Aidan McGennis replaced the self-medication regime with prescribed tranquillisers.

But however unpalatable the notion, all experience is, after all, ultimately a sequence of electro-chemical stimulations; and certainly Fukuyama's idea is relevant to hypomania: could this condition, even in theory, be eradicated by genetic engineering or ongoing medication?

It seems more likely that the post-historical society Fukuyama describes would be more hypomanic than even the present - given its suggested dependence on Prozac or similar drugs, that is, for hypomania is more associated with high self-esteem, as depression is associated with the lack of it. Thus the notion that men like Caesar or Napoleon might not have set out to conquer the world had they had access to Prozac is exactly wrong. It may be that post-Prozac drugs will act like Soma, Orwell's fictitious drug in *1984*, to make people happy in a zombie-like fashion; but such drugs may also, by boosting self-esteem into self-aggrandising delusion, lead to more Caesars and Napoleons.

Fukuyma's claims emerged from his c 1995 examination of the social glue that makes societies work. His discoveries were made after the fall of the Soviet Empire and the end of the Cold War, at a time when people were lamenting the loss of religious or ideological meaning. The moral core that was hollowed out is now filled by a hypomanic trait that is an expression of liberal democratic philosophy, which follows fraternity, liberty and truth, all manic traits. His beliefs were expressed in a new book, *The Origins of Political Order* (2011).

One reviewer observed: "[Futyama] dares to suggest that liberal democracy, rather than being the end point of political evolution, may be a 'fluke'" and that "humans, far from being frontier-busting individualists intent purely on their own gains, have a natural 'sociability'". Indeed, the "presumption that we all start out as individuals and only come to society over time as a result of pursuing self-interest is really not at all the way humans beings developed".[136]

Though Fukyama regards market economics as one of "the biggest intellectual developments of the late 20th century", he believes the emphasis on individual economic rationalism has been deeply flawed by this stage. By focusing on material interest and rationality economists can discount the consequences of human behaviour, which is never entirely predictable and is often capricious. They completely missed the financial bubble because in macroeconomics the field is chaos and bubbles are driven not by rationality but emotion - and by MDI, the high of buying and selling and grandiose delusions.

MDI drives not only the markets but even Liberal Democracy. The emergence of this was not a fluke but the result of the drive of Manic Depressive Illness. In the past people with MDI and paranoid schizophrenia would have been shamans, with a recognised role to play in the community, but they are now controlled in psychiatric hospitals - yet their influence is not entirely discounted. The 1 percent of the population who have MDI drives the 10 percent of the population who are hypomanics and these in turn drive the normal population.

MEN, WOMEN AND EMOTION

Men and women are closer to animals physically than emotionally, but there are significant emotional differences between the sexes, and how they express these emotions. Women like to touch a lot and the greatest mode of emotional expression is our skin. We have the same amount of hair as an ape, but we only have 5 percent of its fur, thereby exposing the greatest amount of nerves to the environment.

Through skin we can sense light touch, deep touch, pleasure, pain, vibration, two-point discrimination, hot, cold and a sense of three-dimensional space which is technically called "propioreception". **The tracts of these senses cross over and back going up the spinal cord**. It is through skin that we become intimate with each other. Lips and hands are the leaders in the touch

---

[136] Richard Woods, *Sunday Times* review, 29 May 2011.

field. In the brain we have two areas: one for touch (sensory use) and one for muscle use (motor use). They lie side by side. In the sense area the lips alone take up one quarter of our brain. The hands take up another quarter. The same is found in motor areas.

It is likely that touch led to language. The exposed skin presented the greatest organ to the environment and the complexities it revealed had to be expressed somehow. That expression is language. Hand-signing led to speech. That past lingers on in the way the Italians and other Mediterranean peoples use their hands when they speak.

One interesting theory as to how we lost our fur is that during a semi-aquatic phase we lived by the sea and took much of our sustenance from it. Fur was of little benefit in this environment so we lost it, just as other animals like pigs and elephants did during their semi-aquatic phase. But we did not lose it from our heads, not so much because we spent more time with our heads above water but because luxuriant head hair provided hand-grip for small children and babies. Hair is most abundant in young women, of child-bearing age; older women lose some of their hair and men lose even more.

Women are more emotional and intuitive than men. At parties they are tuned to understand the relationships between people whereas men register the position of the chairs and the tables. Women "know" by intuition; men discern "facts" by rationality; they each work toward the "truth" in their different and often complementary ways.

Men analyse and break down thought to find the "truth" that women know intuitively. Men and women are physically more similar than the males and females of many other species, **but with the development of emotion they are more complex than other animals**.

Women are more complex emotionally than men. A woman intuitively knows when her child is sick; Professor Donoghue, professor of paediatrics, (National Children's Hospital), says you believe the instinct of the mother. Because of this emotional complexity, women are not primarily rational left-brained, so men can find it hard to "understand" them.

The differences can be accounted for, in part at any rate, by how the emotions of the sexes are wired differently. A man does not play a great part in children rearing because he is away from the home a good deal of the time doing such sometimes-solitary tasks as tracking and hunting, and, after the Agricultural Revolution, herding. This lifestyle might evolutionarily favour those men who are more emotionally free of family involvement. Childrearing, by contrast, is intrinsically emotional, and because it is social as well it lends itself to communal involvement, the sharing of tasks, and of confidences.

Exacerbating the difference is that in the hunting field, or that of war, when men do need to cooperate, the emotional connection between them is of a very different, far more urgent nature. Men's lives may literally depend on others' actions and support, yet those emotions are usually unvoiced - the reticence of war veterans is almost a cliché. In part this male reticence may be a consequence of simply not knowing socially men one may depend on, and a sort of shyness of strangers, coupled to the return, after the temporary cooperation of the hunt or battle, to one's own more isolated way of life. A man may also fail to get to know his companions because these are killed.

Where men did bond emotionally was in the warrior societies of pre-industrial peoples. The American Indians had many such societies and the veteran Marine, Karl Marlantes, believes that such societies served to help warriors transit from peace to war and, most importantly, back to peace. Marlantes believes that many of the problems war veterans have stem from not being able to make the transition back to peace. Training ensures that they are well-prepared emotionally as well as physically and professionally to go to war, but there is no ritual to ease them back out of warrior mode, as there was with burying a war-hatchet.[137]

Emotions obviously play a part in war, but they also dictate all art - without an emotional connection art is lifeless. Maybe the best-known art has been done by men because men do not have as much empathy, the ability to understand emotion, as women tend to have, and therefore need to struggle to express emotion in their art? Men may be moved by art much more than women, and even need it to understand emotion, both being right-brain centred, but their access to understanding is exteriorised and then studied by the left brain. Men see the pattern in cubism and this helps them understand

---

[137] Karl Marlantes, *What It Is Like To Go To War*.

the art. Studies indicate that men are also better at engineering than women. Does this difference come down to hormonal aggression and toughness, cultural ingraining, or is it something hardwired in the sexes?

Cursing comes from the right, musical, side of the brain, so could be associated with artistic expression - perhaps especially when creativity sags. We may speculate that Solomon cursed a lot when he was writing his Psalms. Until recently at any rate, men cursed more than women did, and there is some evidence that intelligent people curse more.

While rugby songs may be an exception, an art form that suits women is singing; it conveys emotional language and since Solomon's time and long before mothers have sung to their children. Children learn their language primarily from their mother and women are often frustrated because the first word of a baby is often "Da".

Until 5,000 years ago almost half the population was left-handed, so they were in touch with the creative side of the brain, which also abhors authority.[138] Today between 10 and 13 percent of people are left-handed, suggesting right-brain dominance. The right brain is concerned with mating: with emotion, intuition, dance, dress, money, numbers and pattern recognition. Most people, up to 90 percent, are left-brain dominant, so right-handed, and for centuries there has been suspicion of people who are otherwise. *Sinister* means not just left-handed but ominous, threatening, dangerous; "the left hand path" is a synonym for evil magic. Until the middle of the twentieth century, left-handed children often had their "good" hand tied to their sides in order to force them to use the right one - "right" in every sense, as far as the teacher was concerned.

The practise of enforcing right-handedness not unusually led to stammering and other problems for the child, as his confidence was, in a single sweep, hugely undermined - imagine a small child suddenly unable to do what he had hitherto been able to do easily, and told that his "right" way of doing things

---

[138] Some authorities claim "there's no evidence that modern man is any different from his ancestors as far as hand preference is concerned" (Rik Smits, *The Puzzle of Left-Handedness*, p. 167), but "the absence of facts and figures doesn't deter professional theorizers" (ibid, p. 258). Left- and right-handed spirals carved at Neolithic sites like Newgrange, and at Aboriginal sites, suggest a more even spread of left-handedness in pre-modern societies.

was "wrong"? 5,000 years ago the wearing down of their teeth was the same on the right and left side (Journal of Evolution) Right Hand 50% = Left Hand 50%.

It's difficult to see why this hostility to left-handedness emerged, but we can guess. It's difficult to see how left-handed people are a threat to modern society but in the past this may have been different. Young boys play at fighting, and this was far more important in the past, when the world was a far more dangerous place and up to 20 percent of people died violently.[139] Men who were quite adept at defending themselves with sword or stave against other right-handed men might be taken by unpleasant surprise by a left-handed opponent. If a great champion was defeated by a perhaps unprepossessing stranger, we can understand how it might be accepted that the defeat could only be explained by infernal assistance.

THE PERFORMER

Manic/hypomanic people tend to be more creative, more intelligent, funnier, and more spendthrift and are more expressive. Some characteristics found in the manic state of manic-depressive illness are also found in performing. Performers express the manic archetypes. They are manic/hypomanic entertainers and people go to the shows because they feel better when they share. Songs on the street then music halls, songs, jokes and dancing i.e. lap dancing, cabaret, radio, TV, video, DVD, porn and the Internet. Entertainers are well paid. Performers need to analyse and thereby seek truth with the left brain and they switch to the right brain to synthesise this truth with their lives and creatively incorporate beauty.

Most songs are about love: love lost, love found and heartache. Fleetwood Mac's *Rumours* album is all about the breakdown of two couples' relationships in the band, as suggested by the songs "Never break the chain" and "You can go your own way". Though the band was in trouble the musicians stayed together to finish the album that sold 60 million albums and went on to record a few more albums; but by now they were mainly a gigging band. The early Fleetwood Mac was dominated by a great guitarist, Peter

[139] Morris, op cit.

Green, who wrote their early hits "Albatross", "Black Magic Woman" and "Man of the World" but he went to a commune in Germany and took too much LSD, developed schizophrenia, had ECT and never came back to the group. Another guitarist, Jeremy Spencer, joined a religious cult in the USA and never came back.

ECT got a bad press from Ken Kesey's *One Flew Over the Cuckoo's Nest*, and came to be perceived as a cruel practice and an intolerable intrusion by power-mad doctors into victim-patients' lives. In the 80's 50,000 people in the UK had ECT and that number is now down to 4,000. For many, many ECT has been far more humane than it is depicted in Kesey's novel and the film of the same, and is often most efficacious, notably in post-puerperal psychosis. Sylvia Plath had ECT in the 60's and more recently Yves Saint Laurent.

Some people with manic traits/archetypes are more successful intellectually/creatively/monetarily than average because they experience a greater breadth of emotion that allows them to express emotional experience in an emotional way. The audience and the performer link in expressed emotion (EE), but EE can be destabilising to people who suffer from schizophrenia, something that may help account for Peter Green's breakdown.

Vowels express emotion and are musical (right brain) - babies can express anguish, distress, excitement, joy long before they can speak - where meaning calls for consonants. Sigur Ros are a unique band from Iceland who sing in meaningless vowels. "It's how I tell 'em" was a punch line of one of Britain's top performers, Tommy Cooper. The Cranberries use vowels in their songs such as La, La, La, Hay, Hay, Hay. Tom York of Radiohead and Van Morrison could sing the telephone directory, they get so much emotion into their songs. Southern Europeans use more vowel sounds than northern Europeans, which may account for why the best operas are from Italy, Spain and France.

Manic/hypomanic people tend to come from socio-economic groups 1 and 2 i.e., the better off. The main aspects that lead to success in adolescence are parental approval and "concerted cultivation", which is more likely to lead to confidence, persistence and success. Concerted cultivation is very much a middle-class phenomenon, and rare in the lower socio-economic groups.

Performers make contact with their emotions and express them in a way their audience can share. The emotion of watching a TV alone is totally different than what a person in an audience shares at a theatre or concert hall - shared emotion.

In any performance, as in a list, the first and the last elements are better remembered as well as the emotion expressed. In the names Curt Cobain, Ian Curtis, Bob Dylan we see both proximity to the start of any alphabetical list and the emotional impact of vowel sounds. The name U2 comes close to the end of the alphabet and had a double-vowel sound that is both musical and emotional and stimulates the right brain; it is probably the best name of a band at the moment.

I told this to Paul McGuiness the manager of U2 in Lillie's Bordello a night club in Dublin one night and suggested that R2 D2 would be a good name. He strongly disagreed and said calling a band after a robot would not work. I beg to differ. In addition to the band's name, Bono and the Edge are excellent names, though the latter is consonantal.

One Direction is a more recent band, whose success may be attributed in part to the vowel sound and number One and the spatial orientation Direction, which comes from the musical right brain. Other connections between music, vowels and numbers can be seen in the singers/groups B52, UB40, L7, 2 unlimited, Six, A1 and 50cent. The big Rock'n'Roll breakthrough east of the Atlantic was "Rock Around the Clock", and it's often been noted that portly, aging Bill Hayley was an unlikely musical idol, but the song's success may lie in "One, two, three o'clock rock".

Changing clothes during a performance is a useful technique, which can improve the emotional connection between performer and audience, and stimulate more creativity. Diana Ross changes her clothes about six times during a concert. "Ross returned in another abundance of fabric, this time in crimson, her ever changing riot of taffeta, saffron, lamé, fur, feathers, fans and sequences were reassuringly expensive in these cash strapped times. Rematerialized in blue, back again as a silver flash," Journalist Andrew Perry, Daily Telegraph, 16th October 2023.

Other musical connotations with clothing can be seen in songs, "Blue suede shoes", "Lady in Red" and the Sultans of Ping's "Where's me jumper?"

Another connection between colourful clothes and emotion is the bright Hawaiian shirts worn by people on – hypomanic - holidays. The phenomenon is recognised in hospitals, where adopting loud clothes may indicate the onset of a manic phase. Hippies famously dressed in colourful clothes, and they also had manic impulses like drug usage and belief in free love and universal peace.

Visualising shapes such as pyramids, cubes and squares, especially in bright colours, stimulates the right musical brain and creativity; the technique was used for this reason by Yeats and others in the Golden Dawn. The connection between maths and music is well documented, though each comes from a different brain-hemisphere. Musical composition may be an example of what the writer EM Forster meant when he said "Only connect the prose and the passion and both shall be enhanced".[140]

The biggest selling single in the UK at 45 million was the Elton John song for Diana, the second biggest selling single at 15 million is One o'clock, two o'clock etc by Bill Haley and the Comets, i.e. numbers the third biggest selling song is "Yesterday" at 1.5million; it has been covered 5,000 times.

Ellie Greenwich was a song writer and producer who died in September 2009. She and her husband Jeff Barry had seventeen singles in the pop charts in 1964. They penned "Da Doo Ron Ron", "Then He Kissed Me", both recorded by the Crystals, and "Do Wah Diddy" recorded by Manfred Mann, which reached number one in the UK, while the Dixie Cups took "Chapel of Love" to number one in the USA. "Be my Baby" was a hit for the Ronettes (great name), and "River Deep, Mountain High" was recorded by Ike and Tina Turner. Ellie considered both "Da Doo Ron Ron" and "Do Wah Diddy", with their vowel sounds, to be rooted in the tradition of nursery rhyme. "Everybody of any age can sing them" she said, "because they are easy to remember."

Such a voluminous output suggests manic energy which no one could sustain. Ellie tried to make a comeback but suffered a nervous breakdown which I presume was manic. She ended up writing and singing jingles, but

---

[140] EM Forster, *Howard's End.*

during her high point she had worked with "Wall of Sound" music producer Phil Spector, who also had a manic edge.

Like Joyce and Freud, Spector was a highly driven manic who suffered from morbid jealousy. Joyce's main character in *Ulysses* was a cuckold, Leopold Bloom, whose father committed suicide; this was possibly a reflection of Joyce's psyche in the novel. He himself was jealous sometimes to the point of paranoia. In Trieste he alternated between accusing a duke of seducing his wife and all but encouraging Nora to cuckold him. His hypomania may have been passed on to his schizophrenic daughter, Lucia - whose illness, incidentally, Joyce refused to accept.

Spector also was morbidly jealous, so much so he had his wife - one of the Ronettes - drive around in his Rolls Royce with a mannequin of himself in the passenger seat so that people would not approach her. In addition to being jealous he was aggressive and paranoid, and likely these traits were exaggerated by the drugs he took regularly. To make matters worse, he liked to play with guns. His mania may have strayed into genuine insanity, if the tales of his toupee are true: allegedly he used to take this off after he turned off the lights at bed time, in a pathetic attempt to conceal his baldness from his wife. At his trial for murder in 2008 he wore different, sometimes outrageous wigs to court, but any insanity was disregarded by the jury who found him guilty of murder and sentenced him to life imprisonment.

Interestingly another music producer, Joe Meek, of "Telstar" fame, was similarly dangerous, and ended up killing his landlord. Meek's paranoia tended to centre on inventions like guitar pedals.

Far more dangerous was Ian Brady, the Moors Murderer, described by a tribunal as being psychotic, paranoid, hallucinatory, and as having a "severe narcissistic personality disorder".[141] Brady died on 15 May 2017, after spending most of his life in prison. Brady's narcissism and manic arrogance were major factors in catching him, but his violence was what scared his brother-in-law into giving him away. Brady was truly mad, bad and dangerous to know.

Dangerous levels of paranoia can be artificially induced, and again the show-

---

[141] Obituary, the *Irish Times*, 20 May 2017.

biz world, with its hypomanic pace and feedback, throws up examples. "When you are on crystal meth it ruins you," testifies Fergi of the Black Eyed Peas.[142] Some days she became insanely paranoid, convinced she was under FBI surveillance and blacking out the windows in her apartment with black rubbish bags.

Man has always danced to music, in ways still seen in primitive tribes in Africa. Pop stars such as Madonna, Take That, Shakira, Boy Zone and Britney Spears dance to music that is both continuity with primitive movement and part and parcel of the music scene today. Dance videos as seen on MTV are much sexualised and they show how sex sells, which is a very manic archetype. Rock groups do not dance but rather pose. Pop dancing was optimised by Michael Jackson who spent months practising his steps with his dancers especially the moon walk which he took from the streets and developed. "Come Dancing" is the most popular program on TV, and Irish dancing, most notably Riverdance and Lord of the Dance, has exploded over the world making Michael Flately worth some €300 million.

More idiosyncratically, ballet has its own unique and punitive training regime. Yet more so, bull fighting is like dancing with the ritual of the matador as he moves in certain ways around his "dance partner", each potentially fatal to the other, in a dance that end with the death of one and sometimes both dancers.

Wagner tried to join up the six elements of culture: Dancing, Acting, Lyrics, Music, Costume and Myth. He did not like opera, which he regarded as snobbish and perhaps too far removed from its *volkish* roots and too Latin for his Teutonic sensibilities.

DANCING

The importance of dancing in our modern pop culture is illustrated by a sample of songs that refer to or invoke it. Thin Lizzy: "Asked You for a Dance"; Bruce Springsteen: "Dancing in the Dark"; Bee Gees: "Dancing to the Music"; Martha Reeves and the Bandellas: "Dancing in the Street"; Roxy Musi: "Do the Strand"; Brendan Boyer: "Do the Hucklebuck"; Little Eva:

---

[142] Interview, *Sunday Times* Magazine, 11 October 2009.

"Do the Locomotion"; Chubby Checker: "Let's Twist Again"; Abba: "Dancing Queen"; Van McCoy: "Do the Hustle"; David Bowie: "Let's Dance"; Joy Division: "Dance, Dance, Dance"; Van Morrison: "Moon Dance"; Pattie Smith: "Dancing Barefoot". That the phenomenon is not merely part of a modern manic phase is shown by much older songs like "The Kerry Dances" and, of course, ballet.

Like music, dance comes from the right creative brain, and dancing has always been important to music, as the title of some of the above songs shows. These days pop bands do dancing routines. Different types of dancing are associated with different types of music, e.g. country and western, Irish, ballroom, rock and roll, hip-hop, rave, disco, punk and R and B. But also, different dances are associated with different cultures, and the music reflects different attitudes. The often-mournful lyrics and themes of country and western songs lend themselves easily to parody by more "sophisticated" sorts, and contrast with the bleak, violent, foul-mouthed lyrics of rap, just as the more flamboyant dance movements of country and western jive contrast with the jerky, spasmodic movement of more modern music.

Is there any connection between a putative increase in hypomania and the emergence of different music and dance forms? People go to night clubs where there is loud music, coloured lights, alcohol, fashion and they dance and try to attract a mate with the intension of having sex. Disco and rave are very manic with beats per minute over 120.

Since the emergence of rock and roll there has been a steady move away from melody toward beat. The pace of this change was accelerated in the 1970s with punk on the one hand, with its angry, hammering beat, and the more subtle, yet still beat-dominated disco music. Amphetamines may have influenced the Sex Pistols' music, given that Sid Vicious was at one point a dealer in drugs, and through the Sex Pistols such a style may have generalised to some extent. Rap reduced the musicality to virtually nothing, and its message is hostile, angry, contemptuous, sometimes racist and even murderous.[143]

---

[143] BBC 2's Newsnight, 17 April 2018, carried a story of armed rap gangs in London threatening each other with murder, and recording the confrontation on their phones. A youth was murdered.

Evidence suggests that society is getting less violent, and there can be no doubt that war, in an almost perverse way, can lead to more peaceful, less suicide, when psychopaths realise they're evil and kill themselves for example in the Liffey (Dr. McGennis RIP), larger political entities whose prosperity is endangered by violence. It is difficult to believe, however, that hypomania is not on the increase, and has been, steadily, for decades, when we look at the changes in music and dance, and objectively murder rates are markedly higher than in the Ireland of the 1950s. Statistics show that the murder and manslaughter rate in 1845-1854 was 24.0 per million population, more than seven times what it was in 1945-54 (3.4 per million). In 1995-2004, however, the rate had quadrupled to 13.7 per million, much lower than in 1845-54, that that was a period of famine, cannibalism, eviction and desperation.[144]

When we look at less violent crimes the picture appears even worse today, and worse still when we consider that many crimes in the past would not even be collated today, far less punished. In the 1945-54 period a youth was sentenced to six months' hard labour in Mountjoy Gaol for stealing the tube from a bicycle in order to get home.[145] Anyone who reported such a "crime" today might be lucky to escape a charge of wasting police time, and one can only marvel at the modern thief's paradise the environs of Croke Park would have been on important fixtures, when literally thousands of bicycles were piled against railings around the stadium.

Dancing is not seen only in humans. It probably emerged from ritualistic display and became a formal expression of acknowledgement or request. Birds use dance in their courtship, but we may see something similar in the ritualistic posturing of rival males showing off their power. Stags confront each other with ostentatious parading of their antlers, and usually the other will defer to the one with the more impressive set. Thus ritual establishes dominance without any actual conflict; the challenger survives without damage to maybe fight another day and perhaps establish his dominance in turn as the older stag becomes more decrepit, and the whole herd better

---

[144] Ian O'Donnell, "The Rise and Fall of Homicide in Ireland" in *Violence in Europe: Historical and Contemporary Perspectives*, eds Sophie Body-Gendrot and Pieter Spierenburg, p. 80.
[145] Recounted by Alice Taylor in *To School Through the Fields*.

conserves its gene pool, to the benefit of all. Stags also express their size by the loudness of their roar.

Dance has been described, not without either wit or truthfulness, as a vertical expression of a horizontal desire. African tribes have different types of courtship dancing and coming of age festivities, and the dancing of pygmies is different from Indian and Chinese dancing, but all express something. In European societies dance was often marked by not just stylized movements but particular dress, which might express both familiarity with society's conventions and also the wealth to indulge in non-essential clothing.

In the past, in Ireland and elsewhere, people tended to meet at dances, and meetings in places like the Galtymore in London led to the marriages of many ex-pat Irish people. Back home, in the heyday of the Catholic Church, priests policed rural dancehalls and patrolled the roads adjacent after the dances ended, flushing courting couples out of fields and hedgerows.

Dancing was, literally, sexy, some dances more than others. In Ireland dance became part of the Gaelic Revival movement, and its stylized movements involved no closeness such as the tango involves; rather, there was something almost puritanical about it, for all its elegance, notably in solo dancing. Troupe dancing, however, had more in common with English dancing - as solo had with Scottish - and with The Lord of the Dance Michael Flatley made Irish dancing sexy and brought it to the wider world. His success may have had something to do with development of Irish self-confidence or the rise of hypomania.

ART

Art, fine or written, is a representation of the human condition; the exteriorisation of emotion. As such it is universal but this universality gives it great potential power. Shelley claimed that the poet is "the unwritten legislator of the world" and proof of this can be found in a very bad novel, which is hardly art yet proves Shelley's point. When Harriet Beecher Stowe met Abraham Lincoln in the White House the president greeted her with: "So you're the little woman whose book started this big war" - and there can be no doubt that *Uncle Tom's Cabin* played a part in the Civil War.

The power of art to express the human condition is a liability to autocratic regimes, which often set out to define what this "really" is. The Nazis banned modern art because it was "decadent", the Bolsheviks because they felt the Dada movement was bourgeois. They wanted revolutionary art; art of the people. Both totalitarian regimes banned and burned books that contradicted their doctrine; the Nazis most famously banned Erich Maria Remarque's All Quiet on the Western Front because it gave a defeatist portrayal of the Germans' "glorious struggle".[146]   Among the Bolsheviks' most infamous book bans were Boris Pasternak's *Doctor Zhivago* and Aleksandr Solzhenitsvn's *The Gulag Archipelago*, both of which revealed the appalling truth beneath the Marxist lies.

More constructively, Stalin used art to represent the Glorious Worker in order to promote the Five Year plans and the Great Patriotic War. Democracy does not tolerate crude interference, but art also was mustered by the West to help defeat its enemies, "Rosie the Riveter" becoming a pin-up of sorts; the earlier Kitchener poster proclaiming, "Your Country Needs You" is the single most successful example of its sort, and created a whole sub-genre.

While there is no book-burning in liberal democracies, individual artists certainly face problems of expression if these challenge the liberal - sometimes faux-liberal - zeitgeist. The Danish "Mohammad cartoons" were criticised by "liberals", even after *Charlie Hebdo* journalists were murdered for reproducing them, on the grounds that they "caused offence" - as if causing offence were not an intrinsic corollary of free speech in any liberal democracy. So anxious not to cause offence to Moslems can the West be that recently the Echo music prize - Germany's equivalent of the Grammy - went to a rapper duo whose songs include "I'm doing another Holocaust, coming with a Molotov".[147]

Historic parallels may be seen with sponsorship of Medieval and Renaissance artists by the Catholic Church, Michelangelo's work on the Sistine Chapel being the best example. As the Renaissance created wealthy merchant princes

---

[146] The Nazis also banned many books that contradicted the false narrative propagated by the *Zenstralstelle für Erforschung der Kriegshuldefrage*, established to discredit the "war guilt clause" of the Treaty of Versailles.

[147] Derek Scally, "Anti-Semitism is alive and well in Germany", the *Irish Times*, 28 April 2018.

these also became sponsors, but seldom added propagandistic conditions to their sponsorship.

Outside of wartime, sponsorship and funding in the West comes not from the state but individuals - though with qualifications. Rothschild and other wealthy Americans patronised the arts and supported artists such as Pollack, who was a modern artist and abstract expressionist, a style later known as "action painting." Though Pollack was thereby supported, his and other Western artists' work was free of control by religion and the state. However, this patronisation was encouraged by the CIA in an attempt to establish a style that was clearly different from that of the USSR. After all, if the Cold War was about culture as much as anything else, a painting, say, by an American, that was essentially indistinguishable from one painted by a Russian, did not reinforce public belief in the need for ongoing competition with the Soviets.

Soviet art was essentially propagandistic and severely constrained within propaganda's requirements; abstract expressionism had an element of random chance to its composition, something that would not have been allowed by the Soviets. Their art portrayed working class heroes, miners and steelworkers, the movers and shifters, in theory at least, of the Revolution of the Proletariat. But as President Kennedy said in 1963, in the United States, "a free society, art is not a weapon.... Artists are not engineers of the soul."

CONTROL

If hypomania is, as I argue, on the increase, how is the hypomanic mood to be controlled so that it does not get out of hand? Hypomanics tend to run into trouble if they become too disinhibited, spending more or indulging in sexual indiscretions and other things they regret. Or is a low-grade hypomania OK?

The increased tolerance for behaviour that would have been deemed criminal sixty years ago suggests that, in certain cases, low-grade hypomania is indeed OK. Some control, however, is needed, notably in clinical settings. In psychiatry the manic mood is controlled with drugs such as Lithium and Largactile tranquillisers, which was developed in the 1950s - and interestingly, local memory of the Central Mental Hospital is that this decade was "when the shouting stopped".[148] In the1980s anti-epileptics like Tegretol and Epilim were used as mood stabilisers. Such medication seems to slow down electrical activity in the CNS.[149]

To some extent medication is a metaphorical sticking plaster, which can cure minor injuries but is no use to a broken leg or a haemorrhage. One needs to go to the core of the problem and try to harness the potential liability toward constructive ends. To stop the mania you should either love yourself or love other people. *Love your neighbour as yourself* does not mean to love everybody (which is not possible) but to love people close to you, to the benefit of all.

The most practical of the "Vienna School", Alfred Adler, realised that people experience problems of various magnitude if they fail to take power over their own lives, but in his *individualpsychologie* full potential and appreciation can only be found in work, community and love. Isolation is always deleterious. Yet love of self and love of others can also turn into the paranoid position, which is often dangerous.

People who love themselves have high self-esteem, but also often high ego. Love of others is an essential requirement of doctors and nurses and other carers, but it's been claimed that up to 40 percent of doctors are unhappy in their careers.[150] In *I'm OK, You're OK*, Thomas Anthony Harris claims to find four fundamental stances taken by people. The first, I'm OK, You're OK, is a healthy situation where the individual likes both himself and others, and likely to be in a healthy "work, community and love" situation. The person who feels I'm Not OK, You're OK, has problems of self-esteem and inadequacy, which can be overcome. The position I'm OK, you're Not OK, is likely to be held by anyone with a superior attitude to a psychopath, often charming, or ruthless criminal, whose justification for what he does may be heightened by hypomania.

Finally, the position I'm Not OK, You're Not OK is occupied by someone who has the potential to project his negative feelings outward without focus and with great violence. Such a person is more paranoid and deeply

---

[148] Anecdotal accounts.
[149] Common knowledge in neurology, and even general practice.
[150] *Irish Medical Times.*

inadequate than psychopathic, the schoolboy who brings an M16 into class, or the jihadist who blows up a nightclub or flies a plane into tall buildings. They are likely to be loners, self-isolation being a logical course taken by one who believes himself to be Not OK, and everyone else the same. The hypomanic milieu, fostered by modern living, is liable to stoke the negativity and nihilism of such people while simultaneously encouraging more grandiose gestures of destruction.

The biggest danger in this country is not so much from either jihadists or National Socialists but from self-denigration. Arnold Toynbee warns that civilisations are not murdered but commit suicide, and it seems possible that Western Civilisation is in the position I'm Not OK, You're OK, *You* being any other civilisation at all, almost. Jihadists or Nazis may deal the death-blow, but self-loathing will allow them to get close enough to strike.

The problem lies with loss of faith in all those institutions in which Western Civilisation once took pride. The Catholic Church set the standard of moral behaviour and when, in the 1990s, two popular and nationally recognised clerics, Fr Michael Clery and Bishop Eamon Casey, were discovered to have been in sexual relationships Ireland was left reeling. The sense of betrayal was worsened when it was discovered that Casey had used diocesan funds to support his son, and when it was remembered that Clery had strongly condemned sexual sin. But worse was to come with the discovery of widespread paedophilia in the Church, and again this was worsened by discovery that these crimes had been covered up and the criminals effectively facilitated by the Church.

In former years society had also been strengthened by respect for schoolteachers, bankers and politicians, respect extended even by those who might not have shared the beliefs of the "pillars of the community". But these pillars too were eroded, by politicians who were exposed as grafters and frauds, and bankers who became more remote from their clients and paid fabulous salaries, even before they failed the country in the collapse of the Celtic Tiger. Respect for schoolteachers declined as egalitarianism proceeded, abetted by individual teachers betraying public trust.

The result of all this loss of faith is a vacuum that is filled by various forces. So far neo-Nazism is not a problem in Ireland, though immigration may give it a foothold, if immigrants gain a large enough mass to constitute a perceived threat, or should jihadism pose a real threat. So far the threat would seem more likely to come from the left than the right, with the emergence of more extreme Socialist groups to replace the Labour Party as this was punished for the economic collapse of 2007-08. Socialism develops in countries that have a sizeable proletariat, and may be propagated more easily where people do not have a good education, especially in science, so as Ireland moved from an agricultural to an industrial economy since the 1960s Socialism has made headway.

Possibly the main danger comes from National Socialism in the shape of Sinn Fein, which since the 1970s has gradually adopted the militant Socialism of James Connolly, and coupled it to the extreme Nationalism of militant Republicanism. Connolly's daughter Nora proclaimed the Provisional IRA to be her father's spiritual heirs,[151] and the danger exists that this green National Socialism, like that in Germany in the 1930s, may become a surrogate religion, now that people do not believe in the traditions of the Catholic Church, nor take solace from its teachings.

The role of charismatic, infectious manic paranoid figures in great revolutionary movements is a perennial historical question. Stalin, Hitler, Mao, Castro and Pol Pot are obvious examples, but here in Ireland de Valera, Charles Haughey and Gerry Adams arguably fit into the pattern. It has been argued that Hitler was not uniquely evil but rather his evil ideas resonated in a particular place at a particular time and circumstances. Every country is vulnerable to such resonance, and when faith in older institutions has failed vulnerability increases. In Germany the old imperial quasi-totalitarianism had been lost and faith in the new democracy did not survive the punitive Versailles Treaty and two economic collapses in the 1920s.

NAMES

Names and labels are emotive; they can be manic. The African freedom cry, *Uhuru!* is a compound of vowel sounds, and vowels express emotions. Names, places and objects are made manic by use of the capital letter that

---

[151] Nora Connolly O'Brien, *We Shall Rise Again*, Mosquito Press, 1981, p. 117.

starts their name: this draws attention to the proper noun and emphasises its importance. A child called Max will be more hyperactive than other children if he feels he has to live up to his name. This may reflect the aspirations of the parents rather than anything intrinsic to the child, but the hypomanic result is the same. To what extent did his name, meaning *pleasure*, drive Freud to fixate on sex as the primary motivator? Jung, named for youth, saw the archetypes grasped in childhood, if only dimly understood, and perhaps rebirth, as the key to understanding human nature. Adler, the eagle, believed power was the key.[152]

SARTRE

Others are more cynical. Existentialists believe that we are defined by our temporary mortal existence rather than any sort of eternal soul; that we exist in a world devoid of moral constructs and one that is vaguely hostile by nature rather than in any way benevolent through divine intervention; that ultimately our existence justifies itself. Obviously this attitude might encourage a hypomanic approach, if only to enable the fittest - who are the survivors - to deal psychologically with a world that is dystopic and is the only one we have.

Jean Paul Sartre used speed when he was writing; one could say that speed (amphetamines) dictated, or at least affected, his thinking about man and nature. This writing would be about the intellectual hit, the magic of the creative moment. Creativity has a manic component, and Sartre's subject matter might seem to necessitate a certain hypomania to engage with fully. In his personal life, too, the philosopher betrays signs of hypomania: he had three girlfriends whom he visited on different days through the week.

LET GO, LET GOD

"Let go, Let God" is an AA saying. It means that one lets go in order to permit the chance of God coming into his or her life. This makes the search for God intuitive, spiritual and right-brained; however, the seeker of logical truth is left-brained. God cannot be questioned as the right brain is concerned

---

[152] See Ian Suttie, *The Origin of Love and Hate*.

with intuitive, creative and synthetic thinking. You have to have faith that you will float in the sea of belief.

Philosophers seek truth by left-brain reasoning whereas intuitive thinkers seek beauty, which is far more difficult to define. As Keats said (quoting Plato): "Beauty is truth, Truth Beauty. That is all you know and all you need to know." This perhaps illustrates the difference between *fact* and *truth*: there may be rhyme in the latter but not always reason. If you are on the same emotional plane as your companion it seems that your thoughts are in tune, if you yourself not psychic. It might not be a fact, but you "know" it's the "truth".

Objectively one can fault this idea. Statistical analysis of how often thoughts are in tune would be difficult though not impossible to quantify, and would likely result in no meaningful correlation. But perhaps this is to miss the real point, which is the subjective feeling of connection, and the meaning this can give to one's life. As more than one poet has observed, no man is an island.

MOON LANDING

After the Russians sent a dog into space the USA had to be first on the moon. No expense was spared to meet the technology challenge and prove the West's will to win was stronger than those Commies'. We're the best. We landed on the moon first. A window was put into the end of the Apollo One so the astronauts could see out even though this was not necessary but it satisfied their egos and provided photographic proof to the Soviets of how far "we" could go from the "pale blue dot" that was our stellar home.

To travel in space is a dream man has had since time immemorial when stars and planets were seen as gods, so the USA built on this dream and achieving it built political and neo-military victory onto mythic achievement. Moon Rock was sent to US embassies in foreign countries and people queued up to see it like I did. Here was proof of what mere mortal man could do.

There was a dark side to the Space Race, aside entirely from the fact that it was part of a proxy war. The *Paper Clip Chase* showed how Nazis who made rockets in Germany to bombard Britain in the last years of World War II were protected and recruited by the Americans at the end of the war, as others were "protected and recruited" by the Soviets. It was "our" Nazis who made the rocket that went to the moon.

The technology necessary to get men to the moon was enormous, however pathetic it seems now, when an iPhone has more computing power. This is one of the spin-offs of the Space Race, but the pace of technological development since then could be described as manic or hypomanic, and evidence that hypomania spawns more hypomania.

A different sort of hypomanic underlies the very impulse to go to the moon: curiosity. People believe that we are learning about space by sending probes to Mars and farther off, but underpinning all this hypomanic activity we want to see if there is anyone out there, or if are we alone. Some people believe that Heaven is in outer space and that when we die our spirit goes there. At other times people have believed our souls become stars; some still do. Others believe - or once believed - that dead souls go to distant lands far to the west where the sun descends: the Isles of the Blest; Tír na nÓg; perhaps Atlantis. The western ocean was once more mysterious than the heavens are today.

Other people believe that rather than go to new home in the sky after we die, we originally came from space. This is a very manic idea. For years man believed there were canals in Mars and that there was a sign of life. It is now believed that there is or was water on Mars so it may once have supported life, in theory anyway. More intriguing is the belief of the African Dogon tribe that humanity came from Sirius, the Dog Star, and that the tribe was aware that this is a binary star. There is considerable doubt about much of this story, and perhaps it says as much about "enlightened" Western fascination with mystery as with actual tribal beliefs. Such fascination is proof of enduring hypomania, however "enlightened" humanity becomes.

Yet Enlightenment, i.e. illumination, is not to be sneered at. The science of astronomy emerged out of astrology in the Renaissance, a great creative time when technology made possible telescopes that penetrated the great spaces of the heavens and allowed men like Copernicus and Galileo to see into what had previously been in the realm of speculation. But telescopes had economic and commercial application too, in allowing Venetian bankers and speculators to spot far off merchant ships coming from the east, and give them a brief advantage in trading stocks and shares.

The Renaissance, which enabled all these advances to be made, emerged out of the great Voyages of Discovery, which had been made possible largely by Arab map-makers. These had developed their skills out of the necessity to know in which direction Mecca lay, so that they could worship facing it and later, *insh'Allah*, make pilgrimage to it. Yet as the Koran, arguably, gave Arabs and then European the maps which led to the Renaissance, the Bible led to the Enlightenment being built on the Renaissance and subsequent Reformation, with its mandating separation of Church and State: "Render to Caesar the things that are Caesar's, and to God the things that are God's". The Koran, by contrast, insists that anything not in it is of the Devil, so the Moslem world could never have seen the Industrial Revolution emerge.

Yet the Moslem world did give Europe something else, which marked the Renaissance: perspective was assimilated from Arab art in Toledo and allowed the great painters and sculptors to do the greatest work art has probably ever seen. This perspective was made possible by Moslems being forbidden to represent the created world and so forced into the abstract. More recently the Dutch painter MC Escher created modern masterpieces like *Night and Day*, *Monks' Work* and *Lobster* with clever use of perspective. Escher based his work on Arabic Tile Patterns in Toledo. Yet perspective antedated Islamic art: Roman paintings in Pompeii that had been protected by volcanic ash and stimulated Picasso's cubist style to develop.

The idea that cleanliness is close to godliness may constitute OCD, a form of hypomania. Arguably, it is more correct to say that creativity is close to Godliness; to create is to play God. When people clean obsessively their children can get asthma because they don't get used to dirt.

JAPAN

The degree to which people "play God" is determined in large part by their social frame of reference. Islamic creativity is unquestionably stunted by the Koranic prohibition on representing anything that God created. In Christian Europe a wariness of "graven images" characterised Protestant countries while Catholic countries, which did not subscribe to this Biblical literalness, gave the world the great art of the Sistine Chapel and much more. Presbyterians smashed the rose windows.

The Japanese view shame as pertaining to the individual, guilt as a broader social construct as in Europeans groups. People feel the need to atone for shame of failure and down through the ages they have committed hara-kiri. Given that many who so died were those who would have been more than usually creative and those who were more than usually ready to take risks, this has diluted the creative gene pool of Japan.

But there are different sorts of creativity. It's said that the Japanese are incapable of original invention but the best in the world at developing the creativity of others, and for decades Japanese manufacture has been regarded, for good reason, as "the best in the world" - to borrow from a Toyota ad. The Japanese save a lot of money and this is reinvested in research and development of technology, which is what has made Japan such a strong economic force today. It has become a world leader notably in electronics and auto manufacture, but also a world centre for finance.

The Japanese are a notably conservative people, but now they are turning to Western ways and increasingly they do not feel shame of the individual but the guilt of the masses. Socio-technological changes are also seeing, for the first time, a generation of unmarried aging children living with their parents and being more influenced by the insular thinking encouraged by social media than by traditional Japanese values. It is only now that the Japanese are spending money especially on brands and this is making them more manic than before.

Japan has for long had quite a manic culture. It has 120 million people squashed into a few islands and this creates enormous pressure. The cost of land is extremely high - about £50,000 for a toilet-cubicle–sized space - high enough to justify digging down four storeys into the basement. The price of rice is four times higher than in other countries, and anyone who can grows a little patch of rice, especially retirees.

Pressure is psychological as well as physical. With such physical pressure on limited resources, social conservatism and a conventional mindset almost have to emerge. To avoid giving unwitting offence, elaborate protocols have evolved, and along with this has grown a deeply-felt sense of honour. Loss of face is almost unbearable for the Japanese, and death seen as both preferable and as a means to redeem lost honour. Suicide is respectable, but like much else, highly ritualised: *seppuku*, or hara-kiri, an extraordinarily painful death by self-disembowelment.

Such behaviour, and the entire *bushido* code, could be called hypomanic - the idea of the emperor as a living god, which survived until 1945, in particular. Bushido, which could be summarised as an oriental code of chivalry, emphasised such virtues as loyalty and honour and also, interestingly, politeness. It helped the Japanese fight with incredible courage and fanaticism in World War II, and accounted for old veterans holding out in the Philippines until the 1970s, but it also helped created the impression of "otherness" in the eyes of their enemies, and probably contributed to the decision to drop atom bombs on Japanese cities.

PASTIMES

People are seeking out more creative lifestyles like music, dancing, drama, singing, comedy, writing, painting and poetry. They want to be more creative and intellectual. Most people wish to write and sing, but few are prepared to make the necessary sacrifices and do the necessary work.

Is there a dumbing-down in society? When people talk derisively of the three-minute attention span of those who watch remote-control TV they do not appreciate that people flick through the channels until they find a channel that is interesting. The moot point is that we are spoiled for choice, but also that a great deal on TV is not interesting. Do we find it not interesting because it is genuinely dull, or because our senses have been dulled by exposure to more and more stimulating experiences? In the early days of cinema one successful film showed nothing but a horse eating hay.

The wide choice of viewing may also suggest that people are no longer willing or perhaps now even able to make the effort to entertain themselves. Before television people read more - Dickens's serialised stories were eagerly awaited every week, crowds often building up on the quays in New York when the latest issue of the magazine was expected. Novels and stories from an earlier time describe soirees where people sing, play the piano, recite poems, to the mutual enjoyment of all. The Thirties and Forties was the golden age of the short story, in magazines like the *Saturday Evening Post*, the *Atlantic Monthly* and *Harper's*. Radio calls for imaginative engagement, notably with radio drama.

This might all seem very stuffy to young people jaded on special effects, but sometimes - at wedding and wakes, for instance - these same young people may express joy and amazement when entertained in this older ad hoc style by grandparents and uncles and aunts. Television spoiled us; it made entertainment a consumer product rather than a participatory activity.

This may reflect another manifestation of hypomania. Many people must work hard and for long hours merely to keep ahead of mortgage payments; when they get home they are too tired to be creative or they think that only professionals can do it. People need to be shown how to be creative. They are scared of ridicule. Anyone can sing, write a story or film or play an instrument. All professionals have learned how to do their specific hob, hobby or entertainment. They started at scratch; that is not to say that certain people are not more talented than others, but everybody can do their bit.

How does this dumbing-down square with the thesis that hypomania does is becoming more prevalent? Surely a society that entertains itself is more hypomanic than one that lethargically sits back to have its entertainment provided to it on its couch? Perhaps; but many aficionados of soaps in particular are all but neurotic about their programme, sometimes taping episodes to watch over and over. Also, the shows themselves are becoming more and more sex-biased, illicit affairs and pregnancies tending to be part of their stock-in-trade, something that would not have been allowed in the early days of *Coronation Street*. The creator of this show once said that it was written for people who have no lives, and arguably those who watch what's supplanted it have lives filled with hypomanic expectations.

REAGAN, KENNEDY AND OBAMA

The president of the USA has to be an icon. He must have the image of being good-looking, healthy, intelligent and a decent guy. Ronald Reagan was charismatic and believable, an actor who became Governor of California and played his part well. Reagan was known for his adverts for General Electric Company during his time as an actor. He was seen as a friendly face of free market economics. He also had a hatred of communism and was one of McCarthy's most famous and successful stooges. Thus he was a good man to sell the Star Wars story to the Russians. Reagan bluffed his way into history; like a good actor, he remembered his lines. **Star Wars forced the USSR to spent 49 percent of GDP on defence and that broke their economy. The USA only spent 8 percent of GDP on defence.**

This seems to beg the question: which is more hypomanic, the country that can generate so much wealth, or the one that so ties itself to a bankrupt ideology that it impoverishes its people to preserve that ideology, even as its failure becomes more and more evident as the enemy makes gains?

The spy Walker caused a lot of damage to the USA. What makes people spy. Is it a grandiose belief in them that they are important and paranoia of their homeland?

Catholics make up 30 million people of 280 million people who live in the USA. There has only been one Catholic President in the USA, John F Kennedy before Joe Biden. Kennedy's father paid the Mafia to rig the Teamster vote in the presidential election against the Republican Nixon. JFK was charismatic but he also had a high sex drive. This might have been due to the amphetamine (speed) injections he got from his doctor for chronic pain. Speed makes you paranoid and this was a dangerous position for a person to be in if he was close to the red telephone.

Both these presidents represent aspects of national hypomania. In Reagan's case paranoia drove his campaign against the tribal enemy, the Reds; in Kennedy's case, the public warmed to the charismatic personality of the youngest ever president and his attractive wife and family, and gave the sobriquet Camelot to his presidency. Even calling it this suggests a post-Romantic yearning for the grandeur of a chivalric past, for the entire political chasm between a medieval kingship and American democracy.

Sally H Jacobs has written a book on President Obama's father called - The Other Obama; The Bold and Reckless Life of President Obama's Father. The review from which this is taken was in the Irish Times on Saturday 30 July 2011 and was written by Bill McSweeney.

Jacobs tells a fascinating "story of a likeable, reckless, talented fool whose dream of himself far exceeded his ability to realise them" all trademarks of the hypomanic.

In his mid-20's in 1959, Obama Snr took a place in the University of Hawaii in Honolulu. In 1961, a report on a black student from the University of Hawaii to the US Immigration authorities stated that the "Subject has been running around with several girls since he arrived here and last summer (the US Immigration and Naturalisation Service) cautioned him about his playboy ways". Subject replied "that he would try to stay away from girls". They could not work out how many wives he had. Obama Snr met Ann Dunham a 17yr old in Hawaii who got pregnant within a few months and the first black President was on his way.

Obama Snr got into Harvard to do a PhD in Economics but the authorities were trying to get rid of him in June 1964 because of his serial relationships with white girls which only became legal in most states in 1967 due to a Supreme Court ruling. Harvard Officials were "going to try to cook something up to ease him out". Even though his mathematical and analytical skills were good he was kicked out in his third year. On returning to Kenya he called himself Doctor and started to drink heavily loosing three jobs and ended up driving into a tree while drunk and dying. He had 7 children, 4wives, 3 of which he left. Onyango Obama (President Obama's grandfather) was supremely confident and arrogant Kenyan which points to hypomania. I would say that Barak Obama has the hypomania gene, charismatic, confident, intelligent and sexually attractive that may develop into paranoia but he is lucky to have a strong wife that hopefully will stop him straying in a sexual way that affected J.F.K. and Bill Clinton. Barak Obama is left handed meaning that he is more creative,musical, emotional, non linear, intuitive, gesture, non verbal and patriotic fever than right handed people.(see left hand right hand).

CLASS

Mania is a middle class illness; it is found in social groups One and Two. Why has mania lasted? If you take a successful family with intelligent parents, there is often a member of the family, as there is in many families, who is a manic failure. In this social group, however, failure is less acceptable than it would be in the working class. Here, too, failure often is overshadowed by the fact that the rest of the siblings have manic traits such as the "work ethic," humour, intellect, creativity, belief, self-esteem, love, money and some paranoia that makes them obsessive so that they do not make mistakes. John F. Kennedy had a sister Rosemary who had a low I.Q. (50-70) a mental age of 8yrs. was manic and attracted to men. Her father made her have a lobotomy. Bobby Kennedy's children descended into chaos, they believed they were the best of the best. Ending up O.D. ing taking drugs, being accused of rape and a plane crash. Bowie had a step brother and James Joyce a daughter who was manic.

The class system exists in all civilisations past and present. Money is the main divider of class in the west but in some cultures it is a blood line class system; for example, in India the caste system depends on what your parents' caste was and in ancient Judaic culture the line of David determined social standing.

In the modern world the nouveau riche dictate culture to a good extent as they have the money to patronise the arts. The artist has an image of starving in a garret, but modern day artists can make a lot of money. For every successful artist there are many failures. Van Gogh only sold one picture in his lifetime. Only two percent of Fine Art College graduates live off their art. Class systems are all about who has the best contact and these are the moneyed people or the upper class. Countries like the UK and the USA are very class driven. As long as you have money you are seen as powerful. The aristocracy is losing its power as the young entrepreneurs take over; this is part of a process that began with the rise of the middle class merchants. In the olden days the aristocracy were the entrepreneurs of their day.

POLICE

Police exist because we're scared and we're paranoid, fearful of the known and the unknown. People respect the police force, uniform and other paraphernalia such as cars and motor cycles. TV programs about the police are popular and have been over the years.

Police are necessary to control manic behaviour that threatens society. They uphold the laws of the land and, in some places still, religion. The Scribes were the policemen of the bible and Judaic law, as the Knights Templar and later the Dominicans were of the Catholic Church. In Soviet Russia there was the Cheka, in Germany the Gestapo and later Stasi in East Germany. The religious police of the Taliban are notorious for their manic and often savage implementation of Islamic law.

But the will to be a policeman is manic too, and history is rife with evidence of policemen who established their own authority - such as when the Dominicans wiped out the Cathar citadel in fourteenth century France. Power does tend to corrupt, and police like their authority; they may think that they are infallible, or at least omnipotent, especially in a police state, i.e. Putin. Their power also tends to their being corrupted in other ways: drug barons can buy the police off, as liquor barons did in Prohibition America.

The police are very quick to act in cases of murder or rape but are slower to act when there is mundane crime such as a housebreak in. This may be because of a lower sense of urgency in the latter case, but it may also have to do with interest level. People complain that, despite the alarming rise in street violence, there are fewer policemen in evidence on the beat. Perhaps police do not like going on the beat or directing traffic, but prefer to work on computers in their offices. If this is so, then it may suggest that the corrupting power of the police allow them to dictate, to an extent at least, the work they are prepared and not prepared to do.

The police were formed in the 1830's by Peel and it was a type of manic control as a result of paranoia of the criminal class. It is probably true to say that the police mainly keep the middle class areas safe.

EUROPE

Northern Europe is cold, uses consonants, wanks, is philosophical and Protestant. Males in rural areas in Norway and Finland that have more manic depressive genes and are in a cold climate have a higher suicide rate than normal. Countries in North-eastern Europe such as Latvia, Estonia (mainly Protestant) and Lithuania have a higher incidence of suicide. Southern Europe is warm, uses vowels, makes love, is emotional and passionate, with much touching and a smaller "personal space," and Catholic. Atheistic countries such as China have a rate of suicide of 20 per 100,00 whereas Italy has a rate of 10 per 100,000. Protestants are found at a distance from Rome, whereas Catholics countries surround the Vatican - except for Ireland, the only non-Protestant country on the periphery of Europe. Irish Catholicism has a special Celtic feel that St Patrick in the fifth century instilled in the early church. The Irish Church was monastically when that of Europe was parochial. At one stage the Pope issued a Bull for St Patrick to go to Rome but St Patrick ignored it. Nicholas Breakspear, Pope Clement IV, endorsed the Norman invasion on the grounds that the Irish Church was heretical and in need of reform, and on condition that the island was administered as a papal fief. The Irish Church has always had a certain independence from Rome but an Irishman, Cardinal Paul Cullen, strongly supported official adoption of the doctrine of Papal Infallibility in the 1870s.

Europe is a very influential place in the world of culture and high finance. It has a cultural mix, and has had it for long. Imperialism drew ex-colonials to the mother-countries, and places like Paris have for long been famous for attracting artists and bohemians from all over the world. Now political and economic refugees are enriching the mix, even in non-traditionally host countries like Ireland, with the potential of causing demographic and cultural problems. How the different nationalities are going to mix is very interesting. There are still old tribal wars being fought e.g. in the supermarkets. The Irish do not like the old enemy of the English companies buying up Irish business and in some cases they shop elsewhere. A friend's father who was a successful business man said the manic movement of a persons hands was an expression of his business acumen.

Intels visionary co-founder Andy Groves motto "Only the paranoid survived" Intel is paranoid enough that its moving into tablets, smart phones and other aspects of computer technology, automobiles and things of that sort. Craig Barret Sunday Times 3rd Feb 2014.

HAIRDRESSING 1

Hairdressing goes back to the Egyptians whose art seems to indicate a high awareness of fashion. Haircuts have differed down through the ages and even differ between classes. The Beatles were seen as having long hair. Monks, skinheads and army personnel have short hair, but where one is pacific the others are aggressive.

People like hairdressing as it is one of the times that the touch taboo is broken down in life. People get their hair washed by hand and the scalp massaged. Then they will have their hair cut as it affects their appearance and they feel good afterwards. Successful hairdressers are often effeminate and the customer feels they appreciate their problems more. They have more empathy. Massage Parlours also break the taboo of touch/tenderness (Ian Suttie: *The Origins of Love and Hate*). Language comes from touch. If you pinch or hit someone they will make a hurt sound "Ouch". If you are caressed lightly you make a "Mmm" sound. These sounds are the basis of language. Vowels express emotion and consonants express meaning.

BANKING 1

In Muslim countries people and banks do not charge interest on money loaned out. They do not believe in usury and this differentiates them from Jews and Gentiles. Money is relatively easy to get through credit cards. ATM machines have made money available twenty four hours a day. Debt keeps us together. Only recently has Britain paid off the dept of the Second World War to America.

The banks own all the beautiful buildings. They have what we want: loans for cars, holidays, insurance, stocks and shares and our castle. Credit is manic. Get insurance so that your family will be safe. It works in the paranoia that death brings. Get your insurance now. You can save for your retirement when people say they will write and sing.

Of course, the credit boom will collapse when banks ask for their money back, as happened notably after Black Monday, 1929, when the world was plunged into a recession that turned into the Depression of the Hungry Thirties. One in every four contemporary Americans 25 yr olds have had a bout of serious depression; in 1955 the figure was 2 percent.

The money system in the major capitalist countries is fuelled by the taking of drugs. Dealers take cocaine and speed and are both buying and selling more and more shares so that they can get more commission. The dealers make hundreds of thousands of pounds in a year. This does not include bonuses.

JOHN BERGER

In the 1970s Australian art critic Robert Hughes did a TV program and book called Shock of the New. John Berger who died in January 2117 did a book called the *Ways of seeing*, a treatise on modern art from a Marxist perspective that was a TV program. Hughes who died in 2012 felt that art students did not paint or draw descriptive scenes enough. Spatial understanding can be used to tune into their creativity. Cubist painting might be more abstract and stimulate the Right brain. Women are not as receptive to spatial painting as men, so is abstract painting a step forward or looking backward for society? Men are better than women at reading maps and following directions and spatial understanding and the lay out or anything from disposition of forces in a battlefield to the layout of furniture in a room. The parietal lobes involved in spatial sense, maps and navigation are larger in men. When a man and a woman walk into a party the women knows intuitively who is getting on emotionally with whom whereas the man knows where the furniture is. The band name One Direction (space) comes from the right creative musical brain.

SCHOOL 1

I have big lips like Mick Jagger with whom I share a birthday, as a well as Stanley Krubeck. I was called Rubber Lips and Smiler at secondary school. Bog the English teacher called me the grinning Gargoyle. I would be slow to get the joke and he would say ah Marshall "the pennies dropped". The maths teacher would say Marshall "think before you speak" because I would ask a question and then when he was half way through explaining the question I would say "it's ok I get it now", which really annoyed him. If we wanted to mess up a class I would say "Sir could you do the Arabic alphabet on the black board" He would do the alphabet and we would eat our sandwiches. Some of the class would talk about dimensions i.e. 10 that went over my head. The teacher had a tin of Zubes on the desk in front of him and there was a temptation to steal one but it rarely happened.

I was embarrassed by my skinny legs and I was called Styks that then became the river of the dead in Roman mythology when I grew up. I was very shy of girls and rarely talked to them. It took drink years later to loosen me up and I became quite good at chatting them up. I went out with quite a few beautiful and intelligent girls whom I learnt a lot from. As like everybody else I got upset when girls broke it off with me.

Ken Livingstone (ex. London Lord Mayor) said that once he adjudicated a debate between a posh school and a working class school and he found that the difference was self-confidence on the part of the posh school.

THE RIDGE

The Grandparents Farm

Waking up to the chant of the forest as wood pigeons sing in the newborn sun. The musty smell of a room rarely used. Condensation in the corner of the windowsill where paint was peeling. Breathe like steam from the cattle but warm beneath the quilted blanket. Blowing on the rust-veined mirror and leaving a mist that you kiss, the imprint of your lips a ghost by evening. Getting dressed with grass-seed on your socks, flies in the room already and sticky yellow Vapona flypaper hanging from the light to catch them. Down the wooden stairs and on with the Wellingtons. Out into the air and down the lane, the hedges netted with cobwebs that catches the dew in beads of light, the ground pocked and muddy with hooves of the cattle and scored by the swing of the gate. Lift the wire loop off the gatepost and into the yard.

The cows are being milked as usual by the hands of Granny and Granddad in the dung-splattered whitewashed cowshed. Granny's cows are placid;

Granddad is stern with the more difficult ones. The swallows swoop through the windows and up into the rafters where a mud-nest is perched. The cat wipes squirted milk from her whiskers and tongues it off her paw. The warm milk is strained into churns that are collected by the creamery-lorry at nine o'clock. Back into the house for a cup of tea, a boiled egg with butter and salt and a few cut slices of white bread with homemade blackcurrant jam.

The Ridge was the name of my Granddad's ninety-acre farm in Carlow, where my father and his thirteen siblings were brought up on. It is on the Castlecomer plateau approximately two miles west of Old Leighin (Cathedral) and St Lazarines well and ten miles south west of Carlow town. The farm was based around a dairy herd and calves. It was once much larger, but my great-grandfather beat his landlord in a horse race and was denied the lease on half the farm as punishment. Every summer my brothers Peter and Philip and I were dumped there for weeks on end, to work and play and blur boundaries.

Feeding calves in the field you call them in: "Suck suck suck" like behavioural therapy. Feeding new calves with milk you put your fingers up the calf's mouth and put the muzzle in the milk and he sucks your finger like a tit and drinks the milk, his coarse tongue rasping your skin an amazing experience. You have to be careful in case they puck the bucket into your face. For older calves you mix musty smelling meal with water, well stirred so there are no lumps. You always have a special favourite calf. Going in at lunchtime, famished, eating bacon with mustard, spuds and cabbage with semolina, rice or sago and home-made jam for dessert. Going out into the fields to unsettle the cattle to see if they had the murrain, blood in the urine a sign of Urinary Tract Infection when they stood up. Finding a cow calving in the far four acres and running to the farmhouse to get Granddad and Granny. They carried the calf with a bag between its legs helping it to walk, watching the cow in case she got angry and charged.

Locking the hens in at night in case there is a fox on the prowl. Granny did not have a cockerel but now and again a hen would have a nest of may be twelve eggs hidden somewhere. The small yellow chicks under a light to keep them warm. Turkeys for Christmas. Rambling up the fields in the evening, relaxed more than tired, somehow energised in the midst of seething nature. The force that drives the flower really did seem to drive life's blood.

Cutting thistles in the well field with worn out sharp spades where the tadpoles develop from the frog spawn in the well. Lazy butterflies in the nettles like scraps of abstract art bobbing in a breeze and the odd ladybird. Climbing trees to look in the nests at the eggs that were sky blue but we left them alone. Getting brown sticky sap on our hands and clothes. Eating the purple frockens (bilberries) on the field ditch and arriving back late from bringing in the cows with the tell-tale purple mouth. The wild strawberries down by the river where you fish for sticklebacks with a jam jar and some twine, as they dart around under the bridge. The young girl you hoped to see by the hill where her granny lived. Getting stung by horse flies and they hurt.

Making a barometer with a jam jar and a mineral bottle with some Indian ink to colour the water. Sneaking a drink of lemon and lime cordial from the press my Uncle had made, while my grandparents were milking the cows. Sitting in the dark at night unless Frank Hall was on or the news and weather forecast at nine o'clock. Playing cards and draughts and building pyramids with the cards. Reading my first book, *Huckleberry Finn* where the boy is dressed like a girl but the lady susses he is not a girl because he threads the needle the wrong way and also when he drops something into his lap he closes his legs whereas a girl would open her legs and catch the object with her taunt skirt. This sort of thinking amazed and fascinated me.

In the summer making cocks of hay and tying them down with twine to season in the sun. Getting caught with my brother smoking hay wrapped in paper by Granddad, as he had caught my father years before. For long unseen, he stood on the field-bank above us where we crouched in the ditch, until he laughed. Bringing the hay cocks in on a low hay cart pulled by Mollie the mare. In the country the weather becomes the major talking point, especially at hay time. Hot sweaty days in the dry heat and in the barn my father throwing up the loose hay with the two pronged hayfork and us trampling it into the corners. Gasping under the corrugated iron roof. Sneezing with hay fever; runny nose and itchy eyes. Drawing water for the stock from the river with Molly in hot weather. Molly was very placid and came to Granddad's "pluh-pluh-pluh" calls without any of the coyness common to field-free horses. Granddad saying, "Are you snug *garcon*?" when he'd sat you down on a shaking of straw in the bed of the cart. We filled the barrels from buckets and covered them with sackcloth tied with twine, but of course gallons splashed through the jute on our way back to the farm, and you had to sit on the front splay-board with your foot on the shaft coming home.

If something went wrong Granddad would say "Bad cess to yeh," or "He's only a pup."

Hearing cars and tractors coming up the road and gawking out the window to see who it was. "There goes Wrigley." The nosiness and gossip of small places everywhere. At noon the postman comes up the back road and Granddad goes in to Granny to read the post and look at the *Independent*. Granddad said that if the swallows flew high then the weather would be good and if they swooped low it would be bad. This was because the flies that the swallows ate flew high in good weather when atmospheric pressure was high. He lived by such lore but he read the weather forecast too. People came from far and wide to get his cure that he made out of plants unknown to us, a cure passed down through the family. He used it for skin diseases such as ringworm. Great aunt Jane brought the cure to America and married a Pharmacologist who worked the cure out and it sold as Wynn's Savlon Cream and made them millionaires. Her grandson Edward visited us one year. Grandad saw his patients in the back parlour that had a painting of dark trees and a gloomy lake done by my great-granny and photos of my uncle who had died young, a tall schoolteacher in a mortarboard and a black gown with red trim around it. He had trained to be a priest but had given it up after a year. He then trained as a teacher.

Granddad worked hard and did not like us petting the dogs as that made them soft and poor at bringing in the cattle. He and Granny got on well and I do not remember one argument between them except when Granny gave tea to a council worker who was working on the road. She had known him when she was young. Granddad was jealous. Granddad would clean his pipe tapping it into his hand and rub the tobacco in his palm and fill the pipe and spit on a piece of paper on the floor by the range. He had a whisky every night before he went to bed, the ritual of pouring it and supping it. He drank tea from his saucer and put bread into his soup along with pepper. He liked brown YR sauce with his cabbage and Smithwicks ale if he was bringing in the hay. He stopped going to both church and pub when he was forty but every Christmas he would go back to the Butts the local pub and win a turkey at cards.

First love when I was 12, I was very naive and did not know about sex. I was up with Bill Daly, a neighbour who lived beside my grandparents' farm. Bill said that they were going to cover the mare with the stallion. I did not know what he was talking about. He brought myself and my older brother Peter down to the stallion and watched him do his thing. The stallion had to be helped to get his penis into the mare's vagina. Later that night when we were getting ready for bed I said to Peter my older brother that I knew what sex was about and he said, "So do I." One night in the night club Lillie's Bordello I meet an American guy whose father ran horses in the Larc de Troimphe. I said what to do was to get a wild fast stallion and an obsessive mare that cleaned herself all day. He said that was what his father did.

One day I was sweeping out the cow shed when Granddad gave off to me for sweeping like I was left handed, a *citeóg*. My father was and my younger brother is left-handed. Apparently it is based on the dominant eye and even though I am right handed my left eye is dominant or so the optician said when he tested my eyes. Left handiness is associated with synthesis, creativity, intelligence beauty and what we call intuition, but to an older generation it was something to be eradicated - probably because of some association between right/wrong, right/left, the connotations with "sinister," meaning originally left. Many unfortunate children were whipped at school for writing with the "wrong" hand, and occasionally the trauma this entailed led to speech impediments and dyslexia. A hairdresser once said that the way my hair grows meant I was left-handed. Some people say that hair grows clockwise or anti-clockwise and this can reflect handedness.

My brother and I spent days-cutting hedges on my grandfather's farm. My grandfather liked the symmetry whereas when my Uncle Sydney took over he let them grow wild. When I was on the farm when I was young I used to go rambling over the fields. I was very shy and enjoyed nature. I fancied my cousins who would call over on Sundays. My aunts and uncles were good to us and gave us unconditional love. I amused them when I wore Granddad's old hats. When I think of Uncle Jack McFeterich I associate him with olives and when I was younger Farley's rusks. I associate Aunt Frances with Rolos we got on a Sunday after church in Old Leighen cathedral. I associate Aunt Maude and Sam with mushrooms that we collected in the morning in the back fields. Sam had a gun that he let Peter shoot but I was too young.

Goose for Sunday lunch - beautiful. Sometimes Uncle Gordon and my cousins would come over in the Morris Minor with the semaphore indicators that stuck out of the door pillar. We'd have tea, home made black berry jam and cinnamon cake - very staid and proper Sunday afternoons. Then Granddad would take a nap on the couch and we'd go out to play in the hayshed. Cousin Linda was very beautiful. Valerie once shocked me with a dirty joke when I was about ten. Granddad would cut you skittles or a cricket bat and you played with Edward, another cousin over from America, who chewed his bones at dinner: "It's good for your teeth." This annoyed Granddad.

DUBLIN

When I was young in Deans Grange during the summer we used to catch bees in jars and put them in a cage. Blowing on the dandelion (the teeth of the lion) clock, 1 o'clock 2 o'clock etc. My older brother and I used to collect rose petals in jars thinking we were making perfume. Days of daisy chains. Playing with clackers and catapulting stones at buses and riding choppers in the park when my father had bought me a big black old-fashioned bike. Putting clothes pegs and cardboard in the wheel to make it sound like a motorbike. Cycling down the hill after David and spotting him in hiding in a drive way, too late, braking hard and going over the handlebars, ending up black and blue. Getting purple iodine on cuts and bee stings. Cutting my finger on glass and going to the doctor and getting stitches and sweets for being good. I was so impressed by the doctor that I decided to become one myself. Another influence was Dr. Wembley M.D. a. program. Good memories. I remember on those long hot days we used to pick the tar on the footpath with lolly pop sticks and one day it got on my vest. That vest was to be found in the hot-press, over and over for years, the stain still there. Ruth, Jane my sisters and Peter my brother used to help me at reading and writing because I was slow.

During French class one day I was reading an essay. I was talking about the crap at the bottom of the pond when I should have said a carp. Roger burst out laughing but I was innocent and did not realise what I had said. Another time we were coming back from a cricket match in a car and I started talking about all the orgasms in the Liffey I did not realise that I meant organisms. Andrew was talking about Concorde being a white elephant which I took literally not knowing how a plane could be an elephant. Walking home from school kicking the autumn leaves on the path where we climbed the horse chestnut tree and throwing bits of wood to knock the chestnuts down. Drying the conkers out in the oven to make them harder and become Champs - tangle tangle one two three. Then there was marbles - the jack and the bull's-eye, ring a ring a rosy. Hopscotch, tig, hide-and-go-seek, British bulldog, catch hand, piggybacks "my partner was the biggest boy Philip who was liked by Jane the girl I loved aged ten". O'Grady says do this. Making a red go-cart and pushing each other down the path. Playing cowboys and Indians and making bows and arrows. Playing football in the park and climbing the trees and robbing orchards and sneaking into the neighbours' garden and eating bitter gooseberries and sweet raspberries. Going to cubs and scouts and camping in Powerscourt. Pitching the tent and gathering wood for the fire and building a lantern. Swapping a chemistry set for a mouse that died and was buried in the back garden.

Playing on the drive with my wind-up train that I took apart and could not get back together. Playing with my red and blue plastic boat in the bath. Being amazed that Stephen could spell *elephant* and *knowledge*. Wondering what nettle soup is like. Remember my sister using ink and nibs and putting blotting paper into the ink well. Running around in the snow with our tongues out as sung by Beth Orton who visited me with Philip my brother.

Parents having parties and the stale smell of beer and cigarettes in the house the next morning. Going to the hospital to collect the new baby Philip. On the pelmet in my mother's bedroom was the red woolly dog that squeaked when you squeezed it and the red money box from Germany that sat beside it. I remember my mother screaming when her father died. It was a heart-rending cry.

Going over to the Tracy's to watch *Batman* because they had a coloured TV. Getting the first stereo and our own coloured TV that replaced the black-and-white one that was always on the horizontal hold. When we went to my cousin's house at Christmas he had comics, the *Victor*, the *Beano* and the *Dandy*. Aunt Vicki made great pavalova and on Christmas day we watched "Top of the Pops" if Granny let us. She did not like long hair on boys and we were not allowed to watch David Bowie. The boys watched *The Alamo* for about ten years running even though the girls wanted to watch "Swan Lake" - just once. Bowie got his name from Bowie in the Alamo.

T.V / Film / Books

During the year we watched "Batman," "Wanderly Wagon," "The Monkeys," "Marcus Welby, MD," "Blue Peter," "John Craven's News round," "Woody Woodpecker" and "Roadrunner," "Alias Smith and Jones." and "Mr.Magoo". I listened to *Oliver* and *Chitty Chitty Bang Bang*. Rolf Harris sang "Two Little Boys." I would watch the Black and White Minstrel Show and Tommy Cooper with my father who died suddenly of a heart attack when I was sixteen. Watching Dave Allen, Billy Conolly and "The Old Grey Whistle Test" and films like *Kes, The Hunchback of Notre Dame, Dr Zhivago, If, The Graduate, Midnight Cowboy "Dustin Hoffman", Midnight Express "John Hurt", The Sting, Marathon Man, Grease, Saturday Night Fever, Apocalypse Now, Blade Runner, Total Recall, Life of Brian, Citizen Kane by Orson Welles.* Orson worked so hard in New York that he had to travel by ambulance to get from job to job. Eraserhead, Twin Peaks and Blue Velvet by David Lynch. The Last Picture Show. Probably the best of them all was "The Night of the Hunter" directed by Charles Laughton starring Robert Mitchum. Low shots of frogs, rabbits and birds. The Name of the Rose (Umberto Eco), Amacord (Fellini) The Yearling, One Flew over the Cuckoo's Nest.

Books I like - Huysman,'s "A Rebour", James Joyce's "Portrait of an Artist as a Young Man", John Berger's "Ways of Seeing" Anthony Burgess. "Film –Clock Work Orange" Mark Twain's "Huckleberry Finn" Oscar Wilde's "Picture of Dorian Grey, De Profundis and Reading Gaol", Tolstoy "Resurrection", Dostoyevsky's "Crime and Punishment", Nietzsche, Marx's "Das Kapital", Satre's " Ad Nausea", Camus "The Outsider", Darren Brown's "Da Vinci Code", J.D. Salinger's "Catcher in the Rye", Anthony Storr's "On Aggression", Edward De Bono,s "The Naked Ape" Kito's "The Greeks", Ian Suttie's "Origins of Love and Hate"(The Taboo of Tenderness),Hermann Hesse's "Siddhartha and Goldmund"(the Hippy bible of the sixties), Arthur Schopenhauer. George Orwell's "1984 and Animal

Farm", Aldous Huxley's "Brave New World", Steinbeck's "Of Mice and Men", James Lovelock "Gaia", Karen Armstrong's "Gospel according to Women" Jack Kerouac's "On the Road", "A day in the life of Ivan Ilovich's" Arthur Miller's "Death of a Salesman", Ernest Hemmingway's "The Old Man and the Sea", John Updike's "Run Rabbit Run", Keats's " Ode to an Nightingale", Patrick Kavanagh's "Raglan Road" "Great Hunger"

TV programs Arena, South Bank Show, Shock of the New, Mr Magoo, Goons, Dave Allen, 3 Stooges, Marxs brothers, Kenneth Clark, History of Civilisation, Bronouski, The Ascent of Man, Buntus Cainte, Fairytales and Myths usually have happy endings i.e. Cinderella, Snow white and Goldie locks i.e. manic. Obituaries are usually positive "Don't speak ill of the dead"

Archetype girls are Kelly Brook and Kate Moss. Sexy, humours, intelligent, confident, ambitious, driven and glamourous all you want in one package.

The paintings I like include Picasso's "Dasmosel de Avingon" and "Guernica"(The Light Bulb),and Lorca's "Brain Cells" and (Light Bulbs), Dali's "Time", Kandinsky, Roden's, "The Kiss", "The Thinker", and "The Ascent of Man" "Balzac", Calder and Moore in Trinity College Dublin, James Barry, Hieronymus Bosch, Jack B. Yeats, Jackson Pollock(backed by the C.I.A.),Andy Warhol, Michelangelo Bunerotti's, "David", "Slaves", "Sistine Chapel" and Moses in the "Chapel of the Viticulares (Chains)"of which I took hundreds of photos. Its base was on a marble floor that reflected the light. It had two horns in it head that symbolised light/spirit. Leonardo da Vinci's "Last Supper", Donatello's, "Bacchus", Francis Bacon's "Pius "11", Escher (Night and Day, Monks Work), Monet, Matisse, and the very manic Van Gogh who painted Sun Flowers and was a very manic preacher and a manic depressive. Sigmund Freud who sent his grandson Lucien Freud pictures by Bruegle.

Friedrich Nietzsche

In order to have art, in order to have any action or any aesthetic contemplation at all, a preliminary physiological condition is indispensable: ecstasy. (Ecstasy is a perfect expression of a manic person S.M.)

Twilight of the Idols.

The title of chapters in Nietzsche's final book Ecce Homo are manic "Why I Am a Destiny"; "Why I Am So Wise"; "Why I Write Such Excellent Books".

"Well and good, very good in fact: after the old God is abolished, I am ready to rule the world" The brilliant son of a German Lutheran minister spent the last 10 years of his life in a lunatic asylum dying in 1900. Probably being manic from General Paralysis of the Insane due to Syphilis in later life but also manic as a young man. *Review by Rob Doyle APRIL 23, 2016*

ANXIETY/PARANOIA

The tinkers were in the field across the way and I was scared of them but a girl I liked talked to them. Their horses made a mess of the front garden. One day when a few of us were in the front garden two itinerants a mother and her 16yr old daughter were passing. The girl ran up the drive shouting and screaming at us and we fled into the back garden. Ian shut the gate and the girl tried to get us. She left us laughing. I was never so scared. I was also scared of the mad woman who walked up and down the road talking and laughing to herself. I confronted my fear by doing Psychiatry. Thinking there was a witch under my bed I used to jump onto it, going down the stairs swinging down the banisters at the fear of the fox I thought was at the top of the stairs in the dark.

FAMILY

The Marshalls (king's farrier) came with the Normans from France. When the Norman knights had to swear allegiance to the King of France they had to kiss his shoes which they did by lifting his foot up, causing the king to fall over. Clearly men with little regard for authority, except their own. William Marshall married Aoife, the daughter of Strongbow the Earl of Pembroke, and tried to make Carlow the capital of Ireland. One daughter married the king of Scotland and his various sons were killed in action or poisoned. He was prince regent to Henry the Third and Marshall to Henry 1, Henry 2, Richard the Lionheart, John whom his granddaughter Eve married and he was buried in the Templar' church in London. With two of his sons. A story has it that he stayed in bed until his early forties, which seems incompatible with his life's achievements. William Marshall was also the name of the soldier who looked after the horses of Julius Caesar. My middle name is William.

Going to St Lazarenes Cathedral in Old Leighlein on a Sunday with Aunt Frances, a nurse. Going to the well of St. Lazarenens. The organ been powered by a man on the bellows and singing to a rickety old record player at the back of the church as there were not enough people to sing. Getting a Mars bar and Rolos on the way home.

To write about myself is such an unusual strange thing that I do not know where to start. Going to schools that were very much based on science and ending up as a Doctor of Medicine and then going into psychiatry. Sometimes I doubt my own existence and I'm left wondering about God and Jesus and Napoleon and the fact that they are dead. That makes me important as I live I exist I emote I feel and I see. I am not in the habit of looking at myself because this involves thought and I'm not good at thinking. I have never really looked at myself and analysed my life. I seem to have drifted along rudderless in a sea of confusion and alcohol. I don't know much about myself or how I work or worked - as infant, child, schoolboy, student, doctor and patient. As I write my story I wonder what I will remember because they say you remember the good things such as the "good old days." Even though I have drifted there seems to be method in the madness. My having drifted into what I call the "manic archetypes" seems to have been dependent on the course I have taken. Going from sport and clean living in adolescence to taking drugs, such as dope and alcohol leading to a slow decline in mental health that often leads to paranoia. Sometimes I wonder what it would have been like if I had not got sick and was a consultant on 150K a year as opposed to my medical pension of 12K a year maybe married with children. If I was to think about my position I would go mad. Drug induced psychosis is not uncommon in people been admitted to psychiatric hospitals. Being a minority religion – Protestant - in a very Catholic country that suffered 30 years of disturbance: with this political disturbance and a scientific background I have looked at Ireland from a certain vantage point that may be unique.

Going up the mountains on Sunday having tried to get the red cherry from the tin of fruit. Racing out into the garden to get on the swing first after lunch. I remember going on car trips with my father playing "I spy." Seeing large rolls of paper the size of a car on trucks and my father would say that they were "Giant's toilet rolls" Fighting in the back of the car and Dad saying "If you don't stop fighting I'll stop the car and you can walk home."

Jane my eldest sister saying that we passed such and such shop in Castle Bellingham. Going to my Aunt Vicky's house in Armagh for Christmas and being fed like royalty. The Christmas tree appeared to be massive. Aunt Vicky's Pavlova was like nectar. A fry with segments of orange every morning. One Christmas Jane and Robert my cousin had a competition to see who could eat the most Brussels sprouts. Jane won after eating 30 sprouts - on top of a Christmas dinner! Trying to stay awake for Santa but we always fell asleep. Comics that we never had the pocket money to buy. "Achtung!" "Schnell, Franz!" Going to the shops to buy sweets for a midnight feast. Opal fruits. The girls always had a better feast. Going swimming and Judy my cousin diving off the high board. I was too scared to even jump off the low board. Getting up on Christmas morning and getting Meccano, carpentry set or chessboard. The usual socks and ties and powder and deodorant and Brut after-shave, Hud talcum powder, sweets and fruit and golf balls and Old Spice for my Father and my Uncle Robin.

Eating and drinking. Sometimes my Uncle Robin, who was a vet, was called out and we would go with him. The smell of the farmyard in the car full of drugs and injections. Holding calves with fingers in their noses. Driving over a hill in South Armagh with a man flagging us down, Uncle Robin put the boot down thinking the worst - an IRA ambush. When we came over the hill there was a flock of sheep on the road. Sigh of relief all around. Hearing British Army helicopters over the house and sometimes there was snow.

My Uncle Robin had a drinks party on Christmas Eve and we were sent to bed. The key was always in the door. Robert (my cousin) driving the car in the back yard and skidding and spinning the car around. Cats all over the place and purring to themselves. The smell of cat piss in the garage.

On Boxing Day we went to see Dungannon play Ballymena at rugby, a yearly fixture. My cousins were very practical and pragmatic. Even though they could have done medicine they went into business. They did not have the guilt factor that my family had. At a wedding in my aunt's when the people had left, the marquee burnt down. Some children had been playing with matches. We cut the connection between the house and the marquee. A cousin had a Downs Syndrome baby, whether or not this was related to a cousin Martin who had Downs Syndrome I do not know. Martin was sent to the best schools and was attending a special school in Switzerland. My late Aunt Roberta, who looked after him, was a born-again Christian and was always preaching that the end of the world is starting in the Far East. She died recently. She expressed the manic trait in our family genes, as does a cousin who has manic depression with religious delusions.

Fiona my younger sister was always the last to finish her ice cream cone. She licked it as slowly and we used to be so jealous having eaten ours so quickly. She played hockey for Ireland since she was a schoolgirl and was a very successful player. Mum says Fiona could organise an army.

One Saturday morning in August when I was sixteen I was upstairs and my father asked me to make him a cup of tea, as he wasn't feeling very well. I went downstairs and put the kettle on, and then I went up the garden to put a tea shirt on the line. When I returned to the house I heard a loud yelp. I ran upstairs and found my dad having a heart attack. I got my older brother Peter and we tried to resuscitate Dad but he was slipping away. I whispered in his ear, "I love you." I rang for an ambulance and when they arrived I was asked was the attack more than three minute's duration. I said," Yes" and as a result they did not try to resuscitate him.

Down to the hospital and one by one the family arrived. I remember praying to God to bring back my dad and saying that I would give up masturbation if he did. When my mother arrived back at the house she let out an unearthly scream and was devastated. The funeral was large and I met people I had not seen for years. I imagined that I saw horses in the clouds during the funeral. Apparently my father was a horse whisperer and when he was twelve he could lead two stallions to the fair.

We did not deal with my father's death properly and the family was easily brought to tears at the mention of his name, like Granny was at the mention of Uncle Bill who died when he was thirty-three in 1959. I had vivid dreams of Dad's death for years and probably had post-traumatic stress disorder.

Madness came slowly or maybe it was always there especially when drink was involved. Like Dick the Edge's brother on Boxing Day asking "Are you mad," while he laughed. Sometimes when I wake up in the morning I wonder what will happen and how the day will go. I realised when Anthony Tobin, a fellow-patient, died of lung cancer that the cigarette I'm smoking might kill me and how stupid I was; but they're hard to give up. Sometimes I look into the mirror and wonder who I am and what I'm here for.

MUSIC

Working in St Brendan's hospital I'd call into Bewley's on Grafton Street (named after the 1st Duke of Grafton the illegitimate son of Charles the second) on the way home and sit in the Mezzanine that overlooked the street sipping coffee. The Duke of Wellington had gone to school upstairs in Bewleys. Meeting Jonathan Philbin Bowman and talking about super realism. He died in 2000. I used to give Jonathan a few pounds - spontaneous generosity is another manic aspect. Jonathan was very funny and also very intelligent. He was a great father to his son Saul and loved the life in town and is greatly missed. His father was heartbroken at his funeral. Jonathan enjoyed working for the *Sunday Independent* through which he met interesting people and he was always a good read and had a wry sense of humour.

I've always been interested in music, and particularly in expressing some of my ideas through song. One night I sat down with Eoin McEvoy from the Eighties band Cactus World News and wrote "Song of love." I recorded it with producer-engineer Paul Thomas and realised that I could do it myself - the songs weren't bad. The first song I recorded was "Howard Hughes" and it is still one of my best ones. I'd read about Hughes and had been taken by some of the lines I had underlined such as "a pool in every mansion but he never swam."

The whole thing was manic-driven. Almost every night I'd buy 25 cans of Heineken in Farm Produce on Baggot Street before going home: ten cans each for Philip, my brother, and Paul Thomas, producer-engineer, and five for myself. Staying up till three in the morning listening to music being made and going to bed and getting up early. Music was it. Then there were the gigs in J J Smyth's and the Baggot Inn. Meeting up on a Saturday afternoon and putting the drums and amps and guitars into the white BMW that we spray-painted at a later date, in imitation of U2's painting of Trabants. Stoned on the aerosol paint fumes from spraying the car and buzzing after two pints. Going to the gig, having a pint, setting up a pint, the gig, and some pints, cleaning up, another pint, bringing the gear home and heading into the Pink Elephant. This was in 1990-92. In a taxi and asking what a Tulip was and the driver said "Fruit and nut case." Those gigs were vital and visceral.

The Mary Janes were good and tight and had a shy front man in Mick Christopher with his dreadlocks. Mick died in Holland after getting head injuries from a fall in 2002 while he was touring with the Waterboys. The Tulips had good songs such as "99 cent breakfast again" "Raging Bull" "Schizo" "Sex Sells." "Insane In Paris" Often new songs were tried out in the sound checks, which as well as the gigs was recorded. Alan Corr putting them in the best ten gigs of the year in the Christmas *RTE Guide*. Barry Egan from the *Sunday Independent* saying they were "somewhat" brilliant. at a gig in Tramore.

One night the rock journalist Bill Graham said to me "Give something back," so I said "It's all numbers and vowels" - i.e. U2 the double vowel with a number that accesses the right musical brain. Bill was good to me and he protected me from people he felt weren't good for me. He was the senior journalist with *Hot Press* - he will, of course, be remembered for introducing U2 to their manager Paul McGuinness and championing them in Hotpress - and at one stage he wanted me to become their scientific correspondent but we never got it together. When I came out of hospital for the first time he gave me a big bear hug. He used to say that I was too soft on bands that I managed. Bill was thinking all the time (when he talked I took notes) and you had to know when to leave him alone.

As I said to Bill Graham of Hot Press, "One Love" is a good lyric because it's a double vowel from the left hand (Emotional, musical) and a number (right hand) that stimulates both sides of the brain. U2 is also a double vowel (emotional, musical) left hand and a number, right hand. The Names Bono and The Edge have double vowels that are musical and emotional. U2, One Love, Bono and Edge are probably the best names in the music business.

Waiting for Bill to turn up at gigs, as he plugged the Tulips and the Mary Janes (who did support for the Tulips in the Baggot Inn) and Roller Skate Skinny. Hanging out with him on the day that the Tulips had played the Junior Common Room in Trinity College. Taking notes on what he said and being brought by him to a book launch in Lily's Bordello where I took the microphone and ranted on about the Tulips being the band to support. Drunk, of course. Without malice Robbie Fox, the manager, kicked me out. I used to meet Bill in Lily's and at gigs and we would talk about everything under the sun - politics, music, and social stuff. One night in Lily's he was leaning against the bar when he fell back onto the ground with a pint of Guinness without spilling a drop. We had not laughed so much for a long time. I will always remember him that night with a big smile on his face.

In May 1993 when I was drunk I tried to stop a fight outside the Pink Elephant where six guys were kicking two guys in the head on the ground. Two of them turned on me and kicked me unconscious. The last thing I remember is seeing Mark my friend over me saying I had been kicked in the head. They do this so you do not remember the attackers faces and after this I was paranoid if I drank alcohol or smoked pot. The chicken and egg: did the beating lead to breakdown, or did incipient breakdown lead to the beating? That year I ended up in a psychiatric hospital, St. Patrick's. I had a vision of the Virgin Mary. Yet I also used to read all the Sunday papers and played innumerable games of chess.

Between beating and breakdown, on Midsummer's Day 1993, I was pissed off with the Tulips and decided to get a band to manage, so I headed to the Rock Garden where a band called Never On Sundays was playing. Their first song was "He thinks he's Jesus but he's paranoid." That struck a chord with my own incipient paranoid manic ideas and I decided this was the band for me. I renamed them The Cans. Within a week we had recorded four songs at the Tunnel Studios. An American video editor friend said these would be perfect for the American market. Later we recorded a song "Sugar" in Lansdowne studio, with Chris O'Brien and Frank Kearnes as producers. It cost £1,000 to get that one song onto digital audiotape but it got played on the Dave Fanning Show that very night. The next day Thomas Black, a talent scout for EMI, rang and he met the band. It looked as if we were going places. We waited, but nothing happened, and after a while I realised I did not agree with the political beliefs of the band. They were too nationalistic and had hard line republican sympathies, so I could not continue to manage them.

The night that Curt Cobain died, in April 94, I went to a gig where the younger brother of a friend Guggi was lead singer with a group called ®. Guggi was in the Virgin Prunes, an art punk band in the early eighties. We sound-proofed the bedroom in my granny flat and ® used to come over at noon, make me coffee and practise until five o'clock. They supported the Tulips on the first Friday of the month in June and July in 1994 and then headlined for September through December in the Baggot Inn. In June I went to a party held by Eva by Lough Dan. There was a band and I got up to sing with the buzz. Connor said that I was great. On midsummer's day in June 1994 there was a Sunflower concert in the Olympia for the Harold's Cross Hospice. At the afters in Blooms Hotel a friends flat mate said "why did Elvis throw it all away" I turned around realising it was a good lyric and Paul Brady was passing and I said the lyric to him and the rest is history (ie. he used it in a song). Around this time, I was driving onto Lesson St from Adelaide road when I was distracted by female ass walking across the road. Needless to say I crashed into the car in front of me and it cost me £400. In the Baggot in October 1994 there were 90 guests and 100 paying gig goers and George Byrne wrote in the *Independent* that ® had played the biggest gig in the Baggot for that year. As a result of this we got a bigger gig in Whelan's. For every gig I designed red black and white posters and flyers, these colours holding certain significance for me, mystical or manic. We taped each sound check and gig and did a hundred studio tapes. We also had printed 70 long sleeved tee shirts which had ® on front and "the best unsigned band in the world / Rolling Stone Magazine" on the back.

For the first gig of 1995 we played on the first Thursday, January 5th in Whelan's with St Jude in support. We got a good crowd even though it was close to Christmas and the New Year. Around this time I relapsed and was readmitted to hospital. Strongman Johnny's brother took over the management of the band The next gig on the first Thursday in February in Whelan's was not well publicised or attended and ® lost the gig spot for

March 1995. The name ® was very hard to sell so they eventually changed their name to Pelvis. As Pelvis they went on to win the best new band in the Heineken Green Energy Festival in May 1995, got a deal for £20,000 with Setanta record company and released a very good single *"Fifteen seconds of Fame"* in September 1995 to early for the album release. They played the Jules Holland Show. They brought out an album in May 1996 that got some airplay on the Dave Fanning show on 2FM and the Tom Dunne show on Today FM. The album cost £19 which is too expensive and sold 1,500 copies, but they have done very little since 2000. I do not know what they are doing now.

My own involvement had ceased shortly after that successful Whelan's gig in early January. Things were heading for a break-up as I was heading for a breakdown. I was on the door that night and let a lot of people in free and the band suspected that I'd been dipping into the takings. I ended up in hospital later that week, January 95, and Strongman, a (Virgin Prune) brother of the lead singer Johnny, became the manager. I had owed the poster printer £200 and the poster company £200 and with me out of the frame Strongman had to pay this. In a subsequent interview with *Hot Press* the band blamed me for their debts and the whole thing turned a bit sour. When they are starting out bands cost money. Also they did not have to pay for the rehearsal space or transport - they practised in my flat and I transported their gear free of charge that all together would have cost £3,000. I had spent three grand in four months' living and covering the expenses for the band. You could say that there was an early manifestation of manic behaviour. I brought a drum trigger machine and a guitar affects machine for R for £800. When I left the band I offered the machines to the vendor but he offered a miserable amount of money. I got a good deal with Sonic Studios that I got time for the machines to record some songs.

As I've explained elsewhere, one of the beneficial aspects of mania or hypomania is sociability. This led me to my making many friends with high-profile public personalities like Bill Graham who was the top journalist with Hot Press. On another night I was in Lillies Bordello another night club with my brother when we meet Jim Steinman whom my brother recognised as the writer for Meat Loaf's Bat Outa Hell. I gave him a line "The God of Sex & Drugs and Rock & Roll" which he put into the song "I'd do anything for love but I won't do that". Jim changed it to "God of Sex & Drums and Rock & Roll." My brother said not to give Jim any more lines. I had got the line Power Sex Money from an interview with Orson Wells on TV which became "Power Sex Money we are Gods set me free" in a song of mine. Another word I came up with was "Californication" that my brother did not like but that the band Red Hot Chilly Peppers use and have the copyright on. An unusual album title was by Jay-Z called Magna Charta Holy Grail 2014. U2 song "One Love," good double vowel and a number.

But it wasn't just the music world. I'd get up late, (noon) have a shower, ring a friend, C, who would call over at two o'clock and we'd head into Café en Seine for coffee and beer. P and D would be there, two of the funniest and most intelligent people that I know.

Pat had taught me what I know about art and appreciation of beauty and had brought me to Paris for ten days when I was twenty. We stayed in the author's room over the shop in the Shakespearean Company bookshop that overlooked Notre Dame on the Seine (a beautiful rose window) where the owner George Whitman who has recently died aged 98 presented us with ice chilled tea. If you slept in the shop at night you had to work in the shop for two hours but myself and Patrick did not have to do this as Patrick had a book published and we stayed for nothing in the writers room for a week. Pat showed me around the galleries and lectured me on the pictures, i.e. The Georges Pompidou Centre. Sylvia Beach who opened the first Shakespeare Company book shop in 1922 published the first edition of James Joyce's Ulysses. Authors such as Henry Miller, Ernest Hemmingway, F. Scott Fitzgerald, William Burroughs and Samuel Beckett were associated with the Shakespeare Company book shop.

On the way home we stopped in Sandymount for some take-away beer. That days band practise sessions by R were taped and Connor and I listened to them as well as playing Oasis "Live Forever "and writing out lyrics and titles. As a name R was impossible to sell.

In Bewley's I drank enough strong Java coffees with Simon Carmody, the charismatic singer with the Golden Horde, to get the caffeine hit shakes. At the time a magazine said, "Why does Simon hang out with a psychiatrist?" Talking about anything and everything but mainly music and my obsession with U2. Then going for a drink to calm down. Most nights I'd go to the Pink Elephant, a club in town, and have a few pints, hoping to see someone famous there, thinking that I might miss something. I used to go up to famous people and hassle them. It was Mike Scott, the singer from the Waterboys, whose song the "Whole of the Moon" was sung by every busker on every corner who told me of James Lovelock's "Gaia" - a great read, worth giving him hassle. Great times. I had gone over to his table in the Waterfront and interrupted his girlfriend and himself. Then he got up to sing and Irene (girlfriend) had to tell me to shut up in a polite way so that she could hear the songs. She said that he was nervous of performing. Guggi and Gavin Friday did the two Biddies. Great fun but mainly driven by my drinking and not without embarrassing moments. Connor Owens my pal used to drive his mother's car and I brought the vino and beer. Connor died in tragic circumstances. We had some great nights together ending up in the Manhattan of Harcourt St for a fry at 2am in the morning. Connor ran his publishing baby The Dublin Event Guide in Temple Bar.

One night I went up to Mick Hucknall and asked him if he was in Simply Red. He turned to me and told me to "fuck off" I deserved it. Another night I waylaid the film director Neil Jordan and told him about my theory about touch and language (language comes from touch) at the top of my voice on the disco floor in the Pink Elephant a night club. "Are you on drugs or what?" he said. But high on drink, embarrassment ran off me like water off a duck's back. It was an "ah what". Another night I went up to Gabriel Byrne the actor who was with his friends and politely asked me to leave him alone to talk to his friends. God what a prick I was.

SONTAG

The same manic energy and reckless confidence impelled me to other places and into the company of other famous people. I met Susan Sontag at a literary meeting at the Royal Marine Hotel in Dun Laoghaire. She was very sexual and charismatic even though she was in her fifties and I was in my 30's. She had a fleck of grey hair in her fringe. I had the confidence to approach her. This confidence was common to other people I approached. I explained my touch theory to her - how touch gave rise to language - possibly to propagate my idea, possibly to impress her. I asked her to write the book and she said in a nice way to write it myself. She put the seed of writing into my mind and changed my life.

At another literary meeting in Earlsford Terrace, National Concert Hall I meet Anthony Burgess a genius who was a very nice man but who seemed to be suspicious if not scared of me. I got him to autograph a few American first editions of his work that I had.

R.D.Laing had a talk in Trinity T.C.D. At the end I stood up (I had three pints) I said that some people were brain cells and some people were liver cells. He agreed with me but the audience were not agreeable they booed. After the talk we went to the students bar the Buttery where U2 had played for 50 pence years before. I sat down beside Laing and explained my touch – language – schizophrenic theory to him. In reality he was only interested in his cheque. Laing wrote "The Divided Self" and he had acquired a licence to give his patients LSD.

On Friday nights I used to go to the Brazen Head with a few psychiatrists from St. Brendan's and then to the Shelbourne Hotel where the movers and shakers used to meet. People like Eamon Dunphy, P. J Mara, the government press secretary, and Paul McGuiness, manager of U2. One night I met Jonathan Philbin Bowman and Malcolm McClaren, manager of the Sex Pistols, and we had a meal in a local restaurant. Malcolm was fascinating and he gave me his address in London but I lost it. Jonathan died around this time. His death was a great loss to the culture of the city. The odd time I went to the Unicorn at noon on a Saturday to have carboniare and wine.

Around this time I was nominated as one of the top fifty bachelors in the country in *Social and Personal* magazine; Nicki Mulcahy called me "incorrigible" in *Phoenix* magazine and in an article on cafés a journalist Orna Mulcahy, noted me as a regular entertainer of females in Bewley's Mezzanine. This reflects the manic energy I was putting into my social life.

Looking back, I'm reminded of a poem by Edna St Vincent Millay, "First Fig":

> *My candle burns at both ends,*
> *It will not last the night.*
> *But ah my foes, and oh my friends*
> *It gives a lovely light!*

A girlfriend's aunt, Rosita Sweetman, had written a few books; 1972 "On our Knees" and 1979 "On our Backs" and some others and the idea to do so probably came from her.

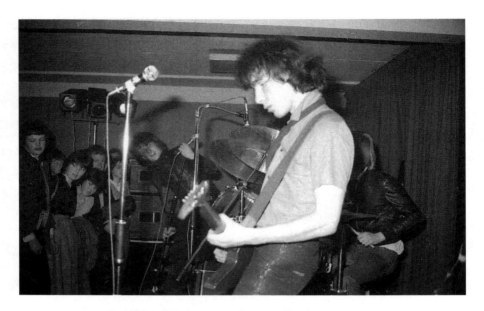

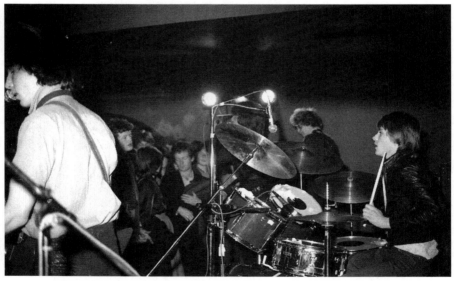

U2 at the Buttery Bar, Trinity College, 3rd of February 1979
Copyright: Patrick Brocklebank.

Buddy Holly died on 3rd February 1959.

BREAKING DOWN

I don't know where to start or what to say. What is on my mind and how this developed over time I do not know. Having been a trainee psychiatrist and now being a patient must or should throw up interesting contrasts and comparisons but I do not see it that way. I am not in the habit of thinking or reflecting on my life even though it might have been lived in strange places. I would not say that I know myself but I hope that by writing I may help myself to understand the outer world and myself. My thoughts and feelings essentially confuse me. I often stand back and say Why this? Why God? Or Why me? Why are we here? What am I doing? Where am I going? This questioning can be tedious and draining. Searching becomes the reason for the search. Not having a God to hide behind and organise my life around. Yet I do believe in a force that comprises electrical, gravitational, magnetic and organic chemistry that has resulted through evolution to our state of mind. I am good at seeing patterns and the Manic Archetypes theory expresses my thinking and feeling. These ideas came to me in various enlightenments/ illuminations that were reflected in my thought patterns, mainly manic and paranoid and this is what I ended up studying. I look at the blank page and I am confused not knowing where I'm going? Or what is going to be said? Often I look into the mirror and say Why? It is not an enjoyable headspace to be thinking of the imponderable question all the time. I ask Why? but I never answer. What will people think of my writing is a headspace I try to ignore. Just go for it and see what happens, where I end up. Where is Caesar where is Napoleon.

Over the next year 1997, I attended a foundation course - computer studies, social skills, writing skills, art therapy and a photography course in Roslyn Park and I started a book. In January 1999 I sent five pages of my book to Eoghan Harris, a journalist. He is an intellectual whom I admire.

My father was and my brother is left handed, a *citeóg*. Apparently it is based on the dominant eye and even though I am right handed my left eye is dominant or so the ophthalmologist said when he tested my eyes. Three percent of people born in 1910 were left handed whereas now in females eleven percent are left handed and thirteen percent of males are left-handed. Left handedness is associated with synthesis, creativity, beauty and what we call intuition.

Once I had a patient who was a professional snooker player in the U.K. who played with Jimmy White and who had said that he himself had taken a lot of cocaine and became paranoid. My patient was diagnosed as a paranoid schizophrenic and put on medication that gave him a shaky hand so that he could not play snooker. I stopped his medication on the grounds that his paranoia was caused by his cocaine use which he had stopped, but he was put back on tranquilizers.

Another patient who was very intelligent and creative was diagnosed as a paranoid schizophrenic. He was more likely a manic-depressive and deserved a chance of going on Lithium but he went missing and was found in Dun Laoghaire harbour six months later.

A great patient who attended Baggot St. Hospital thought he was King George the Fourth. He said that women would stop on the street and point at him and say, "There goes George the Fourth." He also said that he heard confessions and when asked did these people come to visit him he said no that he used to do confessions as they drove past the house.

Another patient got sick when he was 60 years old. His depression seemed to come out of the blue. Eventually it was found that this man, who was a die-hard Catholic republican and nationalist, became suicidal depressed when he found out that his grandfather had been a Protestant.

Once a patient thought she was a vegetable and of all things she thought she was a cabbage. Another thought that the small white spots of toothpaste on the mirror in her bathroom were Jesus' sperm and she wanted to get pregnant by them.

It is not uncommon to get people who have the delusion that they were Jesus or God and that the IRA was after them. About 20% of Guilty but Insane killers have had the messianic delusion.

An unusual use of medication was giving Lithium to mentally handicapped patients who were overactive and it works. i.e mania does not depend on intelligence. Lithium is normally used as a mood stabiliser for manic-depressive patients, many of whom tend to be creative and intelligent. A contradiction here seems to be that hyperactive children are given Ritalin that acts like speed/amphetamines but actually slows the children down. Some people believe that this is because a certain area in the brain lacks blood flow that is remedied by Ritalin's increasing the blood pressure and heart rate.

When I was in rehab in 1997 there was a girl M a lesbian who I had a great laugh with. Unfortunately, she relapsed and killed herself. D a great guy who was depressed also killed himself. M who was a photographer got paranoid and depressed and also killed himself. M used to come up to St. Patrick's Psychiatric hospital where I was a patient and take me out every day. We had a great time going to the Globe, the Front Lounge and Café en Seine for a coffee some cigarettes and the odd pint. I would give him £10 a day with which he went to Lillie's Bordello. Girls loved M, he was very handsome. He used to take photographs of the Tulips my brother's band. He had a great talent.

D, N, R, D ,C and myself would sleep in my flat from 4am to12 noon and then go into Roslyn Park a rehab college we attended for dinner. We would go back to the flat at 3pm and buy beer approximately 10 cans each and cigarettes to self-medicate. For every beer I drank I would take 100 Largactil to stop myself from getting paranoid. I would do the D.J. i.e. the Doors, U2 and Dark side of the Moon and Steve Earle. We would have a Chinese at midnight. And I would go to bed but the others would stay up to play cards until 3am. Professor Clare my doctor in St. Patrick's realised that I was partying in the flat and band me going there. Prof Clare my doctor has since died but he was one of the most intelligent people I knew. He said that psychoanalysis was one of the great cons of the 20th Century. Michael C and Patrick H are also very bright.

PSYCHIATRY

There is almost immediately a problem with terminology. What is abnormal and what normal behaviour? When does circumstance cease becoming a valid cause for normal (exogenous) depression, and the condition become endogenous and "abnormal"? What decides that a patient is manic or schizo-affective or schizophrenic?

Some people feel that they are being controlled and made do and think things. Sometimes they feel that thoughts are being put into their heads. Sometimes they think that the TV and radio are talking to them. Sometimes they think that people can read their minds. These are signs of schizophrenia. The ratio of male schizophrenics to female schizophrenic is 66 to 33. Sometimes their delusions are grandiose and think they are special, i.e. God or Jesus. Religious delusions are normally associated with schizophrenia but I feel they should be associated, at least sometimes, with mania - often messianic delusion is a product of being high, not schizophrenic. Similarly, though paranoia (thinking that people are against you and are evil) is normally associated with schizophrenia, I feel it should be associated with mania if there are other signs of manic traits. Grandiose delusions are seen in both schizophrenia and mania but I feel it is mainly manic.

When you are assessing patients you find out about their family and any illnesses. You talk about their past and how they got on at school and work etc. Then you talk about sleep and appetite etc. If a patient says that they are not sleeping or eating (weight loss, loose clothing) and are depressed you can be fairly sure that they are suicidal even if they deny such a thought. The dangerous time for depression is when patients are coming out of the low mood where they have no energy to do anything to a stage where they are depressed but getting more energy; it is then that they may attempt suicide. This dangerous stage is also found during early medication and soon after ECT.

Schizophrenics feel they are being controlled by people, the radio and the TV, which, they feel, is talking to them and they have cameras in their eyes and microchips under their skin. Their moods do not fit their thoughts and their emotion may be inappropriate e.g. laughing at a funeral.

Manic-depressives in the manic phase are overactive physically mentally and emotionally. They have racing thoughts, labile emotions, they laugh and are funny (over inclusive, intuitive, incongruent) and their mood is infectious. They can be overactive and in the past (before medication) they could die of exhaustion. Even when in a normal mood they feel down compared to their high. They miss the high. When depressed manic-depressives may think they are the devil - more strictly this condition is dysphoric, and it can also happen in the manic phase. They have poor sleep and poor appetite. Their emotion, intellect and physical energy is down. They can be suicidal.

Doctors can assess anxiety as being psychotic. When people go psychotic they can get anxious but being anxious does not mean you are psychotic. Sufferers might complain of fast cognition and that they are hearing voices which can be their own thoughts. With anxiety they might feel they are being controlled and having thoughts taken out of their head. When a new patient with possible psychosis presents he should be put on anxiolytics until he settles which could take a week and then he should be observed before being put on anti-psychotic drugs.

Dr. McGennis (St. Brendan's RIP) felt that new presentations of so called psychosis should be put on a course of Librium and an eye should be kept on them for a few days to observe for any disinhibition or psychosis.

REVELATIONS

St. John wrote the last book in the bible (Revelations) He heard God's voice and saw visions. This would be associated with Paranoid Schizophrenia / Mania especially with Temporal Lobe activity and maybe epilepsy and vertigo. (This also affected St. Paul on the road to Damascus) The writing is very negative and could be associated with dysphoric elation and rapid cyclers. John is the one that Jesus loved. David Corish of the Davidian cult was obsessed with Revelations the end of time and especially the 4 horsemen of the apocalypse. He thought he was Jesus as did his follower's think he was Jesus.

TRINITY U2

In my fourth year doing Medicine in Trinity College Dublin I stayed in rooms that was paid accommodation on campus. I shared my room with Mark Holmes but people thought Mark Hearne shared because he was always there. Mark Prendergast the token black was a frequent visitor. He went on to write "The History of Irish Rock" He is now a respected music journalist in London. My first and only published picture is of the Virgin Prunes taken in McGonagles on south Ann Street in Dublin. It is in this book.

In rooms we would decide in the morning whether to buy cigs or take the bus to the training hospital St. James.

While I was in college I had a job serving meals(commons) to the students, Scols, Professors and Fellows. One of the schols was Brian Lenihan who was the Fianna Fail Minster for Finance in the Fianna Fail / Green coalition. He died of pancreatic cancer in June 2011. There were 5 medical students serving the meals who had better leaving (exam) results than the schols student from the arts because medical schols were rare. Donegan the Minister for Defence in the 1970's was an alcoholic and had been in St. Patrick's a few times and said that the President O'Dalaigh was a thundering disgrace which resulted in O'Dalaigh resigning. I had met O'Dalaigh at Dermot Kinlen's a neighbour summer house in Kerry where he had a small house for the President called the uarchseinne, the President's small house.

When commons was served the students got a free glass of Guinness with their meal. Any excess was imbibed by the waiters, therefore ever night during the week you had a few drinks and you did not feel like studying.

During the year I was in rooms I did not go, to my designated hospital Sir Patrick Dunne's that much and as a result I failed my exams Microbiology and Pathology and I had to repeat the year. For my Microbiology exam I talked to the examiner about Joyce, Wilde and Beckett. He said he had one question for me. What was the medium that Gonorrhoea was grown on. I did not know. He was giving me the exam. It was Stuart's medium. For my exam in Pharmacology we had to write about drugs in pregnancy. I wrote about alcohol and smoking. My teacher said I would fail. I passed.

Ken the Hen as he was known was very bright. He knew a few born again Christians who kept on asking him had he read the Bible which annoyed him. So one summer he read the Bible so he could say "yes he had read it". On New Years Eve 1984 Ken went down to Sandymount strand and read 1984 by George Orwell.

This reminds me of a community psychiatric nurse who said that it was the drug dealers who used people as prawns. Another saying is a packed of Crips or a Hopital or I have a bad Ulster or better the bottle in front of me than a full frontal lobotomy.

In my first year in college the Virgin Prunes, managed by Kieran Ownes and U2, managed by Paul McGuinnes used to hang around the TCD student bar the Buttery. Dick Evans the Edges brother had rooms, he was a schol in Engineering

One afternoon in the Bailey pub on Duke St. this young girl who looked like a school girl came up to me and asked me was Kieran Owens reliable as he had told her she had a good voice when he saw her singing with a band in T.C.D.'s Buttery bar. I said he was trustworthy and a good judge. In retrospect I think it was Sinead O'Connor.

One year at Mark Holme's house on Boxing Day I asked Dick who were the most intelligent people he knew. He said it was a Swiss computer expert and the Edge his brother.

James Mahon used to take photographs of U2 around the college. I remember Bono showing off some of the first posters of U2 and signing a copy for me which I gave away to RTE charity.

The Virgin Prunes did interesting posters and they played events in the Buttery bar, in McGonagle's, Newman House and an exhibition com gig in the Douglas Hyde gallery in TCD. In the Newman House gig there was a table on the stage. Near the end an airport light was shone from the back of the stage and Gavin Friday (Phenom) stood like a crucifix at the front of the stage. In the exhibition in the Douglas Hyde gallery they had a space under the stairs with a net full of leaves of autumn. A toy dog called Pisser stuck to a carpet on the wall. There was loud white sound in a four hanging posters of photographs of breast operations. In another space there was a chair and a gas ring with beans in the pot. This was to show what Guggi's flat was like in Ballymun. In a fenced off area there was a guy on all fours called sheepy with a fleece on his back who was an acid casualty apparently.

A few years previously I had seen U2 and the Virgin Prunes play in the Buttery for 50 pence. The Virgin Prunes played the hate the audience cards. At parties in Mark Holmes house I meet Bono who even then was charismatic and patient. Even then I was overcome by fame and celebrity. I remember asking him who came first the words or the music and he said he did not know which annoyed and confused me. I don't know why but I used to misunderstand Bono when I meet him. He'd be normal and I be like a spoilt child. I remember in 1991 he came to my mother's house before some stag, I think it was Mark Holme's. We were sitting on the couch and I was saying how hard to get a hundred people into the Baggot Inn to see my brothers band the Tulips. He agreed and said he had the same problem which I found hard to understand as he had to sell 40,000 tickets for his gigs in Lansdowne Road. We were out in the garden that evening and we were laughing about Tommy Cooper. Bono did the trick of itchy teeth. This went over my head and it was only the next day that I got the joke. At a dinner that Mark had a few years earlier Bono and myself were talking about favourite films. We got around to talking about "If" and I was wondering about the music and Bono said it was Zairian gospel music. It seems that Bono was always ahead of the posy. The second half of "If" was in black and white not that this had any significance other than the fact that they ran out of money

Later on the night of the itchy teeth we were in the kitchen of my mother's house. A song by U2 came on the radio and you could see the concentration and analysis of Bono's face on the recording. Later someone found a tray of eggs in the fridge. Well boys will be boys. All hell broke loose. Eggs all over the weaved wallpaper that smelt of eggs for weeks. The egg throwing went outside. Ducking and diving, running and attacking. Suddenly Guggi said there was someone at the window upstairs. It was my mother. Every one scattered except me, Mark and Gary who tidied up. Throwing eggs is the best fun. At Reggies stag we made up a concoction that would put Reggie asleep so that we could put a plaster of Paris on his arm. Two women put Imac on Reggies pubes. I said I'd drink his pubes if he drank the concoction. We duly obliged. Nothing happened.

BOOK

Bono has said over the years that America is not just a country but an idea and in my opinion a manic idea that he said in Hot Press was Life, Liberty and the pursuit of Happiness (a very manic idea.) After getting sick I went to a rehab college Roslyn Park. We were set a project to do over six months. I wrote five pages of my ideas. This was the geneses of the Manic Archetypes. Around this time I felt that Eoghan Harris might have a view point on my five pages. I was told that his number was in the telephone directory so I rang him up and we arranged to meet for breakfast. He loved what I had written and he brought me down to a book shop Easons on Dawson St. and told me he wanted to see me selling a book that I was going to write. Eoghan is a great original thinker. I started to write the book in 1997.

During one summer I worked on a building site that was to become the Police headquarters. I was variously asked to get an air hook, a glass hammer, rubber nails, skirting board ladder, a bucket of steam, a long stand, pin stripe paint, left handed screw driver, a long wait and that if I pissed on my hands they would get hard.

BERLIN

One summer in 1981 I went to Berlin with five friends and we worked in an alcohol factory. You could not take alcohol out of the factory because there was a custom stop at the entrance. We worked from early in the morning to the early evening. The underground trains went like clockwork. Some of the time the trains went under East Berlin where there would be an East German guard with a machine gun. The central station, Zoo ban belonged to East Germany but they did not police it and this lead to it being a haven for drug addicts and prostitutes as seen in the film Christen F. While we were in Berlin there were six of us in a room of 25 meters squared. One day we arrived back to the flat and the door was locked from the inside. We picked the lock and found Ian boiling his underpants in the potato pot. He refused to buy a new pot and we eventually used it to cook our food.

Berlin was strange. You had American, French, English and Russian areas. The wall was about 12 feet tall and you could climb up on wooden viewer platforms. Roads and trains lines disappeared under the wall. On the platform you could see the other side with minefields rows of barbed wire and armed soldiers on watchtowers on the East German side with jeeps driving up and down. I threw a rock with a plastic trailer over the wall which freaked my friends. Quells Revolution.

One night we went to a band and I drank too much rum that I had smuggled in to the night club and got sick all the way home. Stopping off to have chips and mayonnaise, as was normal in Germany. The next day a cake was put in front of me but I said "Not today, thanks", It was my 21st birthday and a sign of drinking trouble in the future. I stayed in bed all day with the worst hangover I ever had. G a German friend of my brother Peter was leaving his flat in Berlin to go on holidays and he let me have the flat for two weeks if I looked after his cat. While we were in the flat we had breakfast, cheese, pate, rye bread and granulated coffee. G was broken hearted because he was a communist and his girlfriend had run off with a right wing politician. In the summer of 1978 I was doing my leaving cert exams the equivalent of the UK A levels exams. I fell in love with a girl and I longed to see her every week end. She unknowingly spurred me on to study. I didn't go to school for 4 weeks before the exam. And I studied in the front room using my brother Peter's well written notes. The hardest subject was Honours Maths. She was my first love and I was also broken hearted by this girl who said she was going to holiday in France, in Jean De Lux and that she could not see me to say goodbye the next day. Needless to say I saw her in town the next day and I called her name and she ignored me. Daniel my best friend was with me and he could not understand why she had ignored me. After the exams I went to Tunbridge Wells on a working holiday picking hops and apples and driving a tractor and I had a good time. One day I had a load of hops on the front loader. It went higher and higher and the tractor nearly fell over but luckily I lowered it just in time. I rang the family every week. One evening that year (1978) I got Dermot Kinlen a neighbour (who was a barrister and then a judge and then the Inspector of Prisons who died in 2008) on the phone. He told me I had got A's in honours Biology and Chemistry and a B in honours Physics and fortunately a C in honours Maths. I thought he was joking but he assured me it was true. I had got into Medicine and had come first in school.

Is art good like positive emotion i.e. love or is it a form of domestication that is a form of evolution (natural selection) that is not good. Leave them their libraries then they will not fight.

While we were in Berlin we were obsessed by Joy Division. Leonard Cohen, Bowie, "Heroes" "Young Americans" The Clash, "London's Calling" "All alone in a supermarket", Roxy Music, Iggy Pop, album, "Lust for Life", Lou Reed "Transformer" and "I've seen the light" At home a song I most remember was off This Mortal Coil album called "The Songs of the Sirens" sung by Liz Fraser written by Tim Buckley. Sitting in the back room at 2am smoking and drinking whiskey and listening, it never failed to make me cry at her emotion. Mark gave my Iggy Pop "Lust for Life" and my David Bowie "Heroes" (German version) to a friend.

In Rooms in TCD when I was 22 listening to Pretty in Pink by the Psychedelic Furs and getting up at night to listen to Echo and the Bunny Man's "Over the Wall" and "Songs from under the floorboards" by Magazine and "Torn Curtain" by Television. Listening to Harvest "Mother Nature" by Neil Young, Gang of Four, Bauhaus, "Jailbreak" by Thin Lizzy "Don't believe me", "Rumours" by Fleetwood Mac the Ramones, "Heaven" by Talking heads, Graham Parkers and the Rumour's "Hey Lord don't ask me questions. Ain't no answer in me.". Eyeless in Gaza, Durrieti Column. The Rolling Stones "I Miss You" and "Far Away Eyes" The best debut album in my opinion was The Cure. "Nights in White Satin" Moody Blues. I also listened to The Pogues "summer in Siam", Bob Dylan's "Oh Mercy", Whipping Boy, Nirvana "Teen Spirit" Luke Kelly singing "Raglan Road" by Patrick Kavanagh and the Pixies. My brother's band The Tulips were also great. Patti Smith "Because the night belongs to lovers" Co-written by Bruce Springsteen. U2 were always on my mind. My favourite song being "One Love". "Have you come here for forgiveness? Have you come to raise the dead? Have you come here to play Jesus? To the lepers in your head." "Everybody wants to rule the world" by Tears for Fears. John Lennon "Imagine" "Give me some truth". Johnny Thunders late of the New York Dolls "You can't throw your arms around a memory" (see pages 398-400) Brian Eno. The Cranberries had a song called "In your head" that was the most played song in America for a year. It was about the zombie violence in the North of Ireland and was probably more effective than any politician or journalist even though they probably looked down their noses at it. Donna Summer's "Oh, Love to Love you Baby" "I Feel Love" banned by the BBC as was "Relax don't do it" by Frankie goes to Hollywood" because they were too sexual. Smack my Bitch Up by the Prodigy had a warning and had to be shown after midnight. Censorship of sexuality and violence was and is a way of controlling mania in art whether it is in literature, music or film. e.g. The Life of Brian was banned for ten years in the South of Ireland. Has censorship ended with the explosion of on line media.

On the way back from Berlin I stopped of in London and called into the Colony Room Club in Soho where Francis Bacon used to drink and socialise.

It was up some stairs and it had a steel green door. I knocked on the door. A middle aged man answered and asked me "what do you fucking want". It was Ian Board who died in 1994. A hoarse-voiced, swollen nosed and foul mouthed and a torrent of obscenities I said "I was there to meet Melvyn Bragg." "You stupid Irish git" he told me aggressively to "fuck off and that Bragg had not been there for years." He banged the door shut. I knocked again and waited a while He opened the door and asked "what was wrong with the stupid Irishman, (ME)" I said, "I was there to see Bragg." "Come in," he said. It was like an initiation ritual. The room was small and dark with a bar on one side. I was full of ideas about literature and art. One guy listened and told me to relax and that I would not solve the problems of the world.

Francis Bacon is an example of culture loosing control and getting more aggressive and paranoid. His studio was chaotic as was his mind. On the night of an opening of an exhibition of his paintings in Paris his boyfriend died of an overdose.

Muslim suicide bombers think they will go to heaven and have 72 angels in paradise. What does that say about their culture? They are very controlling and obsessive. Women have to cover up that probably has more to do with men than women. They pray 4 times a day and do not drink alcohol or eat pork.

Do leaders become paranoid such as Hitler / Stalin / Nixon / Kim / Mao / Pol Pot.? Leaders tend to become charismatic manic and paranoid. Politics attract people who want to be leaders and maybe those that are more paranoid succeed. Such as Stalin killing all his enemies. Police are a projection of the middle classes fear in their paranoia of the violence of the working classes. Working class areas are more violent than middle class areas. They can be no go areas to the police who just contain the aggression. Social control was developed in sports such as the Olympics, football, cricket, boxing and hockey and the development of betting mainly in horse racing. Alcohol is also controlled through taxes that make it expensive. Prohibition (1920-1933) was instigated by the puritans who wanted to control what they saw as the breakdown of culture. Illegal clubs started up and the mafia made a lot of money. Around this time J.F.K.'s father made his money that made him the richest Catholic in America. Bruegel painted in the middle ages 1525-1569 and he used to paint people socialising, getting drunk and having sex in public. People drank beer because it was cleaner and safer than water. The upper classes drank beer and the working classes drank gin because it was cheaper. This is the opposite of today's trends. In a similar way in the middle ages rabbit was protected in Warrens. They cost a week's wages. Now nobody really eats rabbits except the French. In ancient Rome the crowd's appetites were controlled in the Coliseum by the gladiators who got more and more vicious whereas in ancient Greece people trained for the Olympics games and a beautiful body. The main sport in the middle ages was jousting among knights where the most successful and powerful knight was William Marshall who ended up being the regent to Henry 3rd. He was called the greatest knight that ever lived and his effigy and that of his two sons is to be found in the Templar church in London.

Knights Templar graves discovered: Researcher Edward Spencer Dyas has found 8 graves of Knight Templar in St Mary's church in Enville, Staffs. The Knights Templar was a wealthy, powerful and mysterious military organisation of devout Christians in the medieval era, formed in 1119 and tasked with providing safety to pilgrims to Jerusalem.

They were rich, many people were jealous of them and they were charged falsely with heresy. The order eventually disbanded in 1308-9. Enville has clear links with William Marshall 1st Earl of Pembroke, who is considered one of the "greatest warriors" England ever produced. One of the knights had once been part of the Templar Order at Temple Mount, Jerusalem. 16th August 2023, Daily Telegraph Reporter.

The social classes are divided by earnings. Socio Economic Class 1 (Upper Class)-and Socio Economic Class 5 (Lower Class). Middle class money is made by Doctors, nurses Policemen, Prison Officers, Lawyers, Barristers, Judges and Business men who rule over the working classes. Doctors are well paid because people are afraid of pain and death. Laws protect possessions and peoples physical well-being.

Working class jobs tend to be manual for example in construction i.e. carpenters plumbers, labourers, brickies, steel workers, jack hammers and electricians.

JOHNNY

Johnny Thunders of the first punk band The New York Doll was in Ireland in 1990 to do a short tour and to appear on RTE's Night Hawks which Thunders was too stoned to play. His Irish contact had no money to buy him food so I, S, Thunders and his minder come saxophone player got into my car and headed for my mother's house which was around the corner. When we got into the car I put on a Bob Zimmerman (Bob Dylan) tape that I had got off E a friend of mine. To my surprise Thunders asked me to turn off the music "I don't like music." "Who is this guy?" I said to myself looking over at S in the passenger seat. At home he asked me for some chocolate ice cream and Coca-Cola (unknown to me as junky food) There was five people in the kitchen and I got their orders for burgers and chips. Miraculously the Spar was open and it had the chocolate ice cream and coke and the chipper Borzas in Sandymount was also open. Thunders was flicking with the TV remote saying, "Don't like politics. Don't like sport. Where's Johnny Carson? I like Hot Rod racing." This became two of my songs. He kept on looking for his guitar as if it was part of his anatomy. "Where's my guitar?"

As he was going he apologised for not playing in the kitchen. The next night he was playing in the Colony a restaurant com small music venue on St. Johns Lane off Grafton St. Thunders blew me away and his capacity to convey emotion was amazing. Thunders had a heckler and at one stage she had to pass him to get to the toilet. Without losing a beat Thunders said with a dry wit "There goes Miss Piggy," laughter all around. Up until this time I had disliked B.P. Fallon for no real reason but when I found out that he had produced a Thunders album I appreciated him.

"You can't put your arms around a memory" by Thunders. Thunders played a gig in the New Inn. The gig was not going to happen 'cos nobody was going to pay him He said "This is for the kids" I was waving my cheque book around but S sorted the situation. Thunders was a small guy but he had loads of attitude. He had purple hair brushed up from his face and purple eyeliner and purple mascara

While in Dublin he went into a chemist and asked for purple mascara and eyeliner. He threw them back saying "they're not purple". Thunders played a gig in the North of Ireland but he was run out of town. He died of a heroin overdose in 1991.

Songs for Johnny

Verse 1

His name was Johnny Thunders, he played a mean guitar (AM D7 M)
He liked hot rod racing, and the smell of burning tyre (AM DM AM E)
He didn't like music, but he knew how to play (AM DM7)
He turned darkness into the light of day (AM E AM)

Chorus

La La Lar
Where is my guitar, where is my guitar (DM7 AM EAM)

Verse 2

Smacked out hero, destined to die young
Not caring who is behind the door, rolling reefer on the floor
Thunder was an angel, That you meet along the way
Makes it all worthwhile, to see the sun at play

Chorus

La La Lar
Where is my guitar, where is my guitar

Verse three

Now that he is gone, to where the sun never sets
He never looked back again, a man with no regrets
Ice cream and coca-cola
A face as white as snow
We should have known, that he wajusta about to go

Chorus

Four legs good, two legs bad X2

Verse 4

A New York doll, purple Barbie man
Hair boufant doud
Full of attitude, Purple eye adored
Boots on the dashboard.

Chorus

La La Lar
Laddeladdelar
Laddeladdelar   Footnote : Keyboard: voice 110, style 0.27, club dance, Tempo 90.

Don't Like

As Johnny Thunders said - This is for the kids

Verse 1

Don't like music, Don't like sport (E D E D)
Don't like politics, don't like papers (E D E D)
Don't like gossip, don't like god (E D E D)
Don't like Jesus, don't like Satan (E D E D)

Chorus

Yeah, yeah, yeah , yeah. (E D E D)

Verse 2

Don't like the CIA, don't like the KGB (E D E D)
Don't like the IRA, don't like the UDA (E D E D)

Chorus

Where is Johnny Carson, where is Johnny Carson

Verse 3

Don't like drinking, don't like dope (E D E D)
Don't like the TV, don't like the pope (E D E D)
Want to be a fireman, wanna be a policeman (E D E D)
Wanna be a doctor, wanna be a thief (E D E D)

Chorus

Yes, yes, yes, yes (Molly Bloom)
Yeah, yeah, yeah, yeah

Verse 4

Don't like heaven, don't like hell (E D E D)
Don't like sex, don't like sin (E D E D)
Don't like school, don't like Stalin (E D E D)
Don't like Mao, don't like Hitler (E D E D)

Chorus

Yeah, yeah, yeah, yeah

Verse 5

Don't like Mussolini, don't like Lenin, don't like Putin
Don't like Franco, Je pense donc je suit
Be thyself,
know thyself,
love thyself
Socialism, Fascism, different sides of the same coin
Hitler and Mussolini, socialists who became fascists
But I love you yeah
But I love you yeah
But I love you yeah

Footnote : Keyboard: Voice 001 or 080, Style 0027, Ibiza, Tempo 130

Chocolate ice-cream and Coca Cola

Where's my guitar
Where's my guitar
Can't have gone far
Chocolate ice-cream and Coca Cola
For those who dare
Propping up the bar
Don't like music
No music in the car
18 hours in the custom's
From Paris to London to Dublin
Checking all the powders
Going around in Par
Car jam in a jar
Covered with feathers and tar
 Going to War
Died a junky in 1991
Under the Sun.

STUART

When I was 15 years old the French teacher asked the class what we wanted to do when we grew up. My friend Michael Fitzgerald put up his hand. I asked him what he wanted to do. He said Medicine. I asked him why. Because it's well paid. I put up my hand and I knew what I wanted to do. Medicine. Around this time, I was in a class play and I cut my hand with a Japanese sword saying "Aye the Abbe of Bayeux" and I cut the tendon in my little finger in my right distal tendon. I had to go into hospital to have an operation. I was put in a room with five old men. I was woken every morning by the rising sun that energised me. When I was a teenager I was very shy of girls and did not talk to them. During 6th year I used to go to the local pub called Crows in Ballsbridge with my neighbour and friend Daniel Mulcahy. Drink set me free from the shyness, suddenly I could talk to anybody and was running around after all the girls. We used to go to Old Wesley disco in Donnybrook where girls danced around their handbags and boys freaked out to "Smoke on the water" and "Child in time" "Knights in White Satin" Where you agonised over slow dances should I ask or should I not ask. Once at a disco I gave my pass to someone and I climbed in through the toilet window and was meet by a bouncer and got kicked out. Me being a do-gooder again.

RUGBY

I was good at rugby playing as a scrum-half. At 6ft 2ins I was one of the tallest scrum-halves in the country. My brother Peter was also a scrum–half as had been my father for Palmerstown R.F.C. Peter was good at rugby but he had a bad back and he had to wear a back brace that limited his movement. In his sixth year he started to play again against the wishes of his doctor.

One Saturday in September when he was eighteen he came home complaining of a sore neck after his first rugby match in years. It told him to go to the hospital which he did on the Sunday (St.Vincents). His neck was x-rayed and he was immediately put to bed with a neck collar. He had a dislocated cervical vertebra.

The doctor said that he was very lucky not to be paralysed. He was let up out of bed but the vertebra slipped out again. He was put in bed with callipers and a water weight coming out of holes in the back of his head for 4 months. He had special glasses made so that he could read while looking up at the ceiling. He used to count the holes in the ceiling to pass the time, 1400 per tile. He was moved out to the Rehab unit on Roche's town avenue, which had other neck injuries from rugby, horse riding, diving, motorbike and car crashes. Peter had a high Tec operation done by Orthopaedic and Vascular surgeons. They fused the two cervical vertebrae 5/6. The operation was a success. He is still a ferverant follower of the game. When Peter came back to school he was made head boy something that my friends thought would happen to me when I went into 6th. I was not even made a prefect and this made me rebel and stand up for myself.

Fishing for pinkie's down at the river at Clonkeen Rd. aged ten at the back of the houses. I caught a big, lovely and colourful pinkie that I put in a jar of water and put it in the outside toilet. The next day it was dead. I was heartbroken and sad. I had killed a beautiful animal. First sign of guilt.

One day my younger sister got locked into the outside toilet and it took all day to get her out. The start of claustrophobia

Dad used to put sweet pea seeds on a tray in the warm boiler house. He kept them on blotting paper which he kept damp. This helped them to germinate and they could be planted early in the spring. When they were in full bloom they covered a wall 10-foot-high and 30 foot wide. A spectacular blast of colour. My father loved gardening especially growing broad beans, purple sprouting, cabbage, peas, potatoes, onions, beetroot and horse radish. In the end we dug up the garden in Clonkeen road where I lived until I was 12 years old and made it into a tennis court. Around this time we sold the house on Clonkeen Rd for 14 grand to which we had built an extension. We bought a house on Merrion Rd in Ballsbridge, the poshest part of Dublin. It was a three story red brick Victorian house with steps up to the front. One day we called to the house soon after buying it. Dad climbed over the garage and let us into the back garden which was big. There was apple, pear and cheery trees. What an adventure. The railings at the front of the house were based on the design of the Fleur de Lye. (Lillie's) The knocker on the ground floor door was a knight. The brass cover on the fire place in the front room was of a sun. The new house needed to be replumed, rewired, repainted and re-wallpapered but it was a beautiful and a bargain. The garden was massive. It was twice the size of the neighbours garden. It was L-shaped. While the house was being done up we lived very frugally. We cooked on an open fire and slept three to a room with extra blankets. Four double rooms on the top floor two on the ground floor with the kitchen and three large rooms on the middle floor. There were very few young people on Merrion Rd. My best friend was Daniel. He had a fish tank but all the fish died and he gave it to me but I did nothing with it because the thermostat was broken. The new house was beside Wanderers Rugby and with my brothers Philip and Peter we played kick the ball over the bar and catch. One point for a punt and two points for a drop ball. We used to play golf in Wanderers, hitting the ball the length of the pitch. Sometimes we made putting greens in the top garden.

Sometimes we went golfing with my father to Foxrock Golf Club. My father was left handed as is my brother Philip. Dad would drive off and when we were out of sight of the club house we would start hitting balls. Eventually a ball would be lost and we would go looking for it and find other balls as the saying goes "a good walk spoilt"

After golf Dad would go into the club house and have a drink and we would practise on the putting green. The changing rooms smelt of grass and deodorant. My father liked Old Spice for which the add was a surfer mainly played on T.V. at Christmas. The smell of cut grass reminds me of my father on a Saturday afternoon cutting the grass in the back garden with the old black mower that kept on breaking down. One evening after swimming lessons in Tara St. baths Mr Kirk collected us and stopped at a chipper in a Martello Tower in Sandymount. This to me was manna from heaven. It was the one and only time I was bought chips when I was young.

Before we went to church on Sundays Ruth my older sister would line us up and see if we had washed properly especially behind our ears. When we were in Clonkeen Rd. we went to Kill O' the Grange Church of Ireland service. On the way home we stopped at the shops to get chewing gum to get footballer cards from the first division for Philip. When we got our pocket money Peter bought Air fix planes and paint to paint them. He used to suspend them from his ceiling along with green balls mobile. I used to collect stamps especially from Hungary as they had unusual shapes such as round, triangular and parallelogram. Mum would run down from the Rotunda where she worked as the chief physiotherapist to the G.P.O. and buy first day issues during her lunch break. On a Sunday Jane used to give out the desert, Angel Delight or lemon meringue or tinned fruit cocktail (She took the cherry). When we had ice cream Jane took the first slice of the block with a wafer and ran outside to get the swing as we watched jealously. We were not allowed to have sweets during the week, but on Sunday afternoon sweets were given out, one for you one for me. I remember Dad coming home with a new car called a Zephyr and then a Peugeot 8-seater. The car of all cars for a family of six children and two parents was the Peugeot 8 carrier. We had a variety of sandwiches for school, peanut butter, lemon curd, sandwich spread, Bovril, Marmite, marmalade and cheese and crisps from Stephen. Another list is Irish things you cannot get in England such as Major cigarettes, Silver mints, i.e. cool Steve (a name a favourite girl friend gave me), Red Lemonade, Tayto, Bulmer's, Fig Rolls, Smoked Cod, Cod Roe, Coddle and Black and White pudding.

On the beach in Brittas Bay 40 miles south of Dublin when mum sat on the deck chair and it ripped and she fell through it. Building sand castles and trying to protect them from the incoming tide. Running in the dunes the feet sinking in the sand, free under the sun.

I remember going to bed with an American girl who had won a holiday to Ireland for being one of the top 10 salesperson for Ford cars in America. She had a tattoo of a butterfly on her bum. She told me how she had been raped by her boss and that she did not trust men. It was at the time of the aids scare and I wanted to have safe sex with her. Unfortunately the Durexs were in the draw on the other side of the room. I did not want to embarrass the girl and was in a dilemma as to what to do. Eventually I got out of the bed and got a durex. A sensible decision with no embarrassment. I had my room covered in pictures of Vogue magazine, a homage to the female form. Once my girlfriend and her friend found my dirty magazines and they were very interested in what pornographic pictures I liked. Once when I was taking some photographs of a girlfriend she pulled down her top and exposed her breasts and pretended it was a mistake. A while later she got annoyed because I had not given the photos to a professional photographer we knew. I found that girls like pictures been taken of themselves in the nude.

When I played rugby for Wanderers, Denis O'Brien and Barry Maloney were the wing forwards on the team 3rd A's they were good friends and used to paint houses for the summer holidays. Denis was the captain of the team. Unfortunately Denis and Barry fell out of friendship. A mistake I made was to give up rugby because a girlfriend said it was too dangerous. The choice was staying in bed with her or playing rugby on a Saturday morning. Another friend who did well was James who set up a very successful shirt business "Thomas Pink" in London which he sold with his brother for 40 million pounds. When he was a student he went from door to door with Willie selling fisheye lens for doors. All they needed was a drill and a screw driver. They were ahead of the posy. Another year they sold springy head pieces.

Con Houlihan said that he had a tear in his eye when the English team came over to play Ireland in Rugby in the early 70's when no other country in the UK would come over because of the troubles and they got a standing ovation.

To show how naive I am Mark and Ken played some tricks on me. One day Mark Holmes said that his Great Grandmother left all her money to a cat's home she was very rich having sold her recipe for ketchup to Heinz. Then Ken said his father developed the mirror in his shed in his back garden using a milk bottle. He only had certain countries under copyright. Suckered again! One night when I was at Mark Holmes house his dad Peter was there. I brought up the ketchup story and he said what are you talking about Mark tried to divert my attention but I now knew that he and Ken had been making fun of my innocence for years. My Grandfather Tom Marshall used to shit under the trees now and again. The well ran dry in the summer and the pump was redundant. Granny used to haul buckets of water up to the toilet cistern on the first floor bathroom so that Peter and myself could use the toilet. But after awhile we copied Granddad by going aux natural. There is a cure in the Marshall family for skin diseases. It was passed down to my Grandfather and my Great aunt Jane. She went to America and married a pharmacist. He worked out the ingredients and sold the cure as Wynn's savlon cream. It made them millionaires.

Finding coal in the Well field when Granddad got someone to dig for water after getting a dowser in to test for water. Granddad told the man to fill the hole where the coal was about 6-foot underground. Granddad's neighbours the Daly's had an old mine 30-foot deep in the back field but it was uneconomical to mine. There was a post box outside Daly's that was painted green over a red box with the royal coat of arms. I remember getting a rabbit skin off Bill Daly and nailing it down on a board. Unfortunately, I had not cleaned it enough and maggots grew on it and destroyed it. I had taken the legs and tail off the skin and brought them home and put them in my treasure box. These were not immune from the maggots and had to be thrown out.

Granddad used to drink his tea from the saucer. There was no coffee in my grandparent's house and the commonest lunch was fatty bacon, cabbage and potatoes with rice, semolina or tapioca for desert and homemade blackcurrant jam. Black currents were a curse to pick very labour intensive. When myself and Peter were ten and eleven years a neighbour who was sixteen played football and rugby with us. He also used to bath us unheard of in the modern world under the cloud of child abuse. The whole relationship between children and adults has changed and everybody is suspicious.

A geriatric patient who said she had two holes in her head for years was seen as being deluded and lacking in insight. One day I put my fingers to her head and low and behold she had two holes from a lobotomy.

Another patient a man in his forties had very severe O.C.D. (Obsessive Compulsive Disorder). It took him 3 hours to get dressed and two hours to get undressed He was assessed by three committees one Irish and two in England where he had the operation. He was given a partial lobotomy that was a success.

The crochet lady was a 75 yr old in St. Davnets psychiatry hospital. She used to crochet napkins which she gave to the nurses and also some to me. She had been admitted as a patient when she was 17 years old for running after boys and had never been discharged. She had probably been manic when she had been admitted. Psychologically there was nothing wrong with her but she died in care in her eighties having been in hospital since she was seventeen. Once I was driving a second hand car in St. Davnets when the steering wheel stuck and I just turned the key in time to get me off the incline where I would have turned over and fallen down a hill.

PHIL SPECTOR

Phil Spector, born December 26th 1939. His father committed suicide when he was 19 years old when he was probably psychotic. When Phil was 19, he had a number one hit and became a millionaire. He worked with different people and then had hits with the Ronettes; "Be my Baby", The Crystals; He's a Rebel", John Lennon; "Imagine", George Harrison "All Things Must Pass". He said in an interview with the Telegraph in December 2002 that he was bipolar and was been treated for schizophrenia. He was found guilty of murder of a model in 2003 when he shot her in the head. Trial ended in 2009.

He was very jealous and kept his second wife Ronney of the Ronettes in the house. She had to run away barefooted. He developed "The Wall of Sound", multiple drums, guitars and vocals. When he went out he carried a gun. Recorded The Righteous Brothers the most played song "You've Lost That Lov'in Feeling" even more than "Yesterday". "It hasn't been a very happy life, I have been a very tortured soul, I have not been happy". Bipolar, Schizpohrenic, paranoid jealous, hypomanic, creative, musical. Died January 2021 from Covid Virus

DOSTOEVSKY

John Walsh review of Alex Cristofis book Dostoevsky In Love (An Intimate Life) in the culture section of the Sunday Times on 3rd January 2021. Fyodor Dostoevsky born in 1821, had three main lovers in his life (hypomania) and Socialism and gambling (Hypomania). Aged 24, he became a literary sensation overnight. Got involved with utopian socialist group that plotted revolt (sign of hypomania) and were betrayed. He got a reprieve from a death sentence and got four years in a Siberian prison. He ended up being a bad gambler. He met the love of his life aged 45 years who was twenty years, Anna Grigorievna Snitkina. They had four children and lived happily together until he died at 61 years and was cheered by crowds at St. Petersburg Streets at his funeral.

ALCOHOL

When you drink you decrease electricity activity in the brain. If you are a heavy drinker and stop drinking you get delirium tremors and are susceptible to epileptic fits and high blood pressure and die in 1:10 cases. The increase in electrical activity can make you more hypomanic and creative (flight of ideas, stream of consciousness) and this means the drinking pattern can express different mood states and end up drowning in their own vomit. Bands drink and take drugs and are creative then they make money, don't have to get up in the morning, don't abuse themselves and become less creative but they don't know why.

MIXED MARRIAGES

Big Tom of the Mainliners came from a mixed marriage. His dad was a protestant and his mother a catholic, a sign of true love. John Hume's grandfather was a protestant who married John's catholic grandmother. A sign of John's hypomania was shown when he studied for the priesthood in Maynooth.

Bono's mother was a protestant and his father was a catholic. There would have been a lot of pressure by family, friends and the religious society against their marriage. These obstacles would have put great pressure on the great love they must have had for each other, true love. Ed Sheeran's grandparents in Wexford, would also have had pressure on their marriage as it was also mixed. Bono's mom had a stroke at her father's funeral, and died three days later, when he was 14 years old. He also married his true love, Ali. Who do you love? Different class, different religion, different colour, different love, true love.

Rosemary Smith the racing driver's father was a Protestant and his mother was Catholic. The nuns would tell Rosemary she would go to hell.

David Byrne's, the singer in the group Talking Heads, parents were a mixed marriage and left Scotland for the U.S.A. to get away from the bigots in Scotland.

DON'T WALK, RUN

Jealousy and paranoia with hypomania is a dangerous thing in a relationship. Even worse than the physical threats in a relationship by a man to a woman is the psychological threats. The dangerous man buys flowers and chocolates and opens doors. But the problem is when he gets jealous of the women talking to other men. You don't like me anymore, you like him. He becomes over controlling. This is a sign of danger, the answer is, Don't Walk, Run "The Blog"

Children of God (COG)

Hope Bastine was brought up in a "free love" community where sexual abuse of children was rife. As her abuser is finally brought to justice, she speaks to Sharon Hendry in the Sunday Times magazine August 9th 2020.

The Children of God (COG) was started by David Berg (the son of strict Pentecostal Evangelist preachers) in Huntington Beach, California in the late 1960's. He attracted the happy counterculture of drug addicts, dropouts to his heady mix of Christianity, radical politics, apocalyptic doom and free love.

By the 1970's there were thousands of (COG) members living in 130 communes around the world. There was distrust of the outside world and of the coming apocalypse. Paranoia.

In 1970's free love, child sexual abuse and illegitimate "Jesus Babies". Control of members with no T.V. or no reading material from the outside world. David Berg wrote 3,000 letters and tapes that were followed by the members.

There was a paranoid view of control by fear of all outside systems, including government, police, doctors and social workers. David Berg hypomania seems to have been inherited from his parents' family devout Christian Evangelists beliefs. Joaquin Phoenix parents left the (COG) in 1977. Fleetwood Mac guitarist Jeremy Spencer left the band in 1971 to join (COG). After Bergs death in 1994 his widow tried to tidy up the cult renaming it The Family International.

Reuters study showed 56% of journalists were left-wing and 18% were right-wing. Value, Voice, Virtue: the new British politics by Matthew Goodwin. Review by Mark Paul, Irish Times: Ticket, 15 April 2023.

ENGLES

Engles said that religion and money came between people who love each other and get married. He was wrong. The most important relationship is between a parent and a child. You can marry anyone but your children have your blood-line, and true love. You need religion and money to pass on true love.

BORIS JOHNSON

Boris's father has written twenty-six books, had affairs, moved house thirty-two times in fifteen years, is relentlessly positive, changes jobs all the time, and has amazing energy, all signs of hypomania. His children have done well at university, and are successful, they are all signs of hypomania. Stanley Johnson, Boris Johnson's father was interviewed by Camila Long in the Sunday Times Magazine on the 14th of June 2020.

Boris is like his father, hypomanic, a serial father, and a social womaniser. Manic-narcissistic, grandiose, looking down at the empire at the end of the tunnel, and over his shoulder, at the paranoia of Brexit and the hard border.

Go forward.
Don't look back.

NUCLEAR WAR

Why we must end our reliance on nuclear weapons, by Eric Schlosser, 2nd of August 2020, Sunday Times Magazine.

Hiroshima was bombed with Little Boy on the 6th of August 1945 a Uranium 98.62% explosion where only 0.7g of uranium 235 was turned into pure energy. A dollar bill weighs more than that. Temperatures of 5500 degrees Celsius were reached and a cloud of 10 miles rose above the city. About

80000 people died immediately and two thirds of the buildings were destroyed. Three days later Nagasaki was bombed with a plutonium bomb and less than a week later on August 15th, the Japanese unconditionally surrendered. An American senator Brien McMahon said the atomic bomb was the most important thing in history since Jesus Christ. Nine countries now possess a nuclear arsenal; the USA, Russia, China, The UK, France, India, Pakistan, Israel and North Korea, and more than a dozen countries have the means to acquire one. US and USSR countries built up 100,000 nuclear bombs many thousands of times stronger than the Hiroshima bomb and that can be carried in a backpack. At least 1200 US nuclear war heads were involved in accidents between 1950 and 1968. Some trivial and some were potentially catastrophic. Until the early 70's, there were no codes or locks to control American bomber crews or missile crews. In the 1962 Cuban missile crisis, there was no proper communication between JFK and Chrushchev over a two-week period. When JFK was asked about the risk of nuclear war years later during the crisis he said it was 'one in three'. JFK did not know there were nuclear submarines around Cuba. Arkhipov, an officer, persuaded a submarine captain not to fire a torpedo with a nuclear war head at a group of American warships above on October 27th 1962. The captain thought he was under attack. The UK plans to spend between 40 and 200 billion re-armourments. The US will spend 2 trillion on nuclear bombers, missiles and submarines. Russia is developing one-man long range submarines. The rudiments of a Nazi atomic weapon show how close Germany came to a breakthrough that could have won the war. Hacking is possible and in 2018 Chatham House said "Yet history has shown the human error, system failure and design vulnerabilities are common occurrences in nuclear weapon systems." Insider threat remains one of the most difficult to thwart. Missile launch officers in the US airforce have in recent years been caught cheating on their exams and using cocaine, ecstasy and amphetamines. All very much in the field of hypomania and paranoia. The manic development of armourments is probably one of the most important ideas in the modern world and needs to be expressed as much as possible.

Armaments have developed from the fist to nuclear bombs.

GEORGE BLAKE

George Blake the spy dabbled with the Dutch Reform church in his early years (as did Van Gogh). He was emotionally complex and was taught Marxist literature while in prison in Seoul that was intellectually complex and satisfied his hypomanic mind. He had approximately fifty allied spies executed.

HITLER'S FATHER

Hitler's father, (Alois), author Roman Sandgruber.

Reviewed by Derek Scally in Berlin by Irish Times 23rd February, 2021.

Nearly eighty years after he took his own life, letters sent by Alois to a friend Joseph Radlegger paint a complex picture.

Alois born in 1837 had two early disadvantages "illegitimate" and no formal schooling. He joined the civil service and rose to the ranks for the customs office (intelligent, focused and hypomanic). First marriage to a woman fourteen years his senior, childless, second wife, eighteen years younger ended with her premature death. Third wife Klara, a distant cousin pregnant when they got married, lost four of six children before she died of cancer ages forty-seven. Adolf was born on April the 20th on 1889. In Braunau am Inn, a small town sixty kilometres north of Salzburg. Author Roman Sandgrubber indicates that Alois had an authoritative personality, arrogant, pig-headedness, and contempt for the church, science and the nobility. Like Adolf his son (signs of hypomania). Alois, in the authors opinion failed as a father, husband and friend. Alois had shared with his son Adolf, a contempt of school knowledge and had the confidence of an auto dictate (hypomanic). Alois said Klara was a smart woman who appears to have been involved in decision making at home "my wife likes to be busy", wrote Alois in 1894 "and has the necessary joy but also understanding for good housekeeping" (hypomanic).

IRA

The thirty-year release of records people in the IRA army counsel were against the socialist elements in Sinn Fein that was found in urban areas.

DEVIL

Paranoid thinking i.e bad, satanic, evil, sick, opposite to love dystopian thinking, paranoid schizophrenia.

Jealousy is also hypomanic. Sinister/left hand.

CLIMATE CHANGE

How to avoid a climate disaster by Bill Gates, Reviewed by Bryan Appleyard, Sunday Times Culture Section, 14ᵗʰ of February 2021.

If we are going to get zero carbon by 2050, we need people like Gates on our side. All the green measures taken by the U.S. will cut emissions by only 5% by 2030. We should focus on the 51 billion tons of greenhouse gases we add to the atmosphere each year. On the other hand, we should all have gone solar by now. Solar panel are ten times cheaper than they were a decade ago. What then must we do? Well, obviously, go nuclear, he thinks. No serious decarbonisation strategy exits that does not include more nuclear power. James Lovelock (Gaia) agrees with this. Cattle emit high emissions of methane, the worst greenhouse gas of all. The equivalent of 2 billion tons of carbon dioxide a year, and 4% of global emissions. Things can be done to reduce this, but obviously the best solution, is to reduce the green premium on artificial meat and sway people to eat it. The Bill and Melinda Gates Foundation originally focused on health, education and poverty. Now these three have been joined by the big beast of climate change. If we do nothing he says, climate change will be as deadly as Covid 19, by 2050, and by 2100 will be five times as deadly. It's hard to think, Gates concludes, of a better response to a miserable 2020 than spending the next ten years dedicating ourselves to this ambitious goal. O.K. he's rich, 122 billion dollars, but come on, he seems nice.

SOCIALISM & FASCISM

Socialism and fascism, different sides of the same coin.

Hitler and Mussolini, socialists who became fascist (Nazi) National Socialist. Hypomanic in the way they went from Socialist to fascist.

Fascia-bundle of sticks held by the speaker in the Roman Senate.

Sinn Fein – Nazi (National Socialist)

Hitler's Nazi Party won less than 3 per cent in the 1928 general elections in which the social democrats got a landslide victory. The catastrophic economic crisis that unfolded in 1929 let Hitler into power.

July 4th 2020 Irish Times Magazine review by Robert Gerwarth of All Against All; The Long Winter of 1933 and the Origins of the Second World War by Paul Jankowski.

Benito Mussolini the world's first fascists prime minister Al Duce and in power since 1922. He had been editor of the Socialist Paper Avanti that he brought from 50,000 copies a day to 250,000 copies a day before he left. Mussolini born in 1883 he was a womaniser and set up the Fascist Party in 1919.

LEADERS & THEIR TARGETS OF LUST

Lust for Power: Roger Ailes, Xi Jinping
Lust for Money: Warren Buffett, Charles Koch
Lust for Sex: John F Kennedy, Silvio Berlusconi
Lust for Success: Hilary Clinton, Tom Brady
Lust for Legitimacy: Nelson Mandela, Larry Kramer
Lust for Legacy: Bill and Melinda Gates, George Soros

Source: *Leaders Who Lust* by Barbara Kellerman and Todd Pittinsky

The above categories follow the architypes of the hypomanic Bipolar Disorder Spectrum.

Emma Broomfield 27th September 2020 – Sunday Times Magazine

Aaker & Bagdonas finding the funny side makes us appear more competent and confident, strengthens relationships, unlocks creativity, boosts our resilience and, very simply, makes us more likeable.

98% of top executives prefer employees with a sense of humour and 84% believe these employees do better work.

300 number of times a four-year old child laughs every day, but it takes an average 40-year-old ten weeks to laugh as much.

Humour has been proven to enhance creativity – research shows that people who watch a funny video before trying to solve a puzzle are twice as likely to be successful.

Journal of Marketing, Daily Telegraph, 21st of June 2022. Joe Pinkstone; A Review. People who took 100mg of coffee spent 50% more money on 30% more items compared too water or decaffeinated drink.

Journal of American Geriatric Society, Hayami Koga (Havard) 9th of June 2022, Telegraph, Review by Sarah Kanapton. Top 25 of optimists live 5 years longer.

Dr. Anna Macin, Why We Love; The New Science Behind Our Closest Relationships. 8th of June 2022, Daily Telegraph. The below hormones are involved in love,

Oxytocin- Hug Hormone
Dopamine- Reward Hormone, makes us feel good
Serotonin- Obsess over the person
Beta Endorphin- Addicts us to the person

Dr Machin says that in a few years we will be able to generate a drug or a hormone for love.

Engel and Marx talked of dialecticism but not of the opposites of emotion (left hand) and analysis (right hand). Marx talked of Private Property buying more and more and selling for Profit and (then being stimulated by the manic archetypes.)

Advertising in the Financial Times shows some of these characteristics.

EYE OF PROVIDENCE

The eye of Providence an Ancient Religious Symbol used variously in the French Revolutions, Declarations of the Rights of Man, The Great Seal of the United States and in freemasonry also found on the dollar bill.

MESSIANIC DELUSIONS

The Messianic delusion is part of the Manic Paranoid Delusion of Mao, Hitler, Lenin, Stalin and Putin. A feeling of superiority where they think they are right and are also paranoid Grandiose Delusions. Socialism and Fascism are different sides of the same coin. Hitler and Mussolini were socialists who became fascists.

JAMES JOYCE

James Joyce an agent in Trieste in 1909 for the Dublin Woollen Mills. That and the Volta Cinema that showed his attempts at being an entrepreneur. Was Jesus a poor entrepreneur? Joyce could have been a singer but it is possible that he was anxious when he sang like John Millington Synge, "Playboy of the Western World," who before shyness and self-doubt dissuaded him from a performing life. Like other creative sensitive artists who get performance anxiety they often use drugs like alcohol, cocaine and heroin to overcome anxiety, i.e., Rory Gallagher, Phil Lynott, Christy Dignam. Maybe Cognitive Behavioural Therapy (CBT) would help as CBT teaches self-relaxation and helps overcomes anxiety.

James Joyce was probably hypomanic writing what is considered the best book in English, *'Ulysses'* His main character is Leopold Bloom a manic advertising salesman who is aware in his paranoia of being cuckolded by Blazes Boylan. Leopold's wife was a singer. Joyce also wrote the very manic 'Finnegan's Wake.' His father was a manic spendthrift slowly sliding down the class scale from upper middle class to almost destitute.

His daughter Lucia was diagnosed as a schizophrenic but was probably a manic depressive inheriting the gene from her father. Joyce thought that his wife Nora liked an Italian aristocrat and he often tried to set them up but Nora was not receptive to Joyce's quasi delusions of morbid jealousy.

'In the Dead' a short story by James Joyce in a collection called Dubliners; the character called Gabriel Conroy is possessive of his wife Gretta Conroy. On New Year's Eve they go to an annual party held by Gabriel's aunts. Gabriel and his wife go back to the hotel after a good evening. Gretta is reminded of a memory of a boyfriend that a song at the party sets off, Michael Furey who had died young. Gabriel asks whether he died of consumption and Gretta says, "I think he died for me." Gabriel was jealous of the boy Michael who died for love and in death was closer than Gabriel was to his wife.

Joyce published 'A Portrait of an Artist as a Young Man' at the end of 1916 with a manic exclamation "going to encounter for the millionth time the reality of experience and to forge in the smithy of my soul the uncreated conscience of my race."

JESUS, ALLAH AND KRISHNA

Key figures in thought and belief deliberately refrained from writing, The Buddha, Confucius, Socrates and Jesus although they lived in a literate culture. Review John Carey, The Written World, Martin Puchner, Sunday Times 12th Nov 2017.

In the West (Christianity) manic paranoiac people mainly male to female 10-1 have the messianic delusion thinking they are Jesus and that someone, often a relative, is evil, i.e., a member of the IRA, the Devil, and bad with some having hallucinations of the face of the devil and approximately 10% hallucinating the smell of burning flesh and they kill them. These people have often seen doctors who prescribed medication and make arrangements for them to be assessed in a psychiatric hospital in a few days. Unfortunately, this is too little too late.

In Arabic countries the messianic delusions focus on Allah. In India the messianic delusion covers many Gods such as Krishna. I have heard of foreigners mainly a German who joined the Hare Krishnas in their own countries and came to India in a very manic state to pray to Krishna. The

Hare Krishna religion attracts manic people and love bombs them making them wanted. David Corish (Waco) and Jim Jones (Guanana) also attracted manic people who thought Corish and Jones were Jesus.

When manic people are high they often think they are Jesus – the messianic delusion. This is often associated with paranoia, thinking someone is evil and this can result in manslaughter often of a family member (N.G.R.I.) Not Guilty by Reason of Insanity.

STALIN, SADDAM AND HITLER

What do Stalin, Hitler and Saddam Hussein have in common? Grandiose Delusions, a manic belief in themselves as being destined to lead and as result of this mania, a paranoia that leads to the "paranoid position" and results in killing without guilt. All three sent their soldiers on what some generals considered to be suicide missions. All three had no sense of remorse and had difficulties with women.

Hitler's paranoia was based on a jealousy of the success of the Jews and would have been compounded by his use of amphetamines, injections of which he got from his doctor. Saddam, Stalin and Hitler killed where there was any dissent including top military and political adversaries and in the case of Saddam, his in-laws. Paranoia and jealousy are emotions that are related to mania and to a lesser extent I believe related to schizophrenia. **Paranoia is made up of the emotions of anger and fear**. Saddam's hero was Stalin and his favourite file was 'The Godfather.' All three had very efficient propaganda organisations with large pictures in public and radio and TV programs and films dominated by their propaganda. All three went on building programs that reflected their Ego's, not unlike the building program of Ramases II in Egypt. Being obsessed with buildings is a very male trait. Hitler spent a long time over his plans for the Third Reich. All three were cruel whether in the Gulags, the concentration camps or the football stadia where Iraqis were executed and Saddam's use of chemical weapons on the Kurds. Was Napoleon another great fascist, mixing socialist dreams with nationalism? In modern Ireland, the manic Messianic delusion (thinking they are Jesus) going forward with the looking back over the shoulder at the paranoia of evil, i.e., Satan and the IRA that can result in killing.

WILLPOWER: Rediscovering Our Greatest Strength, by Roy F Baumeister and John Tierney (Allen Lane Books)

Already a best seller in America, the book asserts that willpower, rather than self-esteem is the essential ingredient for a successful life – and that the lack of self-regulation is "the major social pathology of our time." Baumeister found in a series of comparative tests that, while American eight-grade maths students had exceptional high confidence in their abilities, they scored far below Koreans, Japanese and other students who had low self-esteem. In other words, confidence was not an indicator of success, self-control was.

Other controlled tests in the 1980's supported his conclusions. In the famous marshmallow experiment conducted at a nursery in Stanford University, researchers asked four-year-olds to sit in a room with a marshmallow and told them they could have an extra treat if they resisted eating the sweet for 15 minutes. Tracking these children in subsequent years (between the ages of 27-32 years) they found that the ones who had resisted temptation did better at school, had a better sense of self-worth, perused their goals more effectively, cope more effectively with frustration and stress, went on to get higher paid jobs, and had a lower body-mass-index and better teeth to boot (self-control means regular flossing, apparently.) In middle age they produced "distinctively different brain scans in areas linked to addiction and obesity."

There are two systems at work in the human brain. The limbic system basic emotion such as fear, anger and appetite for food and sex the "hot system" and the "Cold system" the prefrontal cortex that involves planning and analysis. The Marshmallow Test by Walter Mischel (the original experimenter) Understanding self-control and how to master it. Sunday Times, September 28th 2014, reviewer Bryan Appleyard.

When it comes to education, the authors quote Amy Chua, the author of Battle Hymn of the Tiger Mother (2011) with approval. Asian-American toddlers perform better at the marshmallow test than their non-Asian counterparts and, despite being only 4% of the American population, they make up 25% of the students at the Ivy-league schools, despite scoring a little less well on IQ tests. The authors put this down to Asian parenting styles, which emphasise learning self-disciple and real achievement as opposed to giving constant and, therefore, meaningless praise.

Stanford prison experiment where prisoners were controlled by guards taken from a normal population who abused them and caused psychological trauma. In general, what all this leads to is a sense of powerlessness.

BAKER'S VOICE

The pleasing timbre of Baker's voice anchors this album, interrogating and illuminating, bringing various colours – such as the moodiness of the title song, which sounds like Mazzy Star crashing into traditional music, complemented by the atmosphere Crow. (Cinder Well, Irish Times, 21 April 2023, Review by Siobhan Kane)

APOLLINAIRE

Apollinaire coined the term Surrealism, inventing it to characterise a ballet produced by Diaghilev, Picasso Sartre and Cocteau, "a sort of surrealism in which I see the point of departure for a series of manifestations of the New Spirit which... promises to modify the arts and the conduct of life from the top to bottom in universal joyousness." (Mania, SWM) Catherine Flynn, Weekend Ticket Section, Irish Times, Saturday 29 January 2022

LANGUAGE & EATING

Using lips, gums, cheeks, tongue and larynx in the pharynx (not to choke) to eat. Cooked and raw vegetables and meats as well as berries, nuts, corn and rice to get the dirt and stones and the stones in fruit, i.e., oranges, dates, not to be swallowed. This stimulates the touch and muscles around the mouth, lips and throat that helps develop muscles that will be used to make sounds before language has developed over time.

BIDEN

Biden wants republicans to allow an US debt limit of over $31.4 trillion dollars

PHYSICAL BUTTONS VERSUS TOUCH SCREENS

Volvo 17 years old physical buttons adjustments tasks at 78mph done in 10 seconds. Tesla Model 3 touch screen tasks 23.5 seconds. Electric MG Marvel R touch screen tasks 45 seconds more than 4 times the old car distance at 1,372 metres. Pilita Clarke, Irish Times, 8 May 2023 (Financial Times, 2023)

VINYL & CD

> CD is digital: Vinyl is analogue
>
> CD is clean: Vinyl is dirty
>
> CD is ear: Vinyl is brain

My bloody Valentine (Band) interference of radio considered to be one of the greatest song recordings.

Sound waves - CD hears versus Vinyl hears

CD - The interference is cut out.

Vinyl - The brain hears the sound but also the interference, sounds you don't hear but they affect the brain.

Pulp Review by Neil McCormick (Chief Music Critic) who went to Mount Temple School with U2, 29th May 2023, The Daily Telegraph

Britpop is sometimes characterised as a loutish genre but its finest examples (Pulp, Blur, Suede and yes, even Oasis) offered an arty, inventive, slyly seditions illumination of working class British values. The column at which this 1,700 strong audience bellowed every razor sharp line of "Common People" was something to behold. An alternative pop national anthem transforming class anger into righteous joy, 22 years since Pulp released an album and 11 years since they last played a concert.

CHRISTY DIGNAM

Christy Dignam was abused as a child by two neighbours that lead to him being sensitive and ended up with him being addicted to heroin. As a result of this he was kicked out of his band, Aslan. In the end he was serious and focused and entered treatment that was successful only to be stuck down by cancer that he fought with a passion after having re-joined the band.

Lunch with FT Timothy Snyder, Financial Times, 29 July 2023, interview by Sam Jones FT Switzerland and Austria FT correspondent.

Synder is Richard C Levin, professor of history at Yale but lives in Vienna as a research position in the city's Institute for Human Sciences since 1996.

February 2022 was a second '1938 moment' Snyder suggests, referring to the Munich conference of that year, when Britain and France fatally caved in to Hitler's threats over Czechoslovakia. Had Britain and France stood behind Prague, they would have made the second world war impossible – or at least in the form that it took. That Russia wasn't appeased is a sign that I'd like to think we have learnt something.

"Tortured reading of Russia still afflicts Germany and France." "Our misreading of Russia is deep, very deep." Snyder says. Putin like Hitler, MAO and Stalin is hypomanic paranoid. Hypomania covers socialism and fascism (Nazis) at the end of the political circle spectrum. SWM

In the analogy we're talking about Russia in (Nazi) Germany and I think that is generally productive as a comparison, but it's also generally taboo. And the fact that its generally taboo has been one of our problems from the beginning.

People are "weirdly hesitant" to call Putin's Russia fascist, he says but there are many levels on which the analogy (with Nazi Germany) holds.

"He decries our ongoing focus on "pragmatic" solution to the conflict and a conceptualisation of Putin as some kind of cynical, but ultimately relatable, power politician in the western world. Discussion about Putin were shaped by our own ideas about technocracy and pragmatism and stability – categories which I think have already worn out their welcome."

The past, in all its strangeness, often has ways of illuminating the present. Snyder points to our smartphones: symbols of our technocratic triumph over the past. And yet, even Homeric myths has something to tell us about them, "In the Odyssey, the sirens are so irresistible because they have the power to sing to each sailor only about himself. Which is exactly the same algorithmic superpower that that things has," he muses.

Maybe this is my super conservative side but if we all had a little more knowledge of history, we'd be better equipped to read the present."

Financial Times Interview, 12th August 2023 with Christo Grozev with Edward Luce, FT's US national editor.

Grozev is Bellingcats Russia's investigator. Bellincat has been a target of the far right and the far left which seem to have a near identical scepticism about the west's support for Ukraine.

The Kremlin discovered a long time ago they could exploit this "horseshoe coalition" where the extremes meet) by obfuscating the fact that Moscow has a far-right government and there is zero socialism in Russia, Grozev says, "Socialists around the world seem to be oblivious to that. So they are available for free, we only need to bribe the far right in the west because the left is free. They are still our useful idiots.

(Stuart William Marshall)

With hypomania the left wing and the right wing meet under the "horseshoe coalition" where the extremes meet. In six months Prigozhin will either be dead or there will be a second coup.

China President Xi Jinping now apparently spends 10% of Chinas budget on domestic Intelligence services as much as its entire defence budget. Review by Christian Patterson, Culture Section, Sunday Times, 17th September 2023.

SPARKS by Ian Johnson: Sparks: China's underground historians and their battle for the future.

Financial Times Interview, 16th September 2023 by Gillian Tett

Subject: Walter Isaacson and his book on Elon Musk

"He told me he thinks he is bipolar but has never been diagnosed." Do you have to be half crazy to be truly innovative, or a genius? And how do you stop a brilliant mind from spinning out of control?

(Grandiose – he thinks of himself as a historical figure, S.W. Marshall)

Musk goes through manic mood swings and deep depressions and risk-seeking highs and if he didn't have that risk-seeking maniacal personality he would not be the person who launched EV's and got rockets into orbit.

His obsessive addiction to and focus on engineering and has now developed "an anti-establishment populism." (Somewhat paranoid, SWM)

Mania, the paranoid, the venom is simply part of the package of the great man. Walter Isaacson, review by Danny Fortson, Sunday Times, 17th September 2023. The death of his son Nevada, his first child from sudden infant death syndrome, scarred him deeply.

'Zombie' by the Cranberries, written by Dolores O'Riordan and released in 1994 is the most viewed video by an Irish Band on YouTube having over one billion hits, the third best of all time and voted Ireland's greatest hit by 2FM listeners last year. Based on three-year-old Jonathan Ball and twelve-year-old Tim Parry being killed (murdered, SWM) by a bomb in Warrington which was planted by the IRA. O'Riordan felt compelled to express her revulsion after seeing an interview with the mother of one of the children. Dolores says; "I'm not the IRA, they are not me… when it says in the song: "It's not me, it's not my family." That's what I'm saying, it's not Ireland, it is some idiots living in the past.

Dolores died in early 2018 at the age of 46. 'Zombie' is now sung at Rugby matches as one its most popular songs.

Irish Times, 23rd September 2023, Hugh Linehan

RTE Radio, Drive Time, 25th September 2023, Hugh Linehan

'Zombie' has more influence on teenagers and young adults than the hypomanic journalists who think they are important and have anti-establishment views with a taste of paranoia. SWM.

TV Programmes

Happiness levels declined by 4% after watching soap operas such as Coronation Street or Emmerdale. Comedy boosted happiness by 22%, Music programmes by 17% and Art programmes by 14%.

Study called 'The Screen Test' done by researchers from Sussex and Brighton University and in association with the Radio Times.

Reflecting on the last programme they had watched, they reported that their excitement had increased by 10% and happiness by 5% while anxiety went down by 6%.

Reviewed by Flora Bowen, Daily Telegraph 2023.

Band Names:
R2D2, Highbabies, Does God take Lithium, Rhythm.

Band Member Names:
The Kid, Styx, The Marshall.

Lieutenant Colonel Bryan Ray – whenever he heard shouting at night in Somaliland he ordered his men to fire 2inch mortar parachute illuminating flares over the town and this produced satisfactory silence.

Obituary, Daily Telegraph, 27th October 2023.

Right Brain

Mirror Ball

Coloured lights

Mating – making love, disco dancing

Emotions – love, hate, anxious, crying

Girlfriend/boyfriend

Paranoid, lonely, happy

Close/tight

Marriage, divorce

Intuition – over inclusive

Dance - drugs

    -Jive, mosh, pit, ballroom, pogoing, twist

    -One, two, three, four

    -Come in the door

    -Right, left, backward, forward

Money – buy, selling

Number – the only one

    -First Kiss

    -First drink confident social anxiety C.B.T.

Drugs – ecstasy best time

    -Cocaine, speed, hash, LSD – paranoid, alcohol, DTs

    -Attention deficit disorder

    -Ritaline increased blood flow, Pattern recognition

Baby talk – Yeah Yeah Wow Wow

    -Da Da Maha he wowwumyeahyeah

    -Hello Hello

Names – Polly Parton – Joveline, Eileen

    -Caroline, clare

TOP Word

    1st God

    2nd Coca Cola

    3rd Titanic

Motion – scratch eye, rub nose, scratch face, hands behind head, tie shoe laces, hands in pockets, left index finger.

Mobiles – trains, car, plane, airports, hydrofoil

Horse carriage, air ballon, bicycle, truck, glider, air zephlin

Boats, yacht, skiing, running, jumping, pole-vault

Roller-skates, javelin, shotput, long jump

Changing clothes – tee-shirt, jeans, cravat, leather apron

    -Dress trousers, tie scarf, shoes, boots, tie shoelaces

Branding – cross, Jewish cross-6 pointed star

    -Five pointed star, celtic cross

    -Crucifix, army tab

    -Tara broach, clara ring, Claddagh ring

    -Necklace, rings, earring-ex-girlfriend

    -nose piercing, gum piercing, nipple piercing

    -Royal albert

Humour – funny witty

Sexual – Physical/appetite, perfume-ex-girlfriend

Heaven – high, spiritual, forgiveness God Christ

    -Oh holly great brilliant person

Intellect – ideas quick IQ intelligence

Speed/Faster – walking, talking, speeding thought in head

Creativity – ideas, art, beauty, books, painting

    -praise of God – Sistine chapel

    -Michaelangelo

Hey Pal

Hindu – vegetarians, it no alcohol, adopted, serious

    -Sacrifice, incontinent focused twin

    -God Louise the Sun King

    -Turner – God is the Sun: the Sun is God.

Transport, Money, Dress, Synthesis, Cursing, Dance, Names, Numbers, Vowels, Spatial awareness, Emotions, Humour, Spirituality, Intuition, Grandiosity, Sexuality.

Collection of lyrics by Stuart Marshall
Cords by John McElhinney

The Song of dance and illoved (G Am G Am)

Verse 1 (Am)
The beer is cold, the lights are low (G Am C Am G)
The air is sweet, and I wanna go (G C G Am)
Dancing, dancing, dancing (G C G Am)
To the song of dance and illoved (G Am G Am)

Verse 2
Out in the night, under neon light
Oil colours on a pool, taxi taxi, I'm a fool
Kissing, kissing, kissing
To the song of dance and illoved

Verse 3
You turn surprised, eyebrows rise
Stars in the sky, adrenaline flies
Cruising, cruising, cruising
To the song of dance and illoved

Finale
Dancing, dancing, dancing
Kissing, kissing, kissing
Cruising, cruising, cruising
To the song of dance and illoved

Footnote : Keyboard: voice 001, style 027 Ibiza, Tempo 100

LOVE IS ON THE RUN

Verse 1

Love is on the run (G)

And the Devils out on bail (D7)

Lock up your daughters

They might have a soul for sale (G)

Verse 2

Gonna get to New Orleans (G)

If it's the last place she will go (D7)

Shining red leather

Hoping I don't need to know (G)

Chorus

Oh bought and bold, 24 carat gold

Oh bought and bold, 24 carat gold

Verse 3

Got devils in my head (C)

Saying go the whole way (GMG)

Don't know where im being lead (D7)

They've got nothing left to say (G)

Verse 4

It's when he falls in love (C)

With his five o'clock shadow (Gm C)

Hell bent to Gov. (D7)

Never seen the tail of a swallow (G)

Chorus

Oh bought and bold, 24 carat gold

Oh bought and bold, 24 carat gold

Verse 5

One more ticket to nowhere

Hoping hoping enough

Some like it rough

But its going to get tough

Verse 6

Travelling with a red-neck

Heading west toward the shore

They'd kill you in a sec

It's there you find loves a chore

Chorus

Oh bought and bold, 24 carat gold

Oh bought and bold, 24 carat gold

Verse 7

Love is on the run

And the Devils out on bail

Lock up your daughter

They might have a soul for sale

Verse 8

Gonna get to New Orleans

If it's the last place she will go

Shining red leather

Hoping I don't need to know

Chorus

Oh bought and bold, 24 carat gold

Oh bought and bold, 24 carat gold

Footnote: Voice 011, Style: 032, GK, Temp 96

ONE GIRL

Verse 1

One girl one day (Emj Bm7 E)
Going out to play (Em Bm7 E)
Love lost its way
Lay lay De lay (Bm7 E)
Hay hay De hay (Bm7 E)

Verse 2

One girl one day (Emj Bm7 E)
A - OK
Loves lost its way
Lay lay De lay
Hay hay De hay

Verse 3

One girl one day
Up at mdday
Loves lost its way
Lay lay De la
Hay hay De hay

Verse 4

One girl one day
Gonna pray to Rae
Loves lost its way
Lay lay De lay
Hay hay De hay

Verse 5

One girl one day
Oh shessoo sweet
Her hair soo neat
Lay lay De lay
Hay hay De hay

Verse 6

One Queen one seat
Shessoo bright
Loves lost its way
Lay lay De lay
Hay hay De hay

Verse 7

Million dollar voice
Ten cents brain
Comes out at night
She casts a light
Loves lost its way
Lay lay De lay
Hay hay De hay.

LAY ME DOWN

Verse 1

Lay me down, where willows weep (E B7)
Where children cry, where slaves are free (E B7)
Where grown men die, where women love (Gm E Gm E)
Where bells chime (G M E)
Wind whispers..........wind whispers.......wind whispers (B7 E B7 E B7 E)

Verse 2

Where we are friends, where we are one
Where people pray, where templars fight
Where philisophers think, where figs are ripe
When I'm in Zion
Wind whispers.......wind whispers.......wind whispers

Verse 3

Lay me down, where willows weep
Where children cry, where slaves are free
Where grown men die, where women love
Where bells chime
Wind whispers..........wind whispers.......wind whispers

Verse 4

Lay me down where willows weep
When I see love
Where the sun shines forever
When all is forgiven
St. Peter 7 times, Jesus 77 rhymes

VENICE 1

Verse 1

May you kiss the one you love (G Bm Cm D7)
On Friday 13th on a long weekend(G BM C D)
Listening to Nick Caves (G Bm C D7)
Singing straight to you on a wave (G C D7)

Chorus

Baby, baby, baby
Don't say maybe

Verse 2

A genius of a song all right
Wafting through an open window
    on a Venetian night
On a balmy summers evening
    I kissed her
Over a Galoise and a glass
    of Pernod and water

Chorus

Baby, baby , baby
Don't say maybe

Verse 3

Viewing girls in see through frocks
In St. Marks Square by the
    gondolas docks
Like elegant swans in tandam
    forever
Lovers holding hands together

Chorus

Baby, baby , baby
Don't say maybe

Verse 4

And kisses stolen by magic
Caravagio's paintings are tragic
Holding time as it dies
A dog star in my eyes

Chorus

Baby, baby, baby
Don't say maybe

Verse 5

A cold shower in the peak
    of an European day
Taking the gondola out on the bay
In by the Rialto Bridge a dove
Standing on the one I love

Chorus

Baby, baby, baby
Don't say maybe

Verse 6

He got down on his knees
And begged me please
To put on the ring
That would make his heart sing

Chorus

Baby, baby, baby
Don't say maybe
Now she has a baby

COOL

Verse 1 (C/ Em7 / C / D7 /MajG)

You're so cool
Drinking beer
and playing pool
Propped up on a stool
You're such a fool
Black hair Levi's
Build up your thighs
Stocks and shares
She climbs the stairs
Champagne caviar
Got a red sports car
Cowboy boots pin stripe suits
One of the lads, male gonads

Chorus

Boom Boom Boom
You're so cool
Boom Boom Boom

Verse 2

Rich boys, expensive toys
No brains, emotional drains
Stuck in a BMW, label you
Marlborough man
Coke from a can
Got his penthouse suite
One of the elite
Photo in a magazine
One of the has-beens
Brains to burn
Now its your turn

Chorus

Boom Boom Boom
You're so cool
Boom Boom Boom

Don't walk run
Follow the sun
Chocolates and roses
Paranoid poses
Power, Sex, Money
Soil that's stoney
Nose that's runny
Tongue is funny.

Footnote: Voice 080, Style 025, Tempo 130

To Love You (Cords, Stuart W Marshall)

Verse 1

The wind is in the trees (Am)

Begging me please (E)

To love you (C)

The sun is in the sky (Am)

Telling me why (E)

To love you (C)

The moon is in the night (Am)

Shining her light (E)

To love you (C)

The gold is in the chain (Am)

Pouring like rain (E)

To love you (Am)

Chorus

Da DaDa De De Da DaDa

Verse 2

The hot rock car (Am)

Is going far (E)

To love you (C)

The bun is in the oven

Drinking in a coven

To love you

Talk Johnny Carson

Serves like a garson

To love you

The water in the well

Drinking not unwell

To love you

Chorus

Da DaDa De De Da DaDa

Verse 3

Fontain in a car

Smoking a cigar

To love you

A singer on the stage

Emotional rage

To love you

An author and her book

Shes got the look

To love you

Two lovers on a bed

The sweats that's said

To love you

Chorus

Da DaDa De De Da DaDa

Verse 4

As daddy lay dying in his bed

A whisper to his head

I love you

The death of the father of the sun

Under the god of the sun

I love you

It was the last word

Like a songbird

I love you

Footnote: Voice 080, Style 027, Tempo 90.

433

Mine, Mine, Mine

(F C B flat)

Mine, Mine, Mine, one at a time (Am)

My house my food, left hand rude (C Am)

My fridge my car, Going far (G C Am)

Set Me Free, Let Me See (G C Am)

Chorus

Mine, Mine, Mine, 10 dollar dime.

Verse 2

Cut the grass, I'm upper class (G Am G Am)

Put out the bins, One that wins

Tidy your room, Brush with a Halloween broom (Am)

Chorus

Mine, Mine, Mine, I Feel Fine

Verse 3

Are you on drugs, Hate the bugs

Cut the grass, Ah that's bass

Sweep the kitchen, ...

Chorus

Mine, Mine, Mine, let it shine.

Verse 4

Hoover the stairs, 70's flares

This isn't a hotel, It's a Californian hell

Be back at ten, Egg or hen

Chorus

Mine, Mine, Mine, walk the line.

Verse 5

Are you drinking, Are you winking

Give up the cigarettes, Cast your nets

Put the toilet seat up, Lift up the cup

Chorus

Mine, Mine, Mine, bench of pine.

Verse 6

Get your hair cut, Got a mutt
You're day dreaming, You're soo clean
Snap out of it, Turn on your wit

Chorus

Mine, Mine, Mine, drunk on wine.

Verse 7

That's not music,.......That's noise
Do your homework, Young Turk
I didn't ask to be born, Love is torn
Open your mouth, Birds heading south
I'm an aeroplane, Thoughts going insane
Eat your dinner, You're a sinner
I love spam, The band wham
You're a winner, Lights thinner

Chorus

Mine, Mine, Mine, listen to the chime.

Verse 8

Take your tablet, Moses purple velvet
Go to bed, Black white and red
Turn off your phone, Ice cream cone
Turn off the immersion, religious conversion
Don't smoke in the house, The fire douse
Make your bed, Lying what's said
Stop playing those computer games, Your heads in flames

Mine, Mine, Mine, do the time, do the crime.

Get up and go to work, Don't be a jerk
Your drinking too much, You're out of touch
Make the tea, With the Queen dream
You owe me rent, Incense sent.

Footnote: Voice 007/008 style 025 Ebiza tempo 125

Rock and Roll

Verse 1
I wanna be a singer in a rock and roll band
Playing from land to land
Singing with a hairbrush in my hand
Getting the gig rush

Chorus
Rock and roll
From pole to pole

Verse 2
In front of the mirror
Acting like a sooth sayer
Sweeping brush or tennis racket as a guitar
The lead bass and vocal spar

Chorus
Rock and roll
From pole to pole

Verse 3
Plugin the invisible amp
A man, a woman and being camp
Dancing and posing to the music
Eyeing with a group of tricks

Chorus
Rock and roll
From pole to pole

Verse 4
Jumping and shaping on the stage
Turning over another page
Waving and bowing to the crowd
Singing and the guitars are loud

Chorus
Rock and roll
From pole to pole

Verse 5
Posing for the photographs
Signing the audiences autographs
Being dressed in fashionable clothes
The emotion of the music as it flows

Chorus
Rock and roll
From pole to pole

Singularity

In this crazy theory of mine
I feel fine
The Big Bang of another aeon
Nightly lite by neon
Gravity will not let light escape
Painting with masking tape
Singularity
Hilarity
Living for the moment
Fizzy but not content
Now and Always
Mind thinking in a haze
Feel it smell it, Love it aware of it
Think of it, sink it
Buy it, build it
Pray for it, say it
Laugh at it, mind it
Pray for it, say it
Screw it, sexualise it
Talking it, Singing it
See it, hear it
Touch it, taste it
Hot cold pain pleasant
Vibrations soft hard
Two pin pricks, Three dimensions
Elephant dicks, Medical pensions
You can't stop time
There no rules, but rules

What is Love (Cords, Stuart W Marshall)

What is love (D)
I believe in love (F)
I believe in truth (C)
I believe in freedom(E)
Wow wow wow, yeah yeah yeah
What is love (D)
I believe in love (F)
I believe in beauty (C)
Love is art (Am)
Love is art (E)
Love is music (Am)
Love is emotion (E)
What is love (D)
I believe in love (F)
I believe in religion (C)
Love is dancing (Am)
Love is singing (E)
Wow wow wow, yeah yeah yeah
What is love (D)
Thinking positive makes it so
What is love (D)
I believe in love (F)
I believe in kissing (C)
Love is making love (Am)
Love is magic (E)
Love is chaos (Am)
Love is tragic (E)
Wow wow wow, yeah yeah yeah
What is love (D)
Who do I love (E)
As if
Love is a high (Am)
Love is my my Shanghai (E)
Love is an art (Am)
Love is a sweetheart (E)

Love is a hard-on (Am)
Love weighs a tone (E)
Wow wow wow, yeah yeah yeah
Love is sweet (Am)
Love is one of the elite (E)
Love is a whisper (Am)
Love is a name dropper (E)
Love is perspiration (Am)
Love is admiration (E)
Love is looking at the sky (Am)
Wow wow wow, yeah yeah yeah
Love turns and ask why (E)
Love is pure and not a lie (Am)
Love is an undercover spy (E)
Say hello say goodbye (Am)
Wow wow wow, yeah yeah yeah
What is love (D)
I believe in love (F)
Pragmatism is to make life better (C)

Wow wow wow, yeah yeah yeah
What is love (D)
I believe in love (F)
Truth today, lies tomorrow (C)
Truth and ideas is their power to work (C G)
What is love (D)
I believe in love (F)
The first act of love shall be to believe
in love (Am) E AM)

Do you love me
Who's your God?
Who's your Jesus
Mums a virgin
Dads a carpenter
Mary Magdellans his girlfriend.

The Sun

Key of E major

When I saw you (E)
My heart skipped a beat (AE)

You were one (EA)
Of loves elite (E)

Your eyes, your hair, your skin (B7A)
You look soo sweet (B7E)

I knew my heart you would win
Liberty

You walked across the dancehall
Of my 13th trinity ball

Your smiles were so sublime
I was running out of time

Your low cut dress
Made to Impress

Egality
Then our eyes met
It was a two to one bet

Youre face so serene
Like a ship caught in a beam

I knew you were the one
The one and only sun
Fraternity
The one and only one under the sun

You'll be Okay OK OK
Tomorrows another beautiful day

The one and only sun
Under the sun

The Tax Man
Debt will keep us together

The tax man sent me a letter (E A B)
 Things weren't getting any better (E A B)
Saying debt will keep up together (G A)
As changeable as the weather (A Bm E)

Chorus
Debt will keep us together
Sent with love in a letter
Self belief is better
Paranoia rules the world and its director
Cash is king, Bling, bling, bling

Verse 2
You cant afford to leave
Owe to much to believe
Theyre in soo deep
Business lead by a creep

Chorus
Debt will keep us together
Sent with love in a letter
Self belief is better
Paranoia rules the world and its director
Cash is king, Bling, bling, bling

Verse 3
They can never pull the plug
Sweep it under the rug
Don't fall in love with me
Torn between love and what I see

Chorus

Verse 4
I don't want to break your heart
You say we'll never part
Love, politics, culture and art
So beautiful happy and smart

Chorus

Verse 5
Feed the poor
Enlighten the dour
Free the weak
Support the meek
Care for the mad
Punish the bad
Think for the idiots
Straighten the creeps

How can we know the dancer from the dance

How can we know the dancer from the dance (G D7 D7)
The prayer from the preacher Cm C)
The song from the singer (D7 G)
The poem from the poet (D7 G)
How can we know the dance from the dancer (Dm G D7 D7 G)
The dream from the dreamer
The fight from the boxer
The race from the runner
The script from the actor
How can we know the dance from the dancer
The grave from the gravedigger
The bike from the cyclist
The love from the lover
The sword from the fencer
The crime from the thief
How can we know the dancer from the dance
The jockey from the horse
The driver from the car
The menu from the chef
The mother from the child
How can we know the dancer from the dance
How can we know the dancer from the dance
The lover from the romance
The king from the entrance
The shaman in a trance
The billionaire and his expense
How can we know the dancer from the dance
The horror and the suspense
Jesus and the frankincense
The spirit in the séance
The queen from the blue rinse
How can we know the dancer from the dance
Dadda dancer

Follow the money

Follow the money
Bomb the financial city
That's full of honey
We'll have an amnesty, not guilty

Follow the money/another day another dollar
The war is over
But we need your help
In the grass there's clover
Not one more scalp

Follow the money
Bomb cost 1 billion
Government lead by Brooke
They had to stop the rebellion
Took out the chequebook

Follow the money
We have no selfish strategic
Or economic interest in Northern Ireland
Copy of speech given to IRA before speech delivered
It'll be worked out by magic
Said in a way was lectured
Tread gently like an uncut rough diamond

Follow the money
Adams said "Hume was serious"
"So am I" a bit devious
I'm not in the Irish Republican Army
Nor am I their enemy

Follow the money
Adams and Trimble signed the Good Friday Agreement
Both sides stood up and made an endorsement
Put to the vote the majority followed
They kept their hunger and were marshmallowed

Follow the money
25 years later
Celebrating another Easter
The US President and the party leaders
The Peace to which all are crusaders.

Two legs good, Four Legs bad

Just a punk
A neighbourhood drunk/skunk
Rock and roll
A nine inch cockrell called Iggy
One legged rooster

Two legs good, Four Legs bad

Pogo pogo pogoing
Moshin moshin moshing
Freedom of a Norton motorbike
Girlfriend at his back

Two legs good, Four Legs bad

Hair in the wind
Into the headwind
Snake skin boots
Blonde hair black roots

Two legs good, Four Legs bad

Liquorice cigarette papers
Grubby fingered shopkeepers
Lizard in a glass cage
A dead rat in a cage

Two legs good, Four Legs bad

Won at 50 to 1
Lying in the sun
Elbow to elbow
A turbo placebo placebo
A poem by Rimbaud

Two legs good, Four Legs bad

The drugs almost ended
In time we offended
In me killing me or each other
He was my lover.

Does God take Lithium

Does God take Lithium
He took Mummy's little helper
A few tabs a day of Valium
Taken in the innkeeper

His son was Jesus
Who was a manic depressive
He was nervous and rebellious
He was explosive and obsessive compulsive

He had Grandiose delusion
Special charismatic and paranoid
Thought he was a star on television
Had a psychotherapist as talkative as Freud

Lying on the floor drunk
He suffered from delirium tremens
Torn tee-shirt dressed as a punk
Like an angle painted by Rubens

He was known as Linoleum
Man and women vas deferens
Burnt like a bright light magnesium
Killed in Cork the hero Collins

Tall Dark and Handsome

Tall Dark and Handsome
A duellist for a ransom
Love is Hey Hey Hey, Wow Wow Wow
Yeah yeah yeah
What I'd like to be, love is on my wish list, I believe in love
The best of everything that money could buy
Energetic, charismatic, dynamic,
Sporty, healthy, funny, money,
Beautifully dressed, ortho-dentistry.

Love is dancing at lughnasa
Theatre, French literature, educated, cultured,
Poetry, history, witty, film, writing,
Intelligent, independent, art, likes children, kindness.
Vivacity, Christian doctrine, books, food,

Love is lovable, musical, convertible, sociable,
Successful, debates around dinner table,
Dancing, caring, sharing,
Swimming, sailing, playing cards, tennis, football, monopoly,

Love is "no crying is this house,
Waited on hand and foot.
What did your last slave die from?
Price of Camelot, remember where you were
Never forget, crie de Coeur, one lobot, four died 2 shot.

Your clothes are hanging where my clothes used to hang

Your clothes are hanging where my clothes used to hang
Your car is in the driveway where my car used to be
Your pen is writing letters to friends I don't have
I use your coffee maker where I used to make tea
I lie on your futon where I used to lie on my bed
I brush my teeth with your toothbrush in the glass
Where my toothbrush used to be
I would listen to your Rock and roll where my classical music
I would have played
I prune your roses where I used to grow sweet pea
I use your sofa where I used to sit in my rocking chair
I read your guitar magazines on the table where my gardening mags would be
I wear your skull ring where my wedding ring was worn
I watch your 20 sports channels where the news would do me
I write letters to myself because my friends have gone
I use your aftershave where I used to use my perfume
Your food is in the freezer where my food used to be
My family is getting smaller, I ring them and see them when I can
When I fall over no one comes to help
I talk to myself because no one can listen
I read your philosophy books on the shelf where my thrillers would sit
I wear your torn shirt and jeans where my cashmere dressed would do
I use your umbrella where my walking stick would do.